D0992213

FUNDAMENTALS
OF
ORTHOPAEDICS

Second Edition

John J. Gartland, M.D.

*James Edwards Professor of
Orthopaedic Surgery and
Chairman of the Department,
Jefferson Medical College of
Thomas Jefferson University,
Philadelphia, Pennsylvania*

1974
W. B. SAUNDERS COMPANY
Philadelphia • London • Toronto

W. B. Saunders Company: West Washington Square
Philadelphia, Pa. 19105

12 Dyott Street
London, WC1A 1DB

833 Oxford Street
Toronto, Ontario M8Z 5T9, Canada

Library of Congress Cataloging in Publication Data

Gartland, John J
 Fundamentals of Orthopaedics.

 Includes bibliographies.
 1. Orthopedia. I. Title. [DNLM: 1. Orthopedics. WE168 G244f]
RD731.G36   1974   617'.3   74–4563
ISBN 0–7216–4046–X

Fundamentals of Orthopaedics   ISBN 0–7216–4046–X

Last digit is the print number: 9   8   7   6   5   4   3   2   1

Dedicated to

Lynn
Barbara
Jack
Trisha
Meg

*With my love and my
wish that you have happy
and fulfilled lives.*

Preface to the Second Edition

Continued acceptance of *Fundamentals of Orthopaedics* by medical students and practitioners of family medicine has been most gratifying. This acceptance has made the effort associated with writing a textbook worthwhile.

New knowledge concerning musculoskeletal problems has been advanced and dramatic technical progress in the treatment of some of these problems has been made since the first edition was published in 1965. These additions to our understanding of the causes and treatment of musculoskeletal problems have made it essential to rewrite the book to keep the information as timely as possible for the reader.

Press of other duties has delayed my getting to this task for some time, but it has finally been completed. The book has been entirely rewritten. New illustrations have been added and the references made more complete and current. Suggestions made by readers and reviewers, particularly as they relate to content, clarity, and balance, have been carefully considered. My sole intent has been to make the book more readable, more logical, and more timely. A chapter on Orthopaedic Rehabilitation has been written by Dr. Phillip Marone, a member of the American Academy of Orthopaedic Surgeons' Committee on Rehabilitation and a member of the orthopaedic faculty at Jefferson Medical College. The goal of this second edition, however, remains exactly the same as that expressed for the first edition. This is, quite frankly, a basic and introductory book intended principally to acquaint the student with the disorders of the musculoskeletal system and to indicate the scope, the limitations, and the possibilities of this fascinating field of medicine.

My sincere appreciation is extended to Dr. Donald Getz and Dr. Charles Probst for their help in collating some of the newer medical information. Most of the new photographs were made by Walter Katz of our departmental photographic unit. Louise Lang, R.N., has continued to be assistive and supportive and my grateful thanks are extended again. The manuscript was typed and retyped by Nancy Goldenberg, Lynn Gartland, and Ann Louise Smith.

My thanks are gratefully offered to the staff of W. B. Saunders Company for their patience, forbearance, and skillful expertise.

Finally, I would extend my warmest congratulations to my medical university in this their Sesquicentennial Year.

September, 1974

JOHN J. GARTLAND, M.D.
Philadelphia, Pennsylvania

Contents

Chapter One

The Task, the Material, and the Tools

THE TASK

Orthopaedics is that part of medicine directly concerned with the ills that befall the musculoskeletal system. This specialty is surgically oriented and has been formally defined as that branch of medicine especially involved in the preservation and restoration of the function of the skeletal system, its articulations, and associated structures.

With a scope that is constantly broadening, orthopaedics is one of the most rapidly expanding fields in medicine. The task facing the orthopaedic physician now properly encompasses all of the congenital, traumatic, infectious, hereditary, neoplastic, and degenerative processes to which the musculoskeletal system is subject.

The term orthopaedic originally appeared in 1741 in the title of a book, published by Nicholas Andry of the University of Paris, in which certain basic problems in the musculoskeletal development of children were discussed as factors contributing to adult deformity. The word was synthesized by Andry from the Greek roots *orthos* (straight) and *paidios* (child). He submitted the proposition that the prevention of deformed adults lies in the development of straight children. Modern orthopaedics has expanded from this narrow view to apply to patients of all ages and now includes in its scope injuries, diseases, and deformities of bones and joints and their related muscles, tendons, ligaments, and nerves.

Before surgery became safe, the orthopaedist made extensive use of mechanical appliances for the prevention and correction of skeletal

1

deformity. The modern orthopaedic surgeon, though equally concerned with mechanical correction, can now operate with impunity to obtain earlier and more complete correction of a deformity.

The present-day orthopaedic surgeon, in addition to solving clinical problems related to both form and function, has developed a deep interest in the cause of deformity and takes an active part in helping to find answers for unsolved questions. Orthopaedic research laboratories, making use of tools supplied by basic scientific knowledge, are busily engaged in basic research related to musculoskeletal problems. It is hoped that an increasing knowledge of biophysical processes will provide the orthopaedic physician with the key to both the prevention and the cure of deformities and diseases of the musculoskeletal system. Much that is hopeful and exciting in this direction lies on the orthopaedic horizon.

THE MATERIAL

The essential material with which the orthopaedic surgeon must work is bone, a hard, specialized connective tissue with a calcified collagenous intercellular substance. The most striking and obvious difference between bone and all other forms of connective tissue is that bone is the only tissue to contain inorganic mineral deposits within its intercellular matrix space at almost all stages of its normal development (Fig. 1). These mineral salts have a distinct morphologic relationship to the organic elements of the bone matrix, fulfill a definitive mechanical function within this tissue, and are involved in critical metabolic and homeostatic processes that are under stringent physiologic control.

Chemically, the mineral portion of bone is composed of calcium phosphate salts containing a small but significant amount of carbonate (4 to 6 per cent) and very small amounts of other ions, such as sodium, potassium, magnesium, and chloride. It is believed that a large proportion of the calcium phosphate in bone exists in crystalline form, having a configuration very similar to that of the geologic family of calcium phosphate minerals, the apatites.

Bone mineral, then, is an integral part of bone tissue, having individual physical and chemical properties that directly affect those of the tissue as a whole. It is the mineral portion of the skeleton which is involved in the unique role that bone tissue plays in maintaining mineral metabolism and homeostasis. Bone collagen, on the other hand, is relatively inert from a biologic viewpoint. It is a complex, highly insoluble fibrous substance which provides the general mechanical and morphologic architecture of the skeleton.

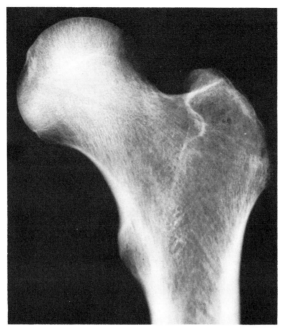

Figure 1. X-ray of dried specimen of adult proximal femur. Mineral content maintains the bone architecture in spite of total cellular death.

Thus it can be seen that bone has two important functions within the body. It serves a *mechanical* function by forming the skeletal support of the body: protecting vital structures, providing attachments for muscles, and housing the bone marrow. It also serves a *physiologic* function related to its mineral content. Bone acts as a storage depot for calcium, and plays a role in meeting the needs of the patient for this element. Abnormal physiologic demands on bone result in pathologic changes in bone tissue.

Belying its appearance, bone is a living tissue in a constant state of physiologic activity. The sequence of bone formation, bone destruction, and new bone formation is repeated many times in the life cycle of a bone. Resorption of bone in one region and deposition of bone in other regions are responsible for the growth changes in the skeleton. This process of resorption and desposition continues throughout the life of the individual in response to various mechanical and hormonal stimuli.

Bone develops by transformation of pre-existing connective tissue. After vascularization of the condensed connective tissue, the cells begin to actively secrete proteoglycans and collagen to form bone matrix (*osteoid*) and bone collagen. The deposition of mineral salts in the

matrix or osteoid tissue probably through the mechanism of direct cellular action begins the process of ossification. Mineral crystals develop
from the calcium and phosphate in the intercellular matrix, and under
the influence of mesenchymal cells, called *osteoblasts*, are deposited
in relation to both the collagen fibrils and proteoglycans of the matrix.
As the calcification progresses, many osteoblasts become surrounded
and embedded within the calcified matrix. These embedded cells are
then called *osteocytes*. The structure of bone tissue is complete at this
point and needs only to mature.

Bone resorption begins while bone formation is in progress. The
two processes go on simultaneously, and their dynamic interaction is
responsible for establishing the final shape and architecture of each
bone. The cells associated with bone removal are called *osteoclasts*.

Bone is also a plastic tissue and is highly sensitive to alteration of
its normal mechanical function. It responds to the forces acting upon it
according to Wolff's law (1870), which states: "Every change in the
form and function of bones or their function alone is followed by certain definite changes in their external configuration in accordance
with mathematical laws" (Fig. 2). Thus, increased skeletal use is ac-

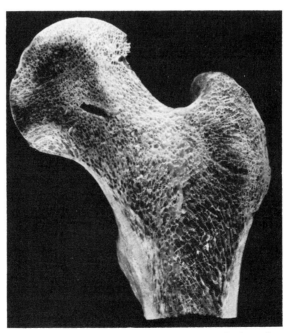

Figure 2.   Dried specimen of adult proximal femur. Thickened cortical bone on
medial aspect of femoral neck and alignment of cancellous trabecular systems illustrates Wolff's law.

companied by bone hypertrophy, with an increase in bone mass. Skeletal disuse results in bone atrophy, associated with a loss of substance.

Biomechanical studies of bone tissue have identified an *elastic phase* and a *plastic phase*. Up to a certain point of loading, bone deforms under load but snaps back to normal shape with release of the load. Beyond this point, bone deforms permanently with load, or if the load is sufficiently high, it breaks or fractures. It has also been shown that bone becomes less elastic or stiffer with age. Putting drill holes or screw holes in bone is known to weaken its structure.

Because of its ability to undergo internal reconstruction in response to external stimuli, bone may, to some extent, be modified at will by surgical and experimental procedures.

Like other body tissues, bone tissue may react to abnormal stimuli in a variety of ways, but these reactions are modified somewhat by its peculiar structure. Fracture healing, for example, consists of stages of inflammation and repair like any wound healing, but has the additional stage of osteogenesis. Infection has a particular effect on bone tissue and periosteum. When an area of bone is completely deprived of its blood supply, local cell death occurs, and this type of response is known as *avascular necrosis* or *osteonecrosis*. The body's attempt to heal the dead segment of bone is known as "creeping substitution."

Bone that remains alive can respond to abnormal stimuli by an alteration of bone deposition, by an alteration of bone resorption, or by a combination of these two processes. Bone deposition involves two stages: the osteoblastic formation of matrix or osteoid, and its subsequent calcification to form bone. Either process can be altered by an abnormal state. As the reader progresses through this book, numerous clinical examples will be noted in which the pathologic bone response is based either on increased or decreased bone deposition, or on increased or decreased bone resorption.

BONE DEVELOPMENT

As already noted, bone always develops by the transformation of embryonic or adult connective tissue into calcified connective tissue. When this process occurs in cartilage, it is called *endochondral ossification*, in contrast to simple intramembranous bone formation. The only difference between the two processes is that the former occurs within a cartilage model which must be removed before ossification can take place, although some of the cartilage matrix may remain as a framework on which bone is deposited. In both instances, actual bone tissue formation is the same.

BONE STRUCTURE

Grossly, bone tissue occurs in two types: *cancellous* (spongy) and *cortical* (compact). Cancellous bone consists of a latticework of interconnecting bony trabeculae surrounding spaces filled with bone marrow. Cortical bone is the outer surface of bone and appears as a continuous hard mass. Almost every bone contains varying proportions of both types of tissue in separate but merging zones. The cortical surface of bone is covered with periosteum. The inner surface of cortical bone is lined with endosteum, which also lines the marrow spaces.

A long bone is divided into several anatomic zones, the names of which are central in orthopaedic terminology (Fig. 3). The zone at ei-

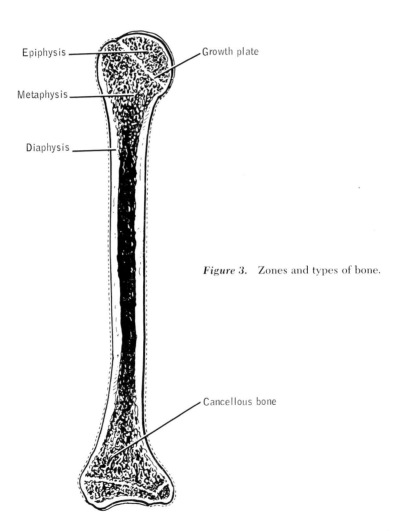

Epiphysis

Growth plate

Metaphysis

Diaphysis

Figure 3.   Zones and types of bone.

Cancellous bone

ther end of the long bone is called the *epiphysis.* This is a mass of cartilage at birth and is joined to the shaft of the bone by a specialized layer of cartilaginous cells known as the *growth plate.* By the time skeletal maturity is reached, the cartilaginous epiphysis has become completely ossified except for its covering of articular hyaline cartilage, and the growth plate has become only a line across the bone. The *metaphysis* is that part of the shaft of the bone immediately adjacent to the epiphysis. The *diaphysis* is the shaft of a long bone.

THE TOOLS

Diagnostic Tools

HISTORY

The history is the story of the patient's condition, related by the patient with the guidance of the examiner. At its conclusion, the examiner should understand clearly why the patient is seeking medical attention.

The story should be built around specific complaints. Disorders of musculoskeletal origin frequently give rise to specific complaints of pain, deformity, and loss of joint motion, or to symptoms of neurologic involvement. The examiner should guide the patient through an exact description in chronologic sequence, questioning him about manner of onset, duration of symptoms, previous symptoms, progress of the complaint, and extent of disability.

It is important to characterize the complaint. Deformity, for example, may be static or progressive, constant or intermittent. Pain may be localized to one area or may radiate to another part of the body. Pain may be described as aching, dull, sharp, or shooting.

Since musculoskeletal complaints are frequently associated with body mechanics, the examiner should determine the effects on the specific complaint of weight bearing, motion of the part, weather change, and rest. The examiner should ask the patient what aggravates the complaint, what relieves it, whether it has ever been treated, and if so, what were the effects of treatment.

PHYSICAL EXAMINATION

The orthopaedic physical examination includes evaluation of the body as a whole in addition to a more detailed examination of the part in question.

GENERAL ORTHOPAEDIC EXAMINATION

The general posture and alignment of the body, both front and back, are observed. It is important to evaluate the patient's body attitude when he is standing, and his carriage while he is walking. The relationships of the feet to the legs and of the hips to the pelvis are noted. The relationship of the upper extremities and shoulder girdle to the upper trunk is observed. The general contour of the spine is evaluated, and its relationship to the shoulder girdle, thorax, and pelvis is noted.

The patient is observed while walking, and any effect upon these various relationships should be evaluated. The manner of walking and the presence of a limp and its type should be observed. Any physical abnormality associated with walking, bending, sitting, or lying should be noted.

LOCAL ORTHOPAEDIC EXAMINATION

Specific physical findings of orthopaedic significance referable to each part of the body are discussed in detail in appropriate sections of the text.

Whenever the complaint refers to an area of either the lower or upper extremity, it is a good plan to examine the opposite side first. This affords the examiner the chance to establish a normal base line for that particular patient.

In general, the local physical examination should include:

Inspection. By inspection the examiner should note contour, appearance, color, or deformity of a part, and its general relationship to the body as a whole.

Palpation. By palpation the examiner should detect tenderness, swelling, muscle spasm, local temperature changes, or gross alterations in shape of the part.

Range of Motion. Each joint has certain characteristic motions that can be measured passively or actively. Motion is normally limited by the resistance of other nearby structures or by actual impingement on the joint by muscles, ligaments, or bone. Motion is abnormally limited by pain and muscle spasm, by inflammation or scarring of the muscles, ligaments, or synovial membrane, or by deformity of the bone.

Joint motion is measured in degrees of a circle (Fig. 4). An extended limb with the bones in a straight line can be said to be either in 0 degrees of flexion or in 180 degrees of extension. This represents the diameter of a circle with the joint at its center. As the joint is flexed from this position, the angle is increased or reduced depending upon

FLEXION and HYPEREXTENSION

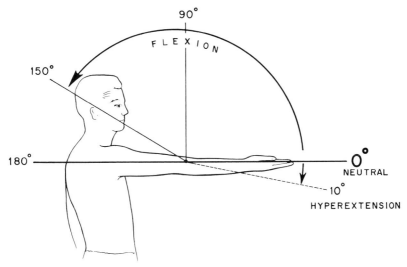

Figure 4. Joint motion is measured in degrees of a circle. (From Joint Motion Manual, American Academy of Orthopaedic Surgeons.)

which style of measurement is chosen, reaching 90 degrees at a right angle.

Passive joint motion is carried out by the examiner with the patient playing a passive role. The examiner tests the range of movements of which the part is normally capable and compares this range with that obtained on the opposite side.

Active joint motion represents the degree to which the patient can, without assistance, move the affected part.

Except in cases associated with muscular weakness or paralysis, the information obtained by testing passive motion is generally more valuable to the physician than the information obtained by evaluating active motion.

Joint Position. There are two important definitive positions that may be assumed by a joint under particular circumstances. The significance of these positions must be appreciated by the examiner.

The *position of function* for a joint is that position which gives the joint its maximum strength and efficiency. The position of function for the wrist joint, for example, is 30 degrees of dorsiflexion and 10 degrees of ulnar deviation. If injury or disease threatens to result in fusion or stiffness of the joint, disability will be minimized if the fusion occurs with the joint in the position of function.

The patient with an injured or diseased joint may assume the *position of comfort.* This is the position in which the joint feels most comfortable to the patient and is usually quite the reverse of the position of function. For example, the position of comfort for the wrist joint is palmar flexion. If the joint remains in this position following injury or disease, the disability that results from fusion or stiffness in this position will be markedly exaggerated.

Patients with damaged or diseased joints will naturally attempt to assume the position of comfort. It is part of the physician's responsibility to make sure that the affected joints are always supported in the position of function.

Measurement.   Atrophy or hypertrophy of a part may be determined by comparing circumferential type measurements with those obtained on the opposite side of the body.

The lengths of the limbs should be measured and compared in order to assess any inequality that may be present.

Neurologic Examination.   The strength of muscle power should be assessed whenever the presence of muscular weakness is suspected.

The quality of the superficial and deep tendon reflexes and the integrity of cutaneous sensation should be determined when indicated.

X-RAY EXAMINATION

Properly exposed and processed x-ray films are an important part of the examination of a patient with a musculoskeletal complaint.

Generally, the most useful views are the anteroposterior and lateral, with the films taken as the patient or the extremity lies upon the x-ray table. Visualization of bone should be in both planes whenever possible. It is frequently misleading and often impossible to attempt to evaluate the extent or character of a bone lesion from a single x-ray view. In certain conditions, it is helpful to obtain these views during weight bearing or while traction or stress is being applied to the part (Fig. 5). In certain instances, oblique x-ray views or films made at other special angles are indicated to obtain special information.

Laminography or body-section radiography is occasionally helpful in locating overshadowed lesions, small cavities, and foreign bodies. It is also useful in determining whether or not a bone graft is firmly united to the host bone.

Scanography is an x-ray technique used to measure accurately the lengths of the long bones. Scanograms are frequently obtained of children with leg length inequality upon whom epiphyseal surgery is contemplated (see p. 83).

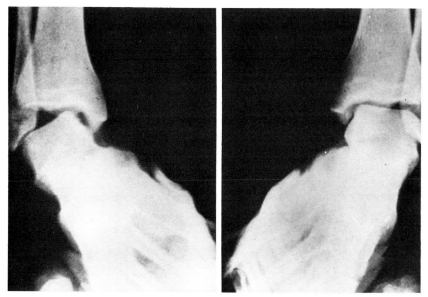

Figure 5.   Stress x-ray of ankle, showing marked talar tilting of right ankle.

LABORATORY STUDIES

The laboratory tests that are of greatest value in orthopaedic disorders are those performed on the blood, urine, synovial fluid, and tissue removed from the involved area.

The red and white blood cell counts, hemoglobin determination, and erythrocyte sedimentation rate are frequently affected in the presence of anemia, blood dyscrasias, infection, and tissue destruction.

The blood chemical findings that are of most significance in skeletal disorders include serum calcium, serum inorganic phosphorus, serum alkaline phosphatase, serum acid phosphatase, blood nonprotein nitrogen, blood sugar, and blood uric acid levels (Table 1).

In certain skeletal conditions, abnormal amounts of calcium and phosphorus may be found in the urine. An abnormal protein (Bence Jones protein) may be detected in the urine of some patients with multiple myeloma. Many of the mucopolysaccharidoses can be diagnosed biochemically by identifying in the urine the specific mucopolysaccharide excreted in excess.

In many pathologic conditions of the musculoskeletal system, confirmation of the diagnosis rests upon the histologic interpretation of tissue removed from the lesion by biopsy.

TABLE 1.   Laboratory Findings in Bone Disease[*]

CONDITION	SERUM Calcium	SERUM Inorganic Phosphorus	SERUM Alkaline Phosphatase	URINE Calcium	URINE Phosphorus
Hyperparathyroidism, primary	↑	↓	↑	↑	↑
Hyperparathyroidism, secondary	N–↓	↑	R ↑	↑	↓
Hyperthyroidism, marked	N	N	↑	↑	↑
Hypothyroidism	N	N	N	N	N
Senile osteoporosis	N	N–O ↓	N	N	N
Rickets (child)	↓	↓	↑	N	N
Osteomalacia (adult)	N–↓	↓	↑	N	N
Paget's disease	R ↑	R ↓	↑	N	N
Multiple myeloma	↑	N–↑	R ↑	↑	↑

CODE
N–normal
O–occasionally
R–rarely
↑ –increased
↓ –decreased
[*]Adapted from table of Dr. James L. Quinn, III. *In* Meschan, I.: Synopsis of Roentgen Signs. Philadelphia: W. B. Saunders Co., 1962.

SPECIAL TESTS

On occasion special tests may be required to aid in establishing diagnosis or proper treatment.

Biopsy.   The term biopsy refers to the removal and examination of tissue from a lesion for the purpose of diagnosis. In many instances, an open operation must be performed to obtain the tissue.

On occasion a core of tissue may be removed from a musculoskeletal lesion by a special type of needle or bore introduced through the skin. This type of biopsy is referred to as aspiration, needle, or punch biopsy. In certain areas of the body, such as the spine, it is necessary to perform aspiration biopsy under x-ray control.

Joint Aspiration.   A joint may be aspirated to relieve pain, to aid in making a diagnosis, or to instill medication. The aspirant obtained may be blood, pus, or normal-appearing synovial fluid.

This procedure must be performed under aseptic precautions and usually local anesthesia. The needle used for aspiration should be long enough to penetrate the joint capsule successfully and of sufficient gauge to allow the withdrawal of thickened fluid.

The joint most frequently aspirated is the knee. This joint may be aspirated through one of two approaches: (1) with the knee joint extended, a swollen suprapatellar pouch may be entered just medial to the superior pole of the patella; (2) with the knee flexed, the joint proper may be entered through the articular cleft just medial to the patellar tendon. This approach is generally the most useful.

Myelography. Myelography is an x-ray technique that allows visualization of the spinal cord by the use of a radiopaque dye injected into the subarachnoid space (Fig. 158). This test may give information if pressure upon the spinal cord or nerve roots is suspected. Herniated intervertebral discs usually either indent the dye column or interfere with the filling of a nerve root-sleeve or both.

Electromyography. Electromyography is a technique in which monopolar or coaxial needles are inserted directly into the muscle for the purpose of studying and measuring the electrical potential change associated with skeletal muscle contraction. Both this test and nerve conduction studies are frequently helpful in the differential diagnosis of neuromuscular affections.

Arthrography. Arthrography is a special type of x-ray examination in which radiopaque dye, air, or both is injected into a joint cavity as a contrast medium to outline soft tissue components of the joint not usually visualized on an ordinary x-ray film. This study is particularly useful in the knee joint as an aid to the diagnosis of meniscal tears or other suspected internal derangements (Fig. 6).

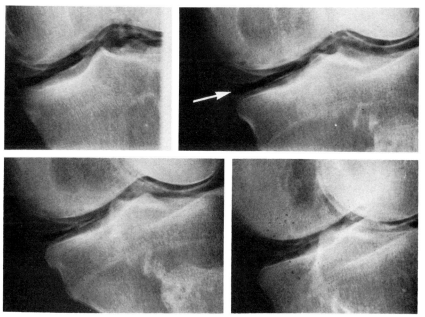

Figure 6. Normal knee arthrogram. Arrow points to triangular-shaped shadow representing a normal medial meniscus.

Arthroscopy. Arthroscopy is the insertion of a specially designed endoscope into a joint cavity under anesthesia for the purpose of direct visualization of the joint's structure and contents. The technique has its greatest usefulness in the knee joint.

Treatment Tools

In the treatment program, the orthopaedic physician makes use of general medical measures, such as reassurance and encouragement, rest, attention to diet, and drugs when needed. He also has special treatment tools available for specific tasks. Among these special tools are plaster bandages, traction devices, braces and appliances, special dressings, orthopaedic surgical procedures, and rehabilitative measures. There should be no hesitation on the physician's part about requesting consultation with other physicians if the information obtained will aid in the diagnosis or management of the patient's problem.

PLASTER OF PARIS

On of the most useful tools available to the orthopaedist is plaster of paris, from which he can make splints, circular casts, and molds of body parts (Figs. 7 and 8).

Plaster is supplied by commercial manufacturers as rolled bandages of varying size wrapped in waxed paper. Plaster of paris bandages are rolls of crinoline bandage impregnated with anhydrous calcium sulfate. When these bandages are soaked in lukewarm water, the anhydrous calcium sulfate absorbs water to recrystallize or set as calcium sulfate dihydrate or gypsum. This process of recrystallization is an exothermic reaction, which makes the plaster feel warm as it sets and hardens. Before the plaster bandages are applied, the part is usually padded with some type of sheet wadding, cotton bandage, or stockinette. Bony prominences should be protected by extra padding.

The types of plaster cast most commonly used include:

Short leg cast, in which the plaster extends from the toes to the level of the tibial tubercle.

Long leg cast, in which the plaster extends from the toes to the upper thigh area.

Short arm cast, in which the plaster extends from the knuckles to just below the elbow.

Long arm cast, in which the plaster extends from the knuckles to just below the axilla.

Hip spica cast, which is used to immobilize the hip joint and

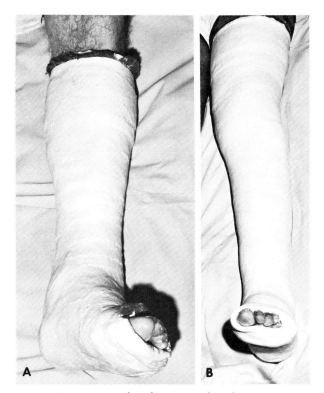

Figure 7. A, short leg cast. B, long leg cast.

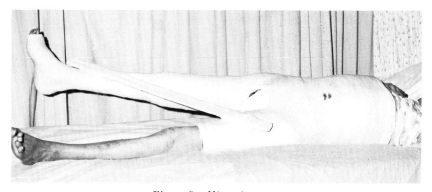

Figure 8. Hip spica cast.

pelvis. A double hip spica cast immobilizes both hip joints and allows the patient to be turned completely without moving the affected part. The plaster extends from the nipple line of the chest to the toes on the affected side and to the knee on the opposite side.

Shoulder spica cast, in which the plaster encases the upper extremity, shoulder region, and trunk. This type of cast is used to immobilize parts of the upper extremity and shoulder joint.

TRACTION DEVICES

Some details regarding skin and skeletal traction devices are given in Chapter 2 (see p. 33).

In addition to its possible use as maintenance traction in the treatment of some fractures, the form of skin traction to the lower extremity known as Buck's extension may be used for any condition of the knee, femur, or hip joint in which partial immobilization with a light traction force is desired. Thus, it may be used for temporary immobilization of a fractured hip or for immobilization following reduction of a dislocated hip joint. It may be used for short periods of time in the treatment of Legg-Calvé-Perthes disease or other causes of a painful synovial irritation of the hip joint to help relieve pain caused by muscle spasm.

BRACES AND APPLIANCES

Braces and appliances may be used to rest a part of the body, to limit or encourage its activity, to aid in correcting or preventing deformity, or to provide mechanical support (Fig. 9).

Braces and appliances may be purely passive supports or may make use of spring devices to become dynamic splints.

SPECIAL DRESSINGS

The Velpeau bandage and Gibney boot are examples of special dressings that find great usefulness in the treatment of some musculoskeletal problems.

The Velpeau bandage binds the arm and shoulder to the chest and is used mostly for immobilization of certain fractures about the upper end of the humerus and the shoulder joint. It is usually constructed from either wide mesh gauze bandages or elastic bandages (Fig. 10). For the treatment of some conditions, a plaster of paris Velpeau dressing may be made.

The Gibney boot is an adhesive tape support useful in the treat-

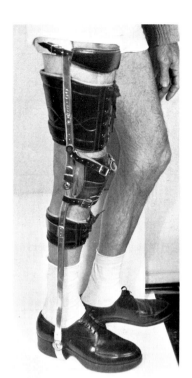

Figure 9. An ischial weight bearing brace.

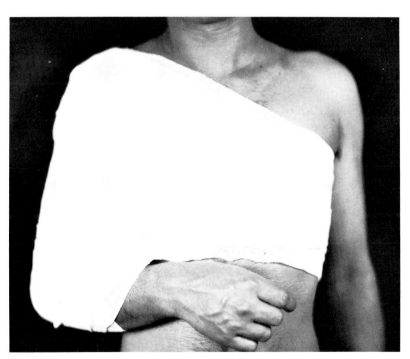

Figure 10. Velpeau dressing.

17

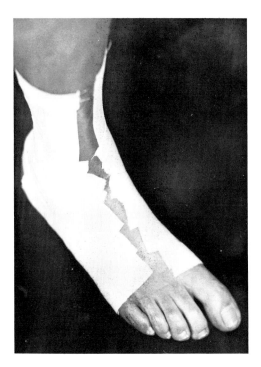

Figure 11. Gibney boot.

ment of sprains and other painful conditions about the ankle joint. The tape is applied by alternate strips in a basket weave fashion (Fig. 11).

ORTHOPAEDIC SURGICAL PROCEDURES

When proper indications exist, the orthopaedist may perform a surgical procedure as a method of treatment. The definitions of these surgical terms are given here. The indications for their use are discussed under the appropriate diagnoses in the body of the text. Orthopaedic surgical procedures may be performed on soft tissues or on bone.

Surgical procedures that are performed on soft tissue by orthopaedists include:

Tenotomy—the surgical cutting of a tendon.

Capsulotomy—the surgical cutting of a joint capsule.

Tendon lengthening—a surgical technique designed to lengthen a shortened tendon without interrupting its continuity.

Tendon transplantation—the surgical relocation of the tendon of a normal muscle to another site to take over the function of a muscle permanently inactivated by trauma or disease.

Surgical procedures that are performed on bone include:

Osteotomy—the surgical cutting of bone in order to correct deformity in the bone or adjacent joint (Fig. 12).

Arthrotomy—the surgical opening of a joint for the purpose of exploring the joint for evidence of disease or removal of injured or diseased tissue.

Arthrodesis—a surgical procedure designed to cause the bones of a joint to grow firmly together or fuse. Arthrodesis, or fusion, involves surgical removal of articular hyaline cartilage and usually the addition of bone grafts across the joint surface. Metallic internal fixation devices may or may not be used. Successful arthrodesis usually results in a stiff, but stable and painless, joint (Fig. 13).

Arthroplasty—a surgical procedure designed to restore motion to a joint deformed by injury or disease. Arthroplasty may involve replacement of part of the joint by a metallic prosthesis. Arthroplasty

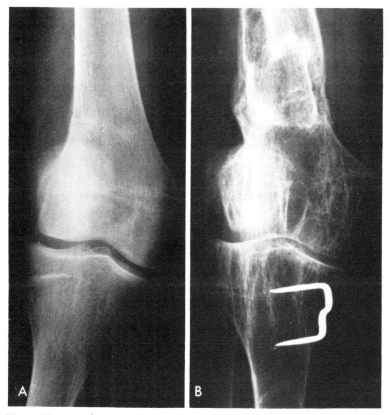

Figure 12. A, valgus angulation of knee in renal dialysis patient. B, appearance after correction of angular deformity by femoral and tibial osteotomies.

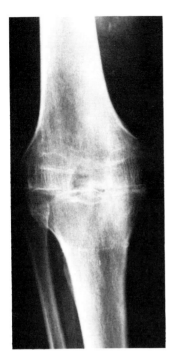

Figure 13.   AP x-ray of a surgically fused knee joint.

may also involve the surgical reshaping of the bones of the joint, and on occasion, the addition of a soft tissue or metallic interposition device between the reshaped bone ends to aid in establishing motion between the bones (Fig. 14).

Total joint replacement — a special type of arthroplasty in which both sides of the joint are replaced by metal or plastic implants anchored to the bone by methyl methacrylate bone cement (Fig. 168).

Bone grafting — the surgical transplantation of pieces of compact or cancellous bone to another location in the body. Bone grafts or transplants are commonly used to fill gaps and defects in bone, to facilitate the healing of fractures that otherwise would not heal, or in which healing would be greatly delayed, and to bring about bony fusion in joints damaged by injury or disease.

The cells in a bone graft die soon after removal from the donor site. The dead bone graft acts as a framework in the host area and is eventually replaced by new bone tissue growing in from the host area.

Bone grafts or transplants are classified according to the source of the material to be grafted: those cut from the individual who will receive them are called *autografts;* those from another individual of the same species are called *homografts;* those from animals of another species are called *heterografts.* Whenever possible, autografts are

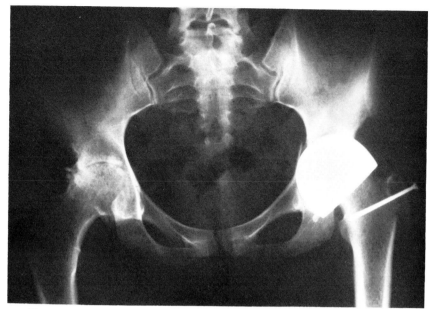

Figure 14.   AP x-ray of hip after arthroplasty utilizing a metallic cup in patient with rheumatoid arthritis of both hips.

used in orthopaedic surgical procedures because they produce no immunologic graft reaction phenomenon. Homografts of stored or "banked" bone are occasionally necessary if large skeletal defects are to be filled. Heterografts are generally unsatisfactory and are seldom used in orthopaedic surgical procedures.

References

Andry, N.: Orthopaedia, Vols. I and II. Facsimile Reproduction of the First Edition in English, London 1743. Philadelphia: J. B. Lippincott Co., 1961.

Bick, E. M. (Ed.): Historical orthopaedics. Clin. Orth. and Rel. Res., *No. 44*, 1966.

Bourne, G. H. (Ed.): Biochemistry and Physiology of Bone, 2nd Edition. New York: Academic Press, 1971.

Boyne, P. J.: Autogenous cancellous bone and marrow transplants. Clin. Orth. and Rel. Res., 73:199, 1970.

Brookes, M.: The Blood Supply of Bone. An Approach to Bone Biology. New York: Appleton-Century Crofts, 1971.

Capener, N.: Surgical implants. J. Bone and Joint Surg., *47-B*:3, 1965.

Chalmers, J.: Transplantation immunity in bone homografting. J. Bone and Joint Surg., *41-B*:160, 1959.

Close, J. R.: Functional Anatomy of the Extremities. Springfield, Illinois: Charles C Thomas, 1973.

Cohen, J., and Harris, W. H.: The three-dimensional anatomy of haversian systems. J. Bone and Joint Surg., *40-A*:419, 1958.

Coventry, M. B.: Development of the human musculoskeletal system. Am. Academy of Orthopaedic Surgeons Instructional Course Lectures, Vol. V:218. Ann Arbor: J. W. Edwards, 1948.

Crenshaw, A. H. (Ed.): Campbell's Operative Orthopaedics, 5th Edition, Vols. 1 and 2. St. Louis: C. V. Mosby Co., 1971.

Duchene, G. B. A.: Physiology of Motion. Translated and Edited by E. B. Kaplan. Philadelphia: J. B. Lippincott Co., 1949.

Ferguson, A. B., Jr.: Orthopaedic Surgery in Infancy and Childhood, 3rd Edition. Baltimore: Williams & Wilkins Co., 1968.

Forrester, D. M., and Nesson, J. W.: The Radiology of Joint Disease. Philadelphia: W. B. Saunders Co., 1973.

Frankel, V. H., and Burstein, A.: Orthopaedic Biomechanics. Philadelphia: Lee and Febiger, 1970.

Frost, H. M.: Bone Biodynamics. Boston: Little, Brown & Co., 1964.

Gardner, E.: The development and growth of bones and joints. J. Bone and Joint Surg., 45-A:856, 1963.

Glimcher, M. J.: A basic architectural principle in the organization of mineralized tissues. Clin. Orth. and Rel. Res., 61:16, 1968.

Green, W. T.: Orthopaedic surgery, yesterday and tomorrow. J. Bone and Joint Surg., 39-A:675, 1957.

Harris, W. H., Salzman, E. W., and Desanctis, R. W.: Prevention of thrombo-embolic disease by prophylactic anticoagulation. J. Bone and Joint Surg., 49-A:81, 1967.

Heiple, K. G., Chase, S. W., and Herndon, C. H: A comparative study of the healing process following different types of bone transplantation. J. Bone and Joint Surg., 45-A:1593, 1963.

Hejna, W. F.: Clinical applications of electrodiagnostic studies. Am. Academy of Orthopaedic Surgeons Instructional Course Lectures, Vol. XIX. St. Louis: C. V. Mosby Co., 1970.

Herndon, C. H.: Principles of bone graft surgery, different methods of operative procedure, and indications for each. Am. Academy of Orthopaedic Surgeons Instructional Course Lectures, Vol. XVII:149. St. Louis: C. V. Mosby Co., 1960.

Howell, D. S.: Current concepts of calcification. J. Bone and Joint Surg., 53-A:250, 1971.

Jaffe, H. L.: Metabolic Degenerative and Inflammatory Diseases of Bone and Joints. Philadelphia: Lee and Febiger, 1972.

Kenney, W. E., and Larson, C. B.: Orthopaedics for the General Practitioner. St. Louis: C. V. Mosby Co., 1957.

McLean, F. C., and Urist, M. R.: Bone: Fundamentals of the Physiology of Skeletal Tissue, 3rd Edition. University of Chicago Press, 1968.

Murray, R. O., and Jacobson, H. G.: The Radiology of Skeletal Disorders. Baltimore: Williams & Wilkins Co., 1971.

Posner, A. S.: Crystal chemistry of bone mineral. Physiol. Rev., 49:760, 1969.

Raney, R. B., and Brashear, H. R., Jr.: Shands' Handbook of Orthopaedic Surgery, 8th Edition. St. Louis: C. V. Mosby Co., 1971.

Rodahl, K., Nicholson, J. P., and Brown, E. M., Jr.: Bone as a Tissue. New York: McGraw-Hill, 1960.

Rosse, C., and Clawson, D. K.: Introduction to the Musculoskeletal System. New York: Harper and Row, 1970.

Salter, R. B.: Textbook of Disorders and Injuries of the Musculoskeletal System. Baltimore: Williams & Wilkins Co., 1970.

Sherman, M. S.: The nerves of bones. J. Bone and Joint Surg., 45-A:522, 1963.

Stein, I., Stein, R. O., and Beller, M. L.: Living Bone in Health and Disease. Philadelphia: J. B. Lippincott Co., 1955.

Tachojian, M. O.: Pediatric Orthopaedics, Vols. 1 and 2. Philadelphia: W. B. Saunders Co., 1972.

Termine, J. D.: Mineral chemistry and skeletal biology. Clin. Orth. and Rel. Res., 85:207, 1972.

Trueta, J.: Studies of the Development and Decay of the Human Frame. Philadelphia: W. B. Saunders Co., 1968.

Turek, S. L.: Orthopaedics. Principles and Their Application, 2nd Edition. Philadelphia: J. B. Lippincott Co., 1967.

Vaughn, J.: The Physiology of Bone. Oxford: Clarendon Press, 1970.

Chapter Two

Principles of Management of Fractures and Dislocations

THE PROBLEM

The problem facing the physician who is called upon to treat a patient with a broken bone or dislocated joint is that of restoring full function to the part, with the bone or joint solidly healed in a position as near to the normal as possible. These results can be obtained only through knowledge and judgment on the part of the physician and cooperation on the part of the patient.

Only principles of management will be given in this chapter. Details regarding particular fractures and dislocations will be found in the chapters dealing with the specific regions involved.

FRACTURES

Definition

The standard definition of fracture is a break in the continuity of bone. However, a fracture is a rupture of living connective tissue and, as such, is more than a broken bone. It ultimately involves all the soft tissues in the injured area as well as the bone. Thus fractures may be accompanied by extensive soft tissue edema, hemorrhage into muscles and joints, dislocation of joints, rupture of tendons, contusions or severance of nerves, and damage to major blood vessels.

23

As might be expected, fractures are most common in males in the 20 to 40 age group, with the bones of the extremities being most often involved. Although the forces causing fractures are no respecters of age or sex, certain fractures show characteristic predilections. Thus, fractures of the clavicle and through the supracondylar area of the humerus are most common in children. Fracture through the surgical neck of the humerus and Colles fracture at the wrist occur most frequently in women. Compression fracture of a vertebra and fracture of the hip show their greatest incidence in the aged.

In normal patients, the healing of fractures is not influenced by the use of vitamins, hormones, or extradietary calcium. Certain disease states, such as hypoproteinemia and severe anemia, delay fracture healing. There is evidence to suggest that certain drugs, such as corticosteroids, Dicumarol, and heparin, also delay fracture healing.

Normally, the age of the patient is no deterrent to fracture healing. Although it is true that fracture repair is more rapid and certain in children, the notion that fractures heal poorly in the aged is erroneous. Age and ability to repair bone are virtually unrelated in the normal adult. Rather, the rate and certainty of fracture healing are in direct relation to the vascularity of the bone and the surrounding soft tissues.

The layman's suspicion that once a bone is broken it is forever weak is not true. Provided normal anatomic alignment of the bone has been obtained, remodeling of the bone tissue after healing has occurred will restore normal strength and structure to the part. However, evidence does exist to indicate that the segment of bone containing the healed fracture does not regain its normal tissue elasticity.

Causes of Fractures

Normal bone with an intact blood supply exhibits a degree of elasticity and can withstand, within limits, compression and shearing forces and, to a lesser extent, tension forces. Bone fractures, therefore, when its capacity to absorb energy is exceeded.

The most common cause of fracture of normal bone is violence. The violence may be applied directly to a bone, as in a fall on the part or when a person is struck by an automobile. Less violent transmitted forces may be applied indirectly to a bone by means of tension strain. Thus torsion injuries to the foot and ankle while skiing may cause an oblique fracture of the tibial shaft, or a fall on the outstretched hand may cause fracture of the radial head at the elbow.

An angulatory force applied to a long bone in a young child may fracture the cortex on the convex side of the bend, but only bend the cortex on the concave side. This is the so-called "greenstick" fracture frequently seen in young children.

Sudden forceful muscle contraction may deliver a shearing force sufficient to break bone. Certain fractures of the patella and os calcis occur in this manner.

Stress or fatigue fractures occur in certain bones in the absence of documented violence. March fractures, seen in the metatarsals, are examples of stress fractures (see p. 404).

Much less violence is required to break a bone in an elderly patient because of accompanying osteoporosis (see p. 175). Evidence indicates that osteoporosis causes quantitative, not qualitative, changes in bone. There is simply less bone present. The bone that remains exhibits no decrease in its strength characteristics or energy absorbing capacity.

A pathologic fracture is a fracture that occurs through an area of bone previously weakened by disease or tumor. In this instance the involved bone is weakened both quantitatively and qualitatively by the underlying disease. As a rule, only minimal trauma is required to induce such a fracture. Examples of disease states that might be associated with pathologic fractures are osteomyelitis, metabolic bone disease, and lytic tumors of bone caused by deposits of metastatic carcinoma.

Classification of Fractures

Fractures may be classified according to the type of fracture sustained, the direction of the fracture line, or the type of bone tissue involved. The proper combination of these terms "describes the fracture."

TYPES OF FRACTURE (FIG. 15)

Closed fracture — a fracture of a bone not associated with a wound extending from the skin surface to the area of bone injury.

Open fracture — a fracture of a bone associated with an open wound extending through the skin surface and down to the area of bone injury. Bone fragments may or may not be protruding through the open skin defect. All open fractures are potentially infected and require emergency surgical care.

Incomplete fracture — an incomplete break in the continuity of bone.

Complete fracture — a complete interruption in the continuity of bone.

Comminuted fracture — a fracture consisting of three or more bone fragments.

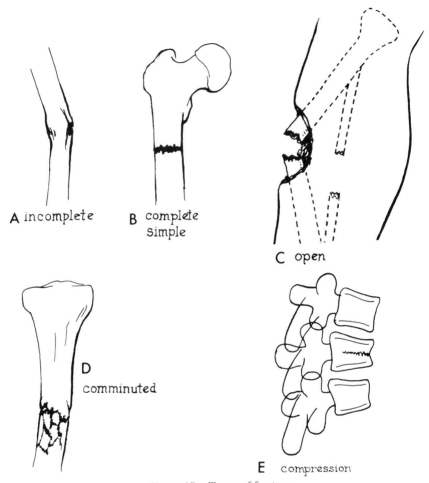

A incomplete B complete simple C open D comminuted E compression

Figure 15. Types of fracture.

Impacted fracture — a fracture in which one fragment is imbedded in the substance of the other.

Compression fracture — a type of impacted fracture characterized by crushed bone tissue.

DIRECTIONS OF FRACTURE LINE (FIG. 16)

As seen on an x-ray film, the fracture line may be described as *longitudinal, transverse, oblique,* or *spiral.* The fracture is said to be *displaced* when the bone fragments have been moved or changed from their normal position; it is said to exhibit *overriding* when the

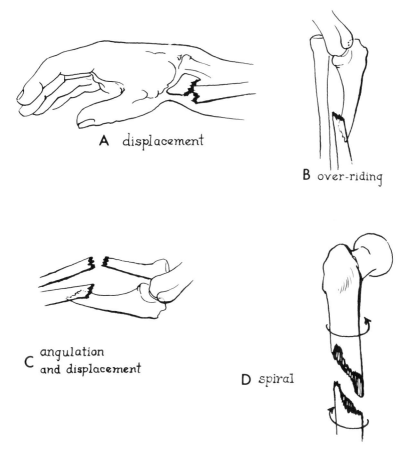

Figure 16. Types of fracture deformity.

fracture fragments overlap, resulting in shortening of the bone. The fracture is said to show *angulation* when the fragments have moved out of a linear relationship into an angular relationship, and *rotation* is present when one fragment has rotated on its axis in relation to the other.

TYPES OF BONE TISSUE

Cancellous bone—Owing to the extremely rich blood supply, fractures involving cancellous bone rarely fail to unite.

Cortical bone—Cortical or compact bone is thick and relatively avascular, enclosing a small vascular medullary canal. Repair of this type of bone tissue is slow.

Healing of Fractures

Most tissues have a common response to injury. This response includes inflammation and repair. Fracture healing is similar to any other type of wound healing, except that osteogenesis occurs to re-establish bone continuity.

Once a bone is broken into two or more parts, each part is thereafter called a fragment. The new tissue that forms at and around the area of the break to join the fragments together for healing is called *callus* or *callus tissue* (Fig. 17). Callus that arises from the periosteum is called external callus. Callus that arises from the endosteum of the marrow cavity and from marrow cells is called internal callus. In suc-

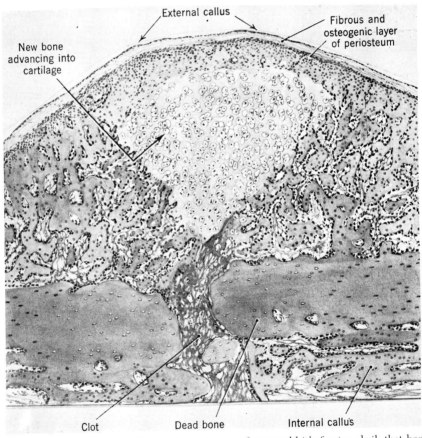

Figure 17. Drawing of part of a section cut from a rabbit's fractured rib that has healed for 2 weeks. This drawing illustrates the external callus to advantage and shows that the cartilage in it is being replaced by bone along a V-shaped line. Some clot, still unorganized, can still be seen. (Ham, A. W., and Harris, W. R.: *In* Bourne, G. H.: The Biochemistry and Physiology of Bone, 2nd ed. New York: Academic Press, 1972.)

cessful healing, the callus is first composed of both cartilage and bone but eventually consists only of bone tissue. In unsuccessful repair, the callus may be composed of dense fibrous tissue that does not convert to bone. If this occurs, the fragments are said to be joined by a fibrous union.

The following steps in fracture repair have been described:

1. The violence that causes fracture results in a tearing or rupture of haversian, marrow, and periosteal blood vessels. Loss of their blood supply leads to the death of bone and periosteal cells in the area adjacent to the fracture line. Bleeding from the ends of a broken bone results in the formation of a blood clot or fracture hematoma between the bone fragments. The normal inflammatory response of the tissue permits gradual removal of cellular debris and fibrin by macrophages. Within 48 to 72 hours, a few connective tissue cells appear in the wound and begin to multiply, having invaded the fracture site from the adjacent vascular connective tissue and marrow. These cells can differentiate into chondroblasts or osteoblasts. The periosteum and endosteum also act as sources of osteoblasts.

2. For the first seven days, the fracture site is similar to any wound, except for the presence of fibroblasts and osteoblasts. The fibroblasts and osteoblasts actively engage in the synthesis and secretion of collagen, which takes the form of fibrils of varying diameter within the wound site. They also synthesize and secrete proteoglycans, which form an integral part of the proliferative connective tissue matrix or callus at the repair site. The callus begins to calcify within 14 to 17 days, and ultimately bone mineral (hydroxyapatite) is deposited in it.

3. External callus grows and develops from osteogenic cells of the torn periosteum as a collar of cartilage and new bone. This collar encircles the fragment, enlarges, and grows toward the collar associated with the adjacent bone fragment.

4. Internal callus, arising from the endosteum of the marrow cavity and from marrow cells, infiltrates the blood clot. The remaining blood clot aids in the joining process by becoming converted into osteoid tissue. Eventually bone trabeculae from each fragment meet and join together.

5. The fracture fragments become firmly united by an external bridge of trabeculated bone and an internal bridge of trabeculated bone. These newly formed trabeculae are joined to living and dead portions of the original bone fragments.

6. Final remodeling of the healed area is the last step in fracture healing. The dead portions of the original fragments are slowly resorbed, and the bone gradually assumes a more normal shape and architecture (Fig. 18).

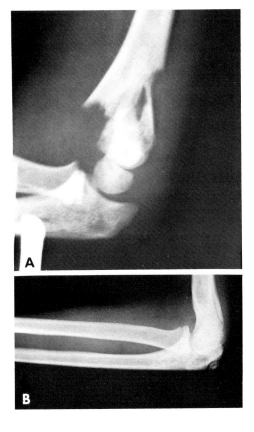

Figure 18. A, supracondylar fracture of humerus treated by skeletal traction. *B*, same area five years later showing final remodeling of bone.

If the healing process is disrupted for any reason — as by loss of fracture hematoma, lack of adequate blood supply to the fragments, poor immobilization, or infection — it is delayed or inhibited completely.

HEALING OF ARTICULAR CARTILAGE

Unlike bone, articular cartilage is very limited in its ability to regenerate. This is of clinical significance when a fracture involves a joint with a splitting of the articular cartilage. Hyaline articular cartilage heals not by hyaline cartilage but by fibrocartilage, which is a form of scar tissue.

If the fracture surfaces of the cartilage are perfectly reduced, the thin band of fibrocartilage is of little clinical significance. If a gap remains between the fragments, however, the fibrocartilage filling the gap will not withstand normal wear and tear stresses, and the joint will eventually show degenerative changes.

FRACTURE MANAGEMENT

Examination

In some patients, fracture of bone may be just one aspect of a multiple injury problem. Under certain circumstances, accompanying soft tissue injury — particularly if it involves brain, spinal cord, thoracic or abdominal viscera, a major artery, or a peripheral nerve — may assume much greater clinical significance than the fracture itself. In these instances definitive fracture care will occupy a lower priority on the treatment scale.

Fracture of a bone may cause physical deformity of the part, resulting in unnatural or impaired motion on careful manipulation. Swelling and local tenderness may characterize the injured area. Exquisite pain is usually produced by active or passive attempts to move the injured part. Protective muscle spasm may be present as a physiologic effort to splint the fracture fragments and to protect against the pain caused by movement (Fig. 19).

Visual examination of the part will determine if the patient has sustained an open wound through the skin surface. Such an open wound may indicate the presence of an open fracture.

The presence or absence of any associated muscle, tendon, blood vessel, or nerve damage must be determined.

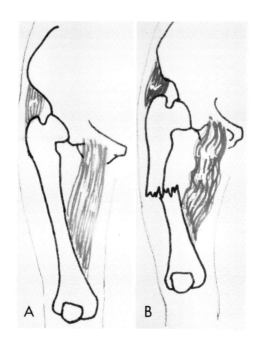

Figure 19. A, normal muscle tension pull on bone. B, after fracture, muscle tension pull may displace the bone fragments.

The general condition of the patient should be evaluated. Extensive hemorrhage or multiple injuries may cause shock, which must be treated and stabilized before the fracture is reduced.

All suspected fractures should be immobilized immediately until adequate x-ray studies have been obtained.

X-ray Examination

The presence of a fracture and its type is confirmed by x-ray examination. X-rays taken for this purpose should always include at least two planes: the anteroposterior and lateral views. Because of the possibility of multiple injuries of the same bone, it is essential to x-ray the joint above and the joint below the bone involved.

Children with suspected joint fracture should also have x-rays of the uninvolved joint on the opposite side for comparison purposes. The variations found in the epiphyses of growing children make it essential to have comparison views if the presence of an epiphyseal injury is to be determined.

Treatment of the Closed Fracture

Once the patient has been examined and the x-ray films reviewed, the physician is in a position to decide on a course of treatment.

The term reduction, as applied to fractures, refers to the means employed to bring the fracture fragments back into close apposition and alignment.

The term immobilization, as applied to fractures, refers to the means employed to maintain the reduction until successful repair of the fracture has occurred.

Successful healing of a fracture is determined to a great extent by three factors: (1) the accuracy of the reduction of the displaced fracture fragments, (2) the efficiency of the immobilization by which the fracture fragments are held in the reduced position, and (3) the local blood supply available to the fracture fragments. Whenever bone has lost its normal blood supply, or when there is serious soft tissue damage interfering with the surrounding invasion of blood vessels, fracture healing is delayed.

Means Employed to Obtain Reduction

The goal of reduction is to bring the fracture fragments into close apposition to each other so that normal position, length, and alignment of the bone are restored. The means employed to obtain reduction are manipulation (closed reduction), the use of traction devices, and open operation (open reduction). The choice depends upon the nature of the fracture and the experience and training of the physician.

Closed Reduction (Manipulation). Closed reduction of a fracture means the manual restoration of normal alignment to the bone. Manipulation is carried out under anesthesia, either general, regional, or local. In most instances, closed reduction consists of manual traction applied by the physician with manual countertraction supplied by an assistant. The physician attempts to lock the ends of the fragments together, thereby restoring normal position, length, and alignment (Fig. 20).

Traction Devices (Reduction Traction). Reduction of certain fractures is best obtained by the use of some type of traction device whose purpose is to restore alignment to the broken bone. In practice, traction is exerted on the distal fragment, aligning it with the less manageable proximal fragment. The traction force necessary to attain alignment is called reduction traction and is usually intense in application but short in duration (see Maintenance Traction, p. 36).

SKIN TRACTION.   A light traction force may be delivered to a bone if pull is exerted on adhesive strips attached to the skin of an extremity. The main disadvantage of skin traction is that it cannot provide more than 8 or 10 pounds of pull to the part, and this limits its usefulness. It is frequently employed for the reduction of fractures in

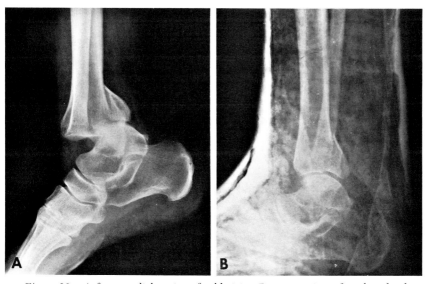

Figure 20.   *A,* fracture dislocation of ankle joint. *B,* same patient after closed reduction and application of cast.

younger children. The most common form of skin traction in use is called Buck's extension.

BUCK'S EXTENSION (FIG. 21).   Strips of ordinary adhesive tape or moleskin are applied to the sides of the leg and attached to a spreader block at the foot. The leg is wrapped with an elastic bandage to improve the purchase of the tape on the skin. A piece of traction cord attaches the spreader block to the weight, which is hung over the foot of the bed. The lower leg is supported on a pillow to reduce friction of the heel against the bed linen. Countertraction is supplied by elevating the foot of the bed on shock blocks.

SKELETAL TRACTION.   A heavy traction force may be delivered to a broken bone by pulling on a metal pin or wire inserted directly into or through a bone. Particularly in adults, strong traction and countertraction are usually necessary for the reduction of transverse and oblique fractures of major long bones showing displacement and overriding. A traction force of up to 40 pounds can be delivered to a bone by means of skeletal traction.

In the lower extremity, the metal pin may be drilled through the os calcis, the distal tibia and fibula, the proximal tibia, or the supracondylar area of the femur, depending on the location of the fracture to be treated.

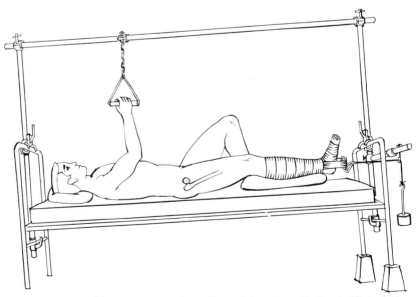

Figure 21.   Buck's extension in place. (From Schmeisser, G., Jr.: A Clinical Manual of Orthopedic Traction Techniques. Philadelphia: W. B. Saunders Co., 1963.)

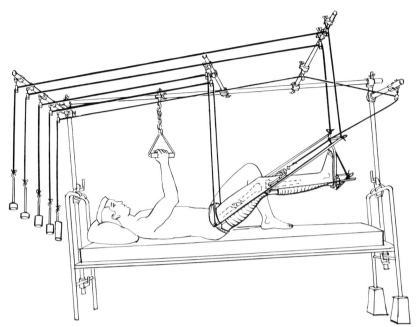

Figure 22.   Skeletal traction with balanced suspension. (From Schmeisser, G., Jr.: A Clinical Manual of Orthopedic Traction Techniques. Philadelphia: W. B. Saunders Co., 1963.)

The pin is drilled through the crest of the ulna below the olecranon when skeletal traction is applied to certain fractures of the elbow or humerus.

A traction bow or yoke is attached to the metal pin, and the traction force is transmitted through a system of ropes and pulleys. The main disadvantage of skeletal traction is the danger of infection developing in or around the pin tract.

A form of skeletal traction currently in general use is called skeletal traction with balanced suspension. This consists of a traction system that supplies the skeletal traction and a suspension system that balances or floats the limb in the traction splint apparatus (Fig. 22).

Open Reduction.   Open reduction of a fracture means the restoration of normal bone alignment under direct vision through an open surgical incision. The decision to employ open reduction should be made only by a physician trained and experienced in fracture management. The main disadvantage of open reduction is the theoretical danger of introducing infection into the bone. In general, open reduction is accompanied by some delay in bone healing time because of loss of fracture hematoma and increased trauma to the fracture fragments by operative manipulation.

MEANS EMPLOYED TO MAINTAIN REDUCTION

Once the fracture fragments have been brought into close apposition and alignment by reduction, some means must be employed to immobilize the bone fragments in position. The goal of immobilization is to maintain the fracture fragments in contact and alignment until successful repair of the fracture has occurred.

The means employed to maintain reduction are external fixation devices, traction devices, and internal fixation devices. The choice of method depends on the nature of the fracture and the experience and training of the physician.

External Fixation Devices. The most commonly used form of external fixation is a plaster cast encircling the injured part to ensure immobilization. Complete fixation of a broken bone with a plaster cast involves immobilizing the joints above and below the fracture site (see Figs. 7 and 8).

Efficient external fixation for some small bone fractures, such as those of the fingers or metacarpals, may be supplied by plaster splints.

Frequently, a combination of closed reduction and plaster cast fixation is employed in the treatment of fractures.

Traction Devices (Maintenance Traction). A fracture that has been reduced in some form of traction device is generally maintained in that traction for immobilization until fracture healing has occurred. Once reduction of the fracture has been effected by the traction force, the weight is reduced to the least amount capable of holding the fragments in apposition and alignment. This is called maintenance traction.

Internal Fixation Devices. An internal fixation device is a metallic pin, wire, screw, plate, nail, or rod that is used to hold bone fragments in apposition and alignment mechanically until successful healing occurs (Fig. 23). These devices may be fixed to the sides of the bone, placed through bone fragments, or, in the case of rods, inserted directly into the medullary cavity of the bone. Although pins and wires may be inserted percutaneously, most of these devices must be applied to bone by means of an operation. Thus the use of internal fixation is most frequently combined with open reduction of the fracture.

A very useful variant of the internal fixation technique is the "pins and plaster" method. In this method, pins are drilled percutaneously into the shaft of the bone at some distance above and below the fracture line and are left protruding from the skin edge. A plaster cast is then applied, incorporating the pins. This type of external skeletal fixation is beneficial in the immobilization of certain unstable fractures of long bones and occasionally in the management of open fractures.

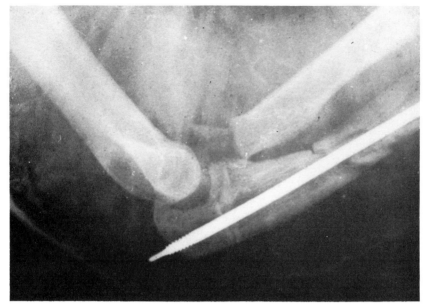

Figure 23. Lateral x-ray of elbow, showing fracture fragments of proximal ulna being held in alignment by an intramedullary pin.

Treatment of the Open Fracture

Open fractures are considered surgical emergencies and demand immediate treatment because of the very serious complication of infection. The skin wound may vary from a small puncture hole to a large lacerated skin defect through which bone protrudes. The wounds are frequently contaminated by road dirt, pieces of clothing, or other foreign material. The soft tissue damage may be quite extensive and the blood loss significant.

Initially the wound should be covered with a sterile dressing, and the part should be immobilized for the patient's immediate transport to the hospital. After hospital arrival, the patient's condition, both general and local, is assessed and stabilized. X-rays of the involved area are obtained, and the patient is taken to the operating room for definitive fracture care. The total time lapse between injury and arrival in the operating room should not exceed eight hours.

At operation, a complete surgical cleansing of the wound is performed. This consists of a very thorough washing and irrigation of the wound with large amounts of sterile saline or Ringers solution, in order to remove dirt and foreign material. This is followed by surgical debridement of the wound, with excision of all devitalized skin, fat, fascia, muscle, and detached pieces of bone. A culture of the wound should be taken at the time of the debridement. A wide spectrum antibiotic is given intravenously during surgery and is usually continued for three to five days postoperatively. If treatment was not unduly delayed or if the wound was not too dirty, an effort should be made to close the skin wound with sutures in order to convert the open fracture into a closed one. If there was treatment delay or if the wound is extremely dirty, it is better to pack the wound open and perform delayed wound closure a few days later if there is no sign of infection.

Following surgery, the fracture is reduced and immobilized with a plaster cast, "pins and plaster," or traction, depending on its type and location. Under ordinary circumstances, internal fixation is not widely employed in the presence of an open fracture.

The patient with an open fracture is at risk in regard to osteomyelitis, tetanus, and gas gangrene. Complete and thorough surgical wound debridement is the best prevention for osteomyelitis. Large doses of penicillin should be administered if there is concern about gas gangrene.

Tetanus is prevented by immunization. If the patient has been previously immunized by tetanus toxoid, a booster dose of toxoid should be given. If the patient has had no previous immunization or if there is inadequate available information, immediate passive immunity can be achieved by the use of 250 units of human tetanus immune globulin. Active immunity with tetanus toxoid is initiated at the same time.

Treatment of Pathologic Fracture

Pathologic fractures, even when accompanying disease states that are ultimately fatal, require treatment in order to spare the patient unnecessary pain and disability. Most pathologic fractures will unite unless the bone resorption rate caused by the underlying disease state is overwhelming. The same principles of management applying to fractures through normal bone apply to the treatment of pathologic fractures.

The single most frequent cause of the pathologic fractures seen in clinical practice is metastatic carcinoma to the skeleton. Internal fixation is usually the treatment of choice when the pathologic fracture is through metastatic lesions in the long bones of the extremities. Mechanical treatment of the bone fracture should be followed by medical treatment of the tumor area, utilizing radiation therapy, hormone therapy, or chemotherapeutic agents as indicated.

If the diagnosis of a metastatic lesion to an extremity long bone is made before fracture occurs, "prophylactic" nailing may be performed (Fig. 24). In this instance the internal fixation device is inserted by means of a more simplified elective operation, saving the patient the pain and misery brought on by waiting for the bone to break.

THE RESULT

UNION OF THE FRACTURE

Successful repair of the fracture will occur in the majority of patients in whom management of the problem has followed established

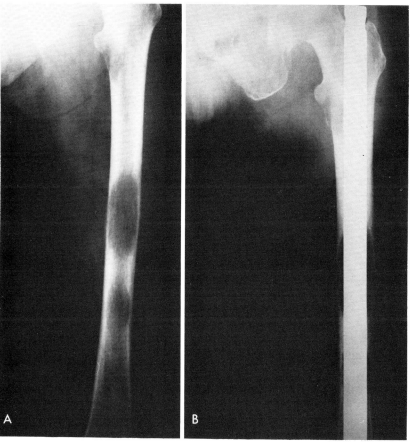

Figure 24. A, multiple lytic areas in femoral shaft due to metastatic adenocarcinoma of the breast. B, same femur after "prophylactic" nailing.

principles. The number of weeks of immobilization necessary for fracture healing will vary according to the type and location of the fracture. However, the mean number of weeks required for each bone to heal in the average patient is known. If the healing period stretches beyond the time normally required, delayed union may be suspected.

It is a well-established fact that most bones appear and feel solidly united before complete obliteration of the fracture line is noted on the x-ray film. This state is known as *clinical union*. Immobilization may be discontinued in most cases after clinical union has occurred.

Internal fixation devices serve no further purpose after the fracture has united successfully. Since modern metallic appliances are completely inert in the body, they may be safely left in place. They may also be removed after the fracture has healed at the election of the physician or if they are causing symptoms in the patient by mechanical irritation due to loosening or migration.

Malunion of the Fracture

Malunion is a term applied to a fracture that heals in a poor or abnormal position (Fig. 25). Two examples of poor position are (1) marked overriding of the fragments with shortening and (2) abnormal angulation of the bone. Malunion frequently interferes with function of the part. The most common causes of malunion are poor reduction and inefficient immobilization.

If malposition of the fragments is detected before complete healing occurs, improvement in the alignment may be obtained by manipulation. If it is not detected until after complete healing occurs, improved alignment can be obtained only by a surgical osteotomy.

Delayed Union of the Fracture

A fracture is said to be showing delayed union when it has not successfully united after lapse of the usual amount of time required for healing of the given fracture.

The most frequent causes of delayed union are large gaps between the fracture fragments, inefficient immobilization, poor blood supply to the fracture fragments, and extensive soft tissue damage, such as might accompany an open fracture.

Figure 25.   A, fracture of tibia and fibula healed in position of malunion. B, osteotomy of tibia to correct malunion. Fragments held with Lottes nail.

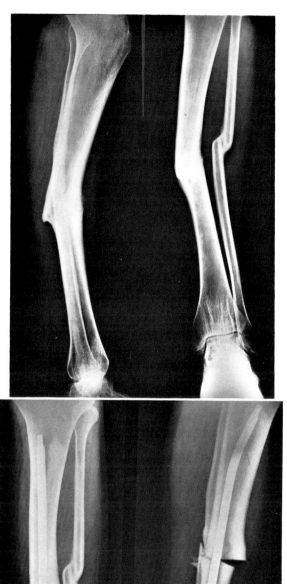

Figure 25. See opposite page for legend.

Delayed union is treated by prolonging complete and continuous efficient immobilization until healing occurs. If healing does not follow this treatment, the fracture is demonstrating nonunion.

Nonunion of the Fracture

Nonunion of a fracture means unsuccessful repair of the break. With nonunion, the callus will be found to be composed of dense fibrous tissue instead of bone. Nonunion of a fracture can be recognized on an x-ray film by the presence of a fracture gap separating rounded, sclerotic, dense bone fragments. The marrow cavity of each fragment will be sealed closed by the dense sclerotic bone (Fig. 26).

The factors tending to cause nonunion include: (1) large gaps between the fragments, (2) poor immobilization, (3) interposition of soft

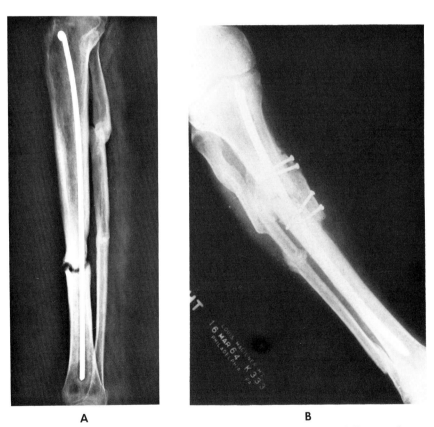

A   B

Figure 26. A, fracture of tibia originally treated with intramedullary Rush pin, now showing complete nonunion. B, nonunion of tibia treated by efficient internal fixation and iliac bone graft.

parts, usually muscle tissue, between the fracture fragments, (4) metabolic disorders, such as hypoproteinemia, (5) extensive damage to soft tissues in adjacent areas, as might occur with open fractures, (6) infection in the bone, and (7) poor blood supply to the bone fragments. Poor blood supply may be an important factor in some fractures of the femoral neck, carpal navicular bone, lower third of the humerus, and lower third of the tibia. These are all areas where nonunion is a common occurrence.

Treatment of nonunion usually involves operative excision of the dense fibrous callus and of the sclerotic bone ends. The marrow cavities are reopened by reaming. Open reduction is then carried out and is usually maintained by some form of internal fixation. Osteogenesis is stimulated by bridging the bone ends with an autogenous bone graft, usually taken from the patient's ilium or tibia (Fig. 26).

DISLOCATIONS

A dislocation is a complete displacement of the bones forming a joint. The cause is trauma and the result is a loss of structural stability of the joint. Varying degrees of tearing of the extra-articular soft tissues accompany traumatic dislocation of a joint. The dislocation may be open or closed (Fig. 27).

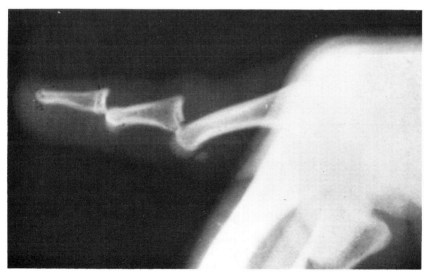

Figure 27. Lateral x-ray of finger, illustrating dislocation of proximal and distal interphalangeal joints.

The patient presenting with a traumatic joint dislocation usually exhibits pain, swelling, deformity of the part, and marked limitation of motion. A careful examination must be performed to detect accompanying damage to a major blood vessel or peripheral nerves. Adequate x-ray study will define the problem as a joint dislocation.

Joint dislocations should be reduced as promptly as possible, preferably under general anesthesia. Most joint dislocations will reduce by means of closed reduction but some may require open reduction. Time of immobilization will vary from three to six weeks, depending on the location of the joint and the time required for soft tissue healing to restore joint stability.

Tearing of various extra-articular soft tissues is associated with joint dislocation and may influence the final result. If the joint capusle tears at the time of joint dislocation, it heals without incident following reduction in the majority of patients. Rarely, a piece of capsule may become trapped between the joint surfaces, effectively preventing closed reduction. In this instance open reduction is needed.

The diagnosis of joint capsule rupture can usually be documented by arthrogram.

Joint ligaments may become stretched and strained at the time of dislocation. These heal uneventfully with immobilization of the joint after reduction.

A joint ligament may also tear or rupture completely at the time of dislocation. If the torn ligament is not perceived and treated, the joint may exhibit permanent instability after reduction. After tearing, the ends of the ligament retract, leaving a gap between the shredded ends. If they are allowed to remain in the retracted position, healing by fibrous scar permanently elongates the ligament and contributes to continuing joint instability.

The presence of a significant joint ligament tear can usually be ascertained by stress x-ray. This involves taking an anteroposterior x-ray of the injured joint while it is being stressed with the patient under general anesthesia. The stress simulates the orginal injury and the x-ray will document joint instability if significant ligament rupture is present (Fig. 5).

It is believed that torn ligaments are best treated by surgical repair in order to restore joint stability.

FRACTURE-DISLOCATION

The most severe form of injury inflicted on a joint is dislocation accompanied by fracture, usually intra-articular in type. This combination is not infrequently seen in the ankle and hip joints (Fig. 28). Because of the violence required to achieve the injury and the accom-

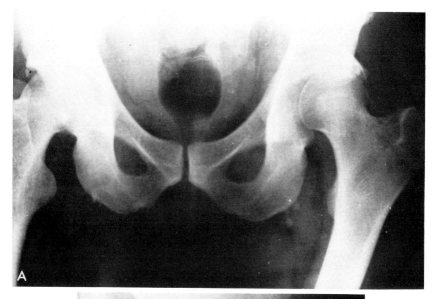

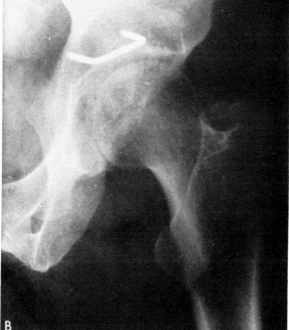

Figure 28. A, fracture-dislocation of left hip. *B*, appearance of left hip after closed reduction of dislocation and open reduction and internal fixation of fracture of rim of posterior acetabulum.

panying articular cartilage damage, the long-term functional results achieved in the patient by treatment may be complicated by avascular necrosis and degenerative arthritis.

Fracture-dislocation of a joint is treated by prompt reduction of the dislocation followed by selective treatment of the fracture, utilizing the most appropriate of the methods discussed under Fracture Managment.

References

Alffram, P. A., and Bauer, G. H.: Epidemiology of fractures of the forearm. A biomechanical investigation of bone strength. J. Bone and Joint Surg., 44-A:105, 1962.

Allen, W. C., Piotrowski, G., Burstein, A. H., and Frankel, V. H.: Biomechanical principles of intramedullary fixation. Clin. Orthop., 60:13, 1958.

Alms, M.: Fracture mechanics. J. Bone and Joint Surg., 43-B:162, 1961.

Anderson, L. D.: Compression plate fixation and the effect of different types of internal fixation on fracture healing. J. Bone and Joint Surg., 47-A:191, 1965.

Blount, W. P.: Fractures in Children. Baltimore: Williams & Wilkins Co., 1955.

Boyd, H. B.: Symposium: Treatment of un-united fractures of the long bone. J. Bone and Joint Surg., 47-A:167, 1965.

Campbell, C. J.: The healing of cartilage defects. Clin. Orth. and Rel. Res., 64:45, 1969.

Cave, E. F.: Trauma and the orthopaedic surgeon. J. Bone and Joint Surg., 43-A:582, 1961.

DePalma, A. F.: The Management of Fractures and Dislocations, 2nd Edition, Vols. 1 and 2. Philadelphia: W. B. Saunders Co., 1970.

Evans, E. B.: Orthopaedic measures in the treatment of severe burns. J. Bone and Joint Surg., 48-A:643, 1966.

Frankel, V. H., and Burstein, A. H.: The biomechanics of refracture of bone. Clin. Orth. and Rel. Res., 60:221, 1968.

Griffin, P. P., and Hamilton, C. M.: Fractures in children. Am. Academy of Orthopaedic Surgeons Instructional Course Lectures, Vol. XIX. St. Louis: C. V. Mosby Co., 1970.

Ham, A. W.: Histology, 5th Edition. Philadelphia: J. B. Lippincott Co., 1965.

MacAusland, W. R., Jr.: Treatment of sepsis after intramedullary nailing of fractures of femur. Clin. Orth. and Rel. Res., 60:87, 1968.

Marmor, L. (Ed.): Management of nonunion. Clin. Orth. and Rel. Res., No. 43, 1965.

Pelltier, L. F.: Fat embolism—A current concept. Clin. Orth. and Rel. Res., 66:241, 1969.

Schmeisser, G., Jr.: A Clinical Manual of Orthopaedic Traction Techniques. Philadelphia: W. B. Saunders Co., 1964.

Wade, E. A. (Ed.): Preoperative and postoperative management of musculoskeletal injuries. Clin. Orth. and Rel. Res., No. 38, 1965.

Wray, J. B.: Factors in the pathogenesis of non-union. J. Bone and Joint Surg., 47-A:168, 1965.

Chapter Three

Congenital Deformities

INTRODUCTION

Congenital deformities are defined as those abnormalities of development that are present at the time of birth. It has been estimated that congenital abnormalities of various types and degrees are responsible for the death of about one-quarter of all human fetuses before or shortly after birth, and handicap a certain proportion of the survivors throughout their life. Defective development of a unit of the musculoskeletal system, while rarely posing a threat to life, might seriously impair the function of the patient as a useful member of society. Significant congenital deformities of the musculoskeletal system are quite common, being exceeded in frequency only by those of the central nervous system and cardiovascular system (Fig. 29).

Some congenital deformities, such as clubfoot and torticollis, are obvious and are readily noticed by the mother, while others, such as congenital dislocation of the hip, may go undetected for a period of time. The remainder may give no clinical evidence of their presence initially until detected by x-ray examination or by the secondary effects their presence may cause. Examples of this group would be deformities of the spine, such as hemivertebra and spondylolisthesis.

It is generally recognized that congenital deformities seem to be more prevalent among the white population than among the other racial groups. Males and females appear to be affected equally, even though certain specific deformities show a definite sex predilection. Multiple births and an older mother seem to be factors in the rate of occurrence. The presence of multiple congenital deformities in the same child is not uncommon and should be constantly borne in mind.

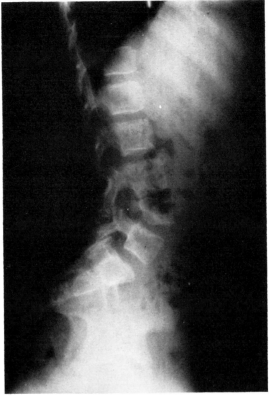

Figure 29. Congenital anomaly of fourth lumbar vertebra in 12 year old female child. There is complete absence of the posterior elements and the body of L4 is "free-floating."

Embryologic development is an orderly step-by-step procedure, and it is thought that most congenital deformities begin early in the life of the embryo when cell division is most active. Although some congenital deformities may be due to uterine malposition, most are believed to be engendered by genetic defects, environmental influences, or a combination of both.

GENETIC FACTORS

The theoretical possibility of having to treat a patient with a congenital musculoskeletal deformity arises as soon as the male germ cell fertilizes the ovum to form the zygote. This act immediately restores the diploid chromosome number for the human (44 somatic plus 2 sex) and establishes the sex of the child. If a male germ cell carrying the X sex chromosome fertilizes the ovum, a female zygote results. If the male germ cell carries the Y sex chromosome, a male zygote is formed. The several thousand genes of each cell nucleus are located on the various pairs of chromosomes. The genes are also paired, one being inherited from the father and the other from the mother. If the genes of a pair are alike, the individual is said to be homozygous; if they are different, the individual is herterozygous.

Genetic defects may be inherited from either parent or from an ancestor, or they may appear initially in a family as the result of a mutation in a chromosome or in one of its genes. The inheritance pattern of abnormalities depends upon whether the abnormal gene is dominant or recessive and also upon whether the gene locus concerned is autosomal or sex-linked. If the abnormal gene is dominant, the resultant deformity is transmitted by direct descent from affected members of a family to some of their children, who transmit it in turn (*osteogenesis imperfecta*). If the abnormal gene is recessive, the resultant deformity may occur in one or more siblings but less often in their children (*Sprengel's deformity*). If the abnormal gene is sex-linked, the resultant deformity is transmitted by clinically normal carrier females but affects only males (*hemophilia*). Gene mutation is also a cause of congenital deformity. If a gene undergoes mutation in the germ plasm, the resultant abnormality will be transmitted.

ENVIRONMENTAL FACTORS

Harmful environmental factors may alter the germ cells of either parent before fertilization, or they may alter the normal development of the fetus during intrauterine life. Extrinsic environmental factors causing fetal insult must pass the placental barrier in order to damage the developing embryo. Fetal insult may be caused by maternal and fetal infections, maternal infection with the virus of rubella, maternal ingestion of certain drugs such as thalidomide, x-radiation, and poor maternal nutrition.

When a congenital deformity has a genetic basis, there is a greatly increased chance that subsequent offspring will be malformed. When a congenital deformity is due to a factor that is not genetic in origin, subsequent offspring should show no greater tendency to malformation than the general population.

CONGENITAL ORTHOPAEDIC DEFORMITIES

Congenital malformations may involve any part of the musculoskeletal system and vary greatly in rate of occurrence and degree of significance. Only the more common congenital deformities are discussed here. The most important and significant congenital deformities of the musculoskeletal system are clubfoot and congenital dislocation of the hip.

CLUBFOOT

Clubfoot is the most frequently encountered of all orthopaedic congenital deformities involving the lower extremity and is estimated to occur once in every 800 births. Family studies of large numbers of children with clubfeet implicate a genetic factor in only about 10 per cent of the children, the rest of the deformities due, presumably, to spontaneous mutation. Clubfoot is also known by the general term talipes equinovarus, which is derived from Latin and makes vague reference to the position of the foot. The deformity affects males twice as often as females and occurs bilaterally in about one-half of the affected children.

Clinical Picture. A foot with this deformity is twisted inward and downward, giving the entire extremity a superficial resemblance to a club (Fig. 30). The foot is tight in its deformed position and resists manual efforts to readily push it back into a normal position. Closer

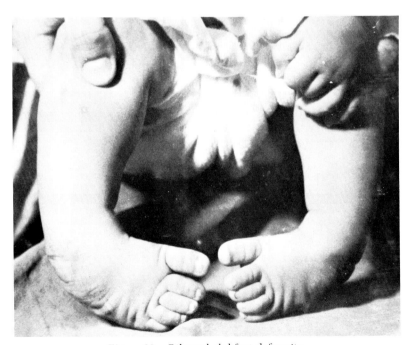

Figure 30. Bilateral clubfoot deformity.

inspection will reveal that there are actually three separate elements to the deformity:

1. *Adduction deformity of the forefoot.* In this instance the forefoot is drawn inward in relation to the rear part of the foot. This motion takes place chiefly in the talonavicular and calcaneocuboid joints.

2. *Inversion Deformity (varus),* which is a turning in of the entire foot and heel. This motion takes place chiefly in the talocalcaneal or subtalar joint. No inversion can occur normally at the ankle joint as the talus is securely locked in the ankle mortise. This element of the deformity elevates the medial border of the foot and depresses the lateral border.

3. *Equinus or fixed plantar flexion of the foot at the ankle joint.* This is related to tightness of the posterior capsule of the ankle joint and the heel cord. In addition, the shaft of the tibia usually exhibits an inward torsion deformity, thus increasing the inward turning appearance of the foot and leg.

The muscles on the posterior and medial aspect of the leg, particularly the calf and posterior tibial muscles, are underdeveloped and shorter than normal. The capsules of all the deformed joints are thick and contracted on the concave side of the deformity. These soft tissue contractures become progressively resistant to correction as time passes, emphasizing the importance of early corrective treatment.

It is generally believed that the bones of the feet are normally formed at first, although deformity of the shape of the talus is almost always noted at birth. The talus, os calcis, navicular, and cuboid are shifted from their normal relationship in the foot by the deformed position assumed by clubfoot. The malposition of these bones can be noted on the x-ray film and their replacement into normal alignment is the x-ray criterion for good correction (Fig. 31). Eventually, all the involved bones may become irregular in shape because of abnormal forces exerted on them by the soft tissue contractures or if the positional deformity of the foot is not corrected by the time walking begins.

Treatment. Successful treatment of clubfoot deformity is based on the principle of first obtaining complete correction of the three elements of the deformity, and then maintaining the correction until all danger of recurrence has passed. All orthopaedists are agreed on this principle but there are, understandably, differences in detail about the methods used to achieve this end.

The most popular methods of obtaining initial correction are the use of stretching plaster casts or the use of the Denis Browne foot plates and bar. Regardless of which treatment method is ultimately chosen, foot exercising is begun immediately after birth. The mother

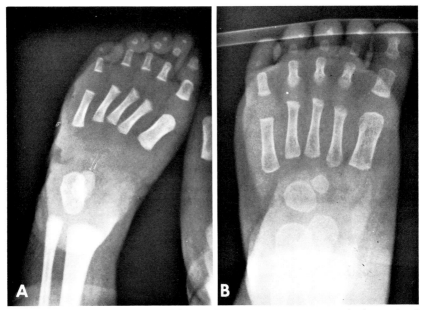

Figure 31. A, AP view of clubfoot, showing superimposition of talus and calcaneus. B, same foot after four months of plaster cast treatment. Talus and calcaneus are
approaching a normal relationship.

is taught to exercise the infant's foot at every feeding period in order
to gain some flexibility over the soft tissue contractures. Treatment
with a plaster cast or foot plate is begun as soon after birth as possible
and certainly within the first four weeks of life. Either method of obtaining initial correction can give good results if the techniques are
mastered. With either method correction must proceed in a certain
sequence. In order to restore proper skeletal alignment between talus,
os calcis, navicular, and cuboid, forefoot adduction must be completely corrected before the heel varus problem is attacked. This, in
turn, must be completely corrected before the equinus component of
the deformity is rectified.

Once initial correction has been obtained, attention must be
given to maintaining it. When all components of the deformity have
been corrected, and x-ray examination shows proper realignment of
the affected bones, a retention cast may be applied for four to six
weeks to hold the foot in the overcorrected position for maximum
stretching of the soft tissues. Initial treatment may take from two to six
months to obtain full correction, depending on the rigidity of the foot.
Daily stretching exercises must be given to the foot after discontin-
uance of the plaster cast or bar treatment. Walking is allowed in clubfoot shoes, which are high-top shoes containing outer heel and sole

wedges. The child should be placed in a foot splint at nap time and during the night to aid in maintaining the corrected position. In an uncomplicated case in which correction has proceded in a progressive manner, the night splint may be left on as long as it is tolerated by the child. With a docile child this could be until at least two years of age.

It must be emphasized again that clubfoot deformity may prove quite difficult to treat. Follow-up studies of large numbers of children with clubfeet treated quite adequately by the methods previously outlined show that only about 60 per cent respond satisfactorily. The remaining 40 per cent prove resistant to this type of treatment for one reason or another and require a change in the treatment program to obtain correction of the deformity.

Treatment of Resistant Clubfoot. In approximately 40 per cent of children with clubfoot deformity, the soft tissue tightness and contracture about the foot is strong enough to prevent complete correction by the cast or foot plate method alone. In these patients surgical release of the contracted soft tissue is required for correction. The most frequently used soft tissue operation is lengthening of the Achilles tendon and section of the posterior capsule of the ankle joint to lessen the equinus deformity. Surgical correction of the varus and forefoot adduction is less often required. In all instances the plaster treatment is resumed after surgery to maintain correction.

After six years of age, soft tissue release operations are ineffective because of the abnormal shape of the bones and surgical procedures on the tarsal bones are required. These procedures are, of necessity, more major than soft tissue release operations and usually result in some stiffening of the foot.

In an occasional patient, the clubfoot deformity may recur some months after appearing to have been corrected by the cast or foot plate method. Although no universal agreement exists on this point, many orthopaedists believe that this type of recurrence is caused by muscle imbalance, principally involving either the anterior or posterior tibial muscles. In these patients, surgical transfer of the involved tendon to the mid-portion of the forefoot restores a balanced foot.

Recently published reports have emphasized performing complete soft tissue release operations on all involved joints of a resistant clubfoot by three months of age. Proponents of this early complete soft tissue surgery are reporting markedly improved results over those obtainable with slower and more conservative forms of treatment.

METATARSUS VARUS

This common deformity of the foot, also known as metatarsus adductus, is frequently mistaken for clubfoot at first glance. Closer examination, however, shows that only the front part of the foot is involved, with the heel and heel cord maintaining normal flexibility. The actual deformity is an adduction of the forefoot in which the forefoot is drawn inward in relation to the rear part of the foot, varying greatly in severity from a flexible to a fixed deformity (Fig. 32). An accompanying internal tibial torsion may accentuate the deformity.

The five metatarsal bones appear normally formed on the x-ray film but show a positional shift to accommodate to the deformity. If the metatarsus varus deformity is not corrected by the time weight bearing begins, adaptive bone deformity of the metatarsals will develop.

Treatment. If the forefoot deformity is flexible and can be manually straightened, correction can usually be obtained by a stretching exercise performed by the mother during the child's feeding periods. If the forefoot deformity is fixed and cannot be manually straightened, correction is obtained by using stretching plaster casts.

Once correction is obtained, it must be actively maintained until

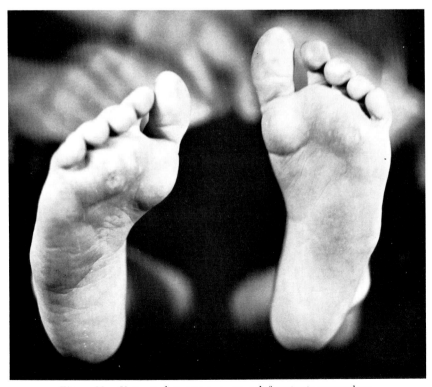

Figure 32.   Untreated metatarsus varus deformity in young boy.

the child begins to walk, because recurrence of the deformity is common. This is accomplished by continuing the forefoot stretching exercises and having the child wear "out-flare" shoes. Occasionally it is necessary for the child to wear a foot splint to bed to prevent his feet from curling under when he lies on his abdomen.

In a child below six years of age, inability to correct the deformity completely by plaster casting is an indication for surgical soft tissue release at the five tarso-metatarsal joints to obtain correction. In a child over six years of age, inability to correct the deformity completely is an indication for osteotomy through the bases of all five metatarsals to obtain correction.

CONGENITAL DISLOCATION OF THE HIP

The hip is the only joint in the body in which congenital dislocation occurs with any degree of frequency. It has been stated that one infant in 60 is born with instability of one or both hips, but 88 per cent of these recover spontaneously in the first two months of life. The remaining 12 per cent, or 1.55 per thousand, demonstrate true congenital dislocation that will persist unless it is treated.

The hip joint is abnormal and underdeveloped in all cases of congenital dislocation of the hip. This developmental abnormality gives rise to a characteristic pathologic, clinical, and x-ray picture (Fig. 33). The dislocation is thought to be present in some children at the time of birth and to occur in others shortly after birth. Although the exact cause is unknown, heredity plays a role in a significant number of cases, with a primary developmental defect suggested by the abnormal development of the femoral head, acetabulum, and ilium.

Congenital dislocation of the hip is about eight times more common in girls and may be bilateral in almost half of the affected children. Since it may cause severe hip disability in adult life, it is absolutely imperative to make an early diagnosis and institute proper treatment. A direct correlation exists between the success of treatment and the age at which it is carried out. Treatment results are good in approximately 90 per cent of children in whom gentle and accurate reduction is instituted during the first three months of life. For this reason examination of both hips should be a routine part of every newborn infant's first physical examination.

Pathologic Findings. The femoral head must lie in correct relationship with the acetabulum for each to develop and grow in a normal manner. If the joint is dislocated, each component of the joint is adversely affected, and growth and development proceed in an abnormal manner. In congenital dislocation of the hip the femoral head is dislocated and lies completely out of the acetabulum. Most often it is

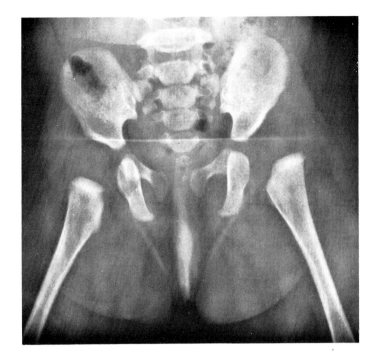

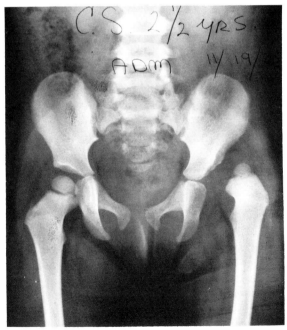

Figure 33. A, congenital dislocation of hip in three month old infant. B, congenital dislocation of left hip in 30 month old child.

found to lie posterior and superior to the acetabulum. The dislocated femoral head ossifies later than in a normal hip and when it does appear, it is always smaller than normal. The roof of the acetabulum is underdeveloped, allowing the acetabulum to assume a shallow shape with its roof sloping steeply upward instead of forming a nearly horizontal shelf over the femoral head.

With the femoral head displaced superiorly and posteriorly, the hip joint capsule becomes stretched and elongated. This capsular tube may become constricted at its midpoint (hourglass contracture), trapping the femoral head in the proximal segment. The ligamentum teres may be quite thick and hypertrophied.

The empty acetabulum is frequently filled with fibrofatty tissue. The cartilaginous limbus forming the rim of the acetabulum may be enlarged and may tend to cover the acetabulur opening. In some children the tendon of the iliopsoas may be displaced laterally, passing across the mouth of the acetabulum.

The unstable hip joint resulting from a congenital dislocation predisposes to weakness of the abductor muscles, particularly the gluteus medius. Their antagonists, the adductors, become tight and contracted from the positional abnormaltiy.

Another factor to be considered is anterversion of the femoral neck (Fig. 34). Normally the femoral neck and upper shaft exhibit an anterior torque angulation of 12 to 25 degrees in relation to the lower

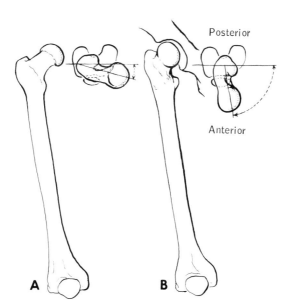

Figure 34. Angle of anteversion of femoral neck.

end of the femur. In congenital dislocation of the hip, the angle of anteversion is almost always increased. This means that the leg on the affected side must be twisted into marked internal rotation in order to seat the head of the femur into a normal relationship with the acetabulum.

Clinical Findings. Abnormal clinical findings in the infant are related directly to the fact that the hip is dislocated and rides upward above the acetabulum. Thus the affected leg may be shorter than the opposite leg. This can be determined by examining the child in the supine position with the pelvis level and with both legs extended, or by flexing both knees and hips to a right angle. In the latter position the presence of shortening will cause the knee on the dislocated side to appear lower than on the normal side (Allis sign, Galeazzi sign) (Fig. 35). Shortening may also be associated with an asymmetry of the skin folds in the buttock and upper thigh area.

Palpation reveals a prominence of the greater trochanter on the affected side and the absence of the femoral head from its normal an-

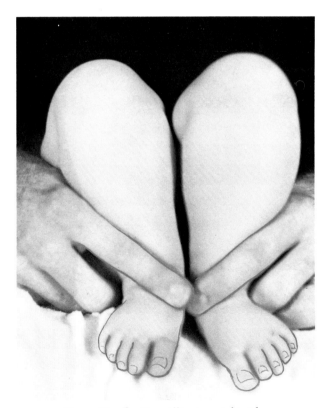

Figure 35. Positive Allis sign, right side.

terior location beneath the femoral artery. When both hips are flexed to a right angle, the motion of abduction is limited on the affected side (Hart's sign) and the adductor muscle can be felt to be tight and contracted. This is frequently noted by the mother when she diapers the child. It is usually possible to internally rotate the affected hip through a greater arc than the normal side because of the increased anteversion.

If the extended thigh on the affected side is pushed toward the patient's head and then pulled back, the greater trochanter and femoral head can be felt to move up and down in the buttock. This is spoken of as "telescoping" or "piston mobility" of the femoral head. In some patients a click may be felt or heard when the thigh is abducted in flexion. The click is caused by the femoral head sliding over the acetabular rim. The click may be repeated when the head slips out of the acetabulum on the opposite maneuver. This is known as Ortolani's click or jerk.

X-ray Findings. The roentgen findings in congenital dislocation of the hip give the impression of underdevelopment or dysplasia involving the entire hip area. The acetabulum appears shallow in depth. This appearance is accentuated by the slanting, poorly formed roof of the acetabulum, which is a reflection of the excessive slope of the ossified portion of the acetabulum. Delayed ossification of the femoral head is associated with the dislocation. The femoral head and neck are displaced upward and laterally in relation to the acetabulum.

The pelvis may appear tilted, and there may be a curvature of the spine in the lumbar region. The ilium on the affected side may appear smaller and underdeveloped.

Most of the abnormalities seen on the x-ray film are illustrated in Figure 36.

Treatment. Treatment must begin as soon as the diagnosis is made and depends, for its success, upon replacement of the femoral head into the acetabulum and maintenance of this relationship until the hip joint becomes stable. It is well established that the younger the patient at the time of treatment the better will be the chance for the development of a normal hip. Thus it is absolutely imperative that the presence of a congenitally dislocated hip be discovered as soon after birth as possible.

Treatment will vary somewhat with the age of the child and may be conveniently considered in four age categories: (1) birth to three months, (2) three months to two years, (3) two years to five years, and (4) over five years.

BIRTH TO THREE MONTHS. This is the golden period as far as treatment is concerned. Every effort should be made to have all affected children started in treatment before this time period has

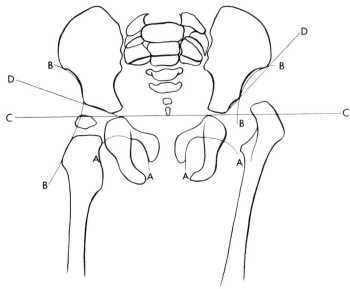

Figure 36. Certain lines may be traced on the x-ray film to assist in establishing diagnosis of congenital dislocation of hip. *A,* Shenton's line lies along the upper margin of the obturator foramen and continues outward and downward along the undersurface of the femoral neck. *B,* line running along lateral margin of ilium and outer edge of acetabulum and extending along upper margin of femoral neck. Normally these two lines form even curves, but they are interrupted in a hip dislocation. *C,* line running horizontally through the triradiate acetabular cartilage. Normally the femoral epiphysis and metaphysis should lie below the level of this line. *D,* line drawn along roof of acetabulum to meet line C. These lines form acetabular angle, which is relatively obtuse in presence of congenital dislocation. Note absence of capital femoral epiphysis on dislocated side.

passed. The results are good in approximately 90 per cent of children in whom gentle and accurate reduction is carried out during the first three months of life.

During this early period of life, the dislocated hip can usually be reduced by a very gentle manipulative reduction followed by maintenance of the reduced hip in a position of flexion and abduction. This position is maintained by a type of splint-brace or a plaster cast for a period of time sufficient to allow the joint capsule to tighten and the joint to become stable. Usually between four and six months are required. Successful reduction is followed by stimulation of the femoral head and acetabulum to grow and develop in a more normal manner.

Some authorities favor reduction by gentle prolonged traction instead of by manipulation. Several weeks of skin traction, with the leg in increasing abduction, frequently result in reduction of the dislocation. The reduced position of the hip is then maintained as previously described.

THREE MONTHS TO TWO YEARS. If the diagnosis is not made until the child is in this age range, it will be noted that the hip dislocation is associated with an adduction contracture. This will require a preliminary period of traction, usually skeletal in type, in order to lengthen the contracted adductor muscles before an attempt at closed reduction is carried out. Subcutaneous adductor tenotomy, followed by gentle manipulative reduction, frequently results in successful reduction of the dislocation.

If closed reduction is unsuccessful, open reduction should be performed and the hip immobilized in a plaster spica cast for an average period of six months (Fig. 37).

TWO YEARS TO FIVE YEARS. If the diagnosis is not made until the child is in this age range, adequate treatment becomes exceedingly difficult. By this time the child is walking and will exhibit a typical limp. If the dislocation is unilateral, the child's trunk will lurch to the side of the dislocation with each step. The gait will resemble a waddle if the dislocation is bilateral. Weight bearing will tend to accentuate the soft tissue shortening and tightness about the hip and may cause secondary bony changes about the hip joint.

Several weeks of preliminary skeletal traction and a subcutaneous adductor tenotomy are required before an attempt at closed reduction can be made. It is more likely that an open reduction will have to be carried out. In this age range, the problem most frequently encountered is the difficulty of maintaining the reduction, because joint mal-

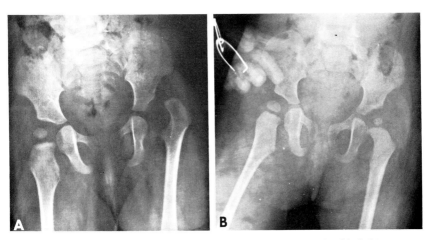

Figure 37. A, congenital dislocation of left hip in 18 month old child. B, same patient nine months following open reduction of left hip.

formation has rendered the joints unstable. It is frequently necessary to perform an osteotomy through the innominate bone in order to redirect the entire acetabulum to sit more squarely over the femoral head like a hat. Once accurate reduction of the joint has been obtained and maintained, immobilization must be continued for a period long enough to insure joint stability.

OVER FIVE YEARS OF AGE.   Satisfactory hip function is almost impossible to achieve if treatment is not started until the child is in this age range. By this time severe secondary bone changes have occurred in association with shortening and extensive soft tissue contracture. Reduction is either inadvisable or impossible to achieve in many of these children.

Occasionally a combination of extensive soft tissue release and skeletal traction will restore some of the leg length. Some bony stability at the joint can be obtained by constructing a bone shelf over the dislocated head or by performing an osteotomy of the femur below the neck. Most children in whom the diagnosis is not made until this age range will develop painful hips in early adult life and will require secondary reconstructive hip operations for relief.

Complications.   Avascular necrosis of the capital femoral epiphysis may occur as a complication after reduction, possibly because of damage to or compromise of the blood supply. Immobilization of the hip in an extreme or forced position of abduction or internal rotation is probably the most important cause of avascular necrosis of the femoral head. Its x-ray appearance and subsequent course will closely resemble the appearance and course of Legg-Calvé-Perthes disease (p. 85) and, as in the disorder, weight bearing is not permitted until the femoral head has reconstituted itself.

If the child is left with incongruity of the joint surfaces after treatment is completed, it is possible that the hip joint may develop secondary degenerative arthritis in adult life. The stresses of weight bearing and everyday activity on incongruous joint surfaces may precipitate articular cartilage degeneration.

SUBLUXATION OF THE HIP

A newborn infant may be seen in whom the motion of abduction at the hip is limited and the adductor muscles are felt to be tight and contracted. X-ray examination may disclose a shallow acetabulum and a small capital femoral epiphysis but no actual dislocation. In this instance the hip is considered unstable, with the femoral head lying at the lateral edge of the acetabulum but not actually out of the joint. Because there is no dislocation, there is no shortening of the leg. This situation is called subluxation, partial dislocation of the hip, or acetabular dysplasia.

Because there is no dislocation, no reduction is required. It is necessary, however, to seat the femoral head more squarely into the acetabulum so that pressure will influence each to develop normally. This is accomplished by the use of a device to keep the baby's legs abducted, gradually loosening the tight adductor muscles. Double diapers, a Frejka pillow splint, or various types of abduction braces are used for this purpose. X-ray examination is repeated at intervals until a normal appearance of the joint is seen. As a rule this condition is corrected quite readily.

SPRENGEL'S DEFORMITY (CONGENITAL HIGH SCAPULA)

During embryonic life, the scapula develops in the neck region and normally descends to its thoracic position during early development. If this descent fails to occur, the child is born with the scapula lying in the lower cervical and upper thoracic regions and is said to have a Sprengel's deformity. The condition is sometimes bilateral and may be associated with congenital anomalies of the cervical vertebrae and upper ribs.

As a consequence of this malformation, the scapula appears short and squat as compared to its counterpart, and the inferior angle is usually rotated medially. The supraspinous portion of the scapula tends to hook forward beneath the trapezius muscle (Fig. 38). In about 25 per cent of children the scapula is connected to the cervical spine by a band of fibrous, cartilaginous or bony tissue called the "omovertebral bone."

Clinical Picture. Because of the abnormal location of the scapula, the entire shoulder area may appear higher and forward when compared to the normal side. Frequently the hooked supraspinous portion can be palpated beneath the fibers of the trapezius muscle. In most patients the malrotation of the scapula greatly restricts abduction of the shoulder.

Treatment. Treatment is always surgical and is justified only in an attempt to obtain more shoulder motion or improve a severe cosmetic deformity. Two procedures for correction are in popular use. The first procedure calls for removal of the "omovertebral bone," if present, plus a large part of the upper portion of the scapula, including the spine and supraspinous portion. However, no attempt is made to pull the scapula down to a lower position on the chest wall.

In the second procedure, the scapula is entirely freed of its muscular attachments by subperiosteal dissection and is pulled down to approximate the level of the opposite scapula. The muscles are then repositioned to provide anchorage for the scapula in its new location.

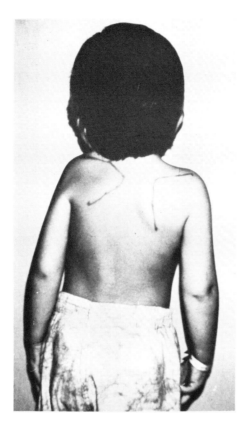

Figure 38. Sprengel's deformity, left. (Courtesy Dr. Roshen Irani, Thomas Jefferson University Hospital, Philadelphia, Pa.)

Because of the traction on the nerves that results when the scapula is pulled down from its elevated position, this procedure may be complicated by a temporary partial brachial plexus palsy.

Spina Bifida

Spina bifida is a relatively common (1 to 2 per 1000 births) congenital anomaly of the spine characterized by a developmental gap or cleft in one or more of the posterior vertebral arches. The laminar defect may range from the presence of small deformed laminae separated by a midline gap to complete absence of laminae over a wide segment, such as the entire sacrum and lumbar spine. Although this developmental defect may occur at any level of the spine, it is most frequently found in the lumbosacral region. If the gap is large enough, the contents of the spinal canal may protrude posteriorly in the midline beneath the skin of the back with grave neurologic, urologic, and orthopaedic consequences for the affected child.

When this posterior sacular herniation contains meninges and cerebrospinal fluid, the condition is called *spina bifida with meningocele*. When the sac contains spinal fluid, spinal cord, and nerve roots, the condition is called *spina bifida with meningomyelocele*. The term *myelodysplasia* is more general and refers to defective development of the spinal cord.

The extent of the neurologic deficit depends on the level and the severity of the spinal defect. It is generally more severe in meningomyelocele than in meningocele and may vary from mild muscle imbalance and sensory loss in the legs to complete paraplegia. The paralysis in the lower extremities may be flaccid, spastic, or mixed, depending on the level of involvement. Extensive sensory disturbance may result in distressing trophic ulcers. Certain of these children with spina bifida may have an associated hydrocephalus. Bowel and bladder incontinence, exstrophy of the bladder, and imperforate anus may also be associated complications of spina bifida.

Orthopaedic deformities associated with spina bifida depend to a great degree on the level of the lesion in the spinal cord and whether or not the resulting paralysis is flaccid or spastic in type. The most common orthopaedic deformities are clubfoot, dislocation of one or both hips, and malformations of the spine with varying degrees of scoliosis, kyphosis, and lordosis.

Treatment.   In recent years, the use of an aggressive team approach among neurosurgeons, urologists, and orthopaedists has resulted in a dramatic decline in mortality rate associated with a significant rise in the functional level attained by many of these severely handicapped children.

Closure of the sac by the neurosurgeon within the first hours of life has been shown to prevent progression of the neurologic defect. Appropriate shunting operations will decompress hydrocephalus and prevent irreversible brain damage. Urologic treatment is aimed at control of urinary incontinence and prevention of ascending urinary tract infections.

The goal of orthopaedic treatment is to allow the patient to become ambulatory if possible so that he may gain a measure of functional independence. In the severely involved patient, aids to ambulation such as crutches, leg or spine braces, or both may have to be utilized, along with gait training to facilitate independent ambulation.

Specific orthopaedic deformities associated with the paralysis of spina bifida, such as clubfoot and dislocation of the hip, will require correction in order to make ambulation with brace support a reality. Such treatment may require the use of casts, braces, surgery, or some combination of these. Any associated sensory disturbance must be constantly borne in mind during treatment so that serious pressure sores can be avoided.

Clubhand

If there is defective development of the radial elements of the limb bud, a child may be born with a partial or complete absence of the radius (Fig. 39). If the radial defect is substantial, the associated ulna is short and curved, causing the hand to be carried in a position of marked radial deviation. A similar primary defect in the ulna is possible but less common. If a primary ulnar defect is present, the hand is carried in a position of ulnar deviation.

A radial clubhand may be accompanied by absence of the thumb, the first metacarpal, and some of the carpal bones. The humerus and scapula may be smaller than normal. Various muscle defects may be present, including absence of some arm and forearm muscles and abnormal insertions in others.

Clubhand is usually a very difficult deformity to overcome. Correction requires replacement of the hand over the remaining forearm bone by stretching with plaster casts, combined usually with both soft tissue and bone surgery. This position then must be maintained by protective splints for a long period of time.

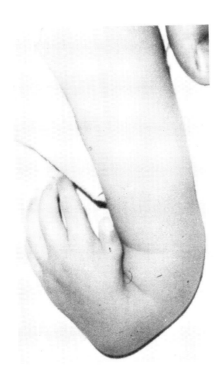

Figure 39.   Radial clubhand deformity. (Courtesy Dr. James Hunter and Dr. Lawrence Schneider, Thomas Jefferson University Hospital, Philadelphia, Pa.)

Syndactyly (Webbed Fingers)

Congenital webbing of the fingers is said to be the most common congenital anomaly of the hand. It is thought to be an inherited trait and is often bilateral. It may occur in association with webbing of the toes and other foot deformities. The abnormality may range from simple skin webbing between two fingers to severe webbing of all the fingers, with incomplete segmentation of the bony parts and multiple joint deformities. The thumb is seldom involved.

Treatment is surgical and is undertaken only after careful study of the degree of involvement. The optimum time for treatment is thought to be between the second and fifth years of life.

Polydactyly (Extra Digits)

Extra digits is an inherited deformity often accompanied by other congenital malformations. The degree of deformity may vary from a small extra soft tissue mass not attached to bone to a complete extra digit containing all elements and attached to an extra metacarpal or metatarsal.

Extra fingers usually cause no functional difficulty, particularly in the early years of life. Extra toes may cause a shoe fitting problem.

Treatment is based upon the degree of difficulty caused by the deformity and could include surgical excision of the extra digit. Frequently, small extra skin tabs noted at birth are ligated by the obstetrician or pediatrician and allowed to slough.

Congenital Pseudarthrosis of the Tibia

This very disabling but fortunately rare abnormaltiy is characterized by fracture of one or usually both bones of the leg shortly before or shortly after birth. The significant difference between this abnormality and an ordinary birth fracture is that in this condition the bone at the fracture site is abnormal and will not heal. The usual area of fracture is the lower third of the tibia and fibula, but fracture may also occur in the clavicle, humerus, ulna, first rib, and femur.

The cause of the condition is unknown but may be related to a congenital deficiency of bone production or to neurofibromatosis. The bone in the area of the fracture is defective in quality and surrounded by a sleeve of dense connective tissue. On an x-ray film, the bone ends characteristically appear atrophic and tapered, bearing a resemblance to a sucked candy stick (Fig. 40). The false joint between the bone ends may vary from a fibrous tissue cuff to a jointlike arrangement with sclerotic bone ends, cartilage, and a joint cavity.

When the tibia is involved, anterior angulation of the leg may

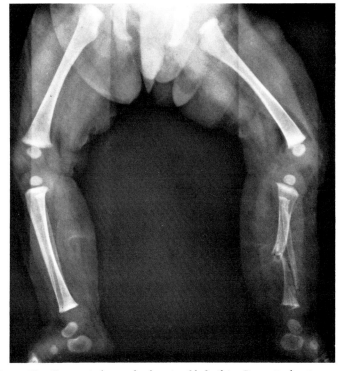

Figure 40.   Congenital pseudarthrosis of left tibia. Opposite leg is normal.

occur through the false joint. Shortening of the extremity may be extreme.

Treatment is aimed at securing bony union across the fracture site by the use of bone grafts and frequently internal fixation devices. Unfortunately this happy state is quite difficult to achieve, and multiple attempts at bone grafting are the rule. Not infrequently repeated failures of bone grafting procedure leave the patient with a shortened deformed leg that is best treated by a below knee amputation.

ARTHROGRYPOSIS MULTIPLEX CONGENITA

This extremely disabling condition is characterized by multiple congenital contractures in many limb joints, particularly in the hips, knees, elbows, and wrist (Fig. 41). The trunk is usually unaffected, as is intelligence, but scoliosis may be present. Clubfeet, clubhands, and dislocated hips are frequently associated with this disorder. Some of the joint contractures are in the direction of flexion but some, like the elbows and knees, may be in extension. Characteristically the joints are fixed, with extremely limited motion.

The term "arthrogryposis" derives from the Greek and means "curved joint." The condition has also been called amyoplasia congenita and myodystrophia fetalis.

The cause of the condition is unknown, but it is not thought to be genetically determined. Defective formation or degeneration of the anterior horn cells of the spinal cord has been reported.

Although joint stiffness is the main characteristic of arthrogryposis, the joints themselves appear normal except for their limited motion. The major pathologic changes appear mostly in the extra-articular soft tissues. The joint capsules are thickened and contracted. The muscles may be decreased in bulk or entirely absent, being replaced by fat. Excessive fibrous tissue infiltration is found in the periarticular soft tissues as well as in the subcutaneous fat. The skin is tight and inelastic.

The goal of treatment is to make these severely handicapped children as self-sufficient as possible. For that reason each joint is treated on an individual basis with the idea of correcting the deformity and gaining motion if possible. The aim of treatment in the lower extremity is to obtain stable well-aligned joints suitable for weight bearing. Because of the inelastic nature of the pathologic changes and the lack of muscle power, the results of treatment are often disappointing. In many instances institutional care is required for these children.

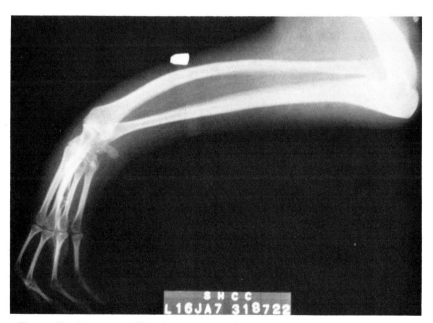

Figure 41.   Forearm and hand in patient with arthrogryposis multiplex congenita.

References

American Academy of Orthopaedic Surgeons Symposium on Myelomeningocele, October, 1971. St. Louis: C. V. Mosby Co., 1972.

Barlow, T. G.: Early diagnosis and treatment of congenital dislocation of the hip. J. Bone and Joint Surg., *44-B*:292, 1962.

Boyd, H. B., and Sage, F. P.: Congenital pseudarthrosis of the tibia. J. Bone and Joint Surg., *40-A*:1245, 1958.

Coleman, S.: Treatment of congenital dislocation of the hip in the infant. J. Bone and Joint Surg., *47-A*:590, 1965.

Colonna, P. C.: Capsular arthroplasty for congenital dislocation of the hip: Indications and technique. J. Bone and Joint Surg., *47-A*:437, 1965.

Duthie, R. B., and Townes, P. L.: The genetics of orthopaedic conditions. J. Bone and Joint Surg., *49-B*:229, 1967.

Frantz, C. H., and O'Rahilly, R.: Congenital skeletal limb Deficiencies. J. Bone and Joint Surg., *43-A*:1202, 1961.

Gibson, D. A., and Urs, N. D. K.: Arthrogryposis multiplex congenita. J. Bone and Joint Surg., *52-B*:483, 1970.

Hass, J.: Congenital Dislocation of the Hip. Springfield, Illinois: Charles C Thomas, 1951.

Irani, R. N., and Sherman, M. S.: The pathological anatomy of clubfoot. J. Bone and Joint Surg., *45-A*:45, 1963.

Kite, J. H.: The classic: Principles involved in the treatment of congenital clubfoot. Clin. Orth. and Rel. Res., *84*:4, May 1972.

Kite, J. H.: The Clubfoot. New York: Grune and Stratton, 1974.

Lloyd-Roberts, G. C.: Pitfalls in the management of congenital dislocations of the hip. J. Bone and Joint Surg., *48-B*:66, 1966.

Mayer, D. M., and Swanker, W. A.: Anomalies of Infants and Children. New York: McGraw-Hill, 1958.

Nance, W. E., and Engel, E.: Human cytogenetics. J. Bone and Joint Surg., *49-A*:1436, 1967.

O'Rahilly, R.: Morphological patterns in limb deficiencies and duplications. Am. J. Anat., *89*:135, 1951.

O'Rahilly, R.: A survey of carpal and tarsal anomalies. J. Bone and Joint Surg., *35-A*:626, 1953.

Patten, B. M.: Human Embryology, 3rd Edition. New York: Blakiston, 1968.

Ponseti, I. V., and Becker, J. R.: Congenital metatarsus adductus: The results of treatment. J. Bone and Joint Surg., *48-A*:702, 1966.

Rosen, S. von: Diagnosis and treatment of congenital dislocation of the hip joint in the new-born. J. Bone and Joint Surg., *44-B*:284, 1962.

Salter, R. B.: Innominate osteotomy in the treatment of congenital dislocation and subluxation of the hip. J. Bone and Joint Surg., *43-B*:518, 1961.

Settle, G. W.: The anatomy of congenital talipes equinovarus: Sixteen dissected specimens. J. Bone and Joint Surg., *45-A*:1341, 1963.

Siffert, R. S., Ehrlich, M. G., and Katz, J. F.: Management of congenital dislocations of the hip. Clin. Orth. and Rel. Res., *86*:28, 1972.

Smith, E. D.: Spina Bifida and the Total Care of Spinal Myelomeningocele. Springfield, Illinois: Charles C Thomas, 1965.

Vesely, D. G. (Ed.): Clubfoot. Clin. Orth. and Rel. Res., No. 84, 1972.

Chapter Four

Epiphyses

INTRODUCTION

At birth, cartilage masses called epiphyses are found at each end of a long bone. The name is derived from the Greek words *epi* (upon) and *pausis* (growth). The epiphysis consists of a central bony nucleus surrounded by a mass of hyaline cartilage and, with growth, enlarges by endochondral ossification of this adjacent cartilage. The part of the cartilage that lies between the bony nucleus and the metaphysis constitutes the *growth plate*, which is the source of longitudinal growth in a long bone (Fig. 42). At the completion of bone growth at the time of skeletal maturity, the growth plate and epiphysis are completely ossified except for the layer of cartilage that surrounds the epiphysis and persists as adult articular cartilage.

Two types of epiphyses are found in the extremities: *pressure epiphyses* and *traction epiphyses*, also called *apophyses* (Fig. 43). Pressure epiphyses are found at the end of long bones and are considered articular elements. They are subjected to pressures transmitted through the joint of which they are a part. The growth plate of pressure epiphyses provides for longitudinal growth of the long bone. After skeletal maturity is attained, pressure epiphyses persist as joint components covered with articular cartilage. Examples are the femoral and humeral head epiphyses.

Traction epiphyses or apophyses are the site of origin or insertion of major muscles or muscle groups and are therefore subjected to traction rather than pressure. They do not enter into the formation of joints and hence are not covered with articular cartilage. Traction epiphyses contribute to bone shape but not to longitudinal growth of the bone. Examples are the tibial tubercle, lesser trochanter of the

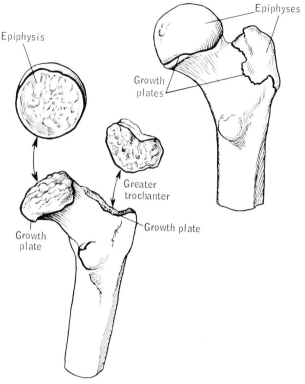

Figure 42.   Upper end of femur, showing capital femoral and greater trochanteric epiphyses.

femur, and humeral condyles. In the two types of epiphyses the growth plate has the same anatomic appearance and responds to the same physiologic influences.

Bone Growth

Longitudinal growth of bone is primarily a function of the growth plate of pressure epiphyses. Affections of bone growth, therefore, are essentially those of the growth plate. The basic controlling and monitoring mechanism of growth is hormonal. Although there are underlying genetic limitations to skeletal stature, many aspects of growth, such as maintenance of rate, growth spurts, and time of cessation, are regulated primarily by anterior pituitary function. The gonads and thyroid, either by their direct effect on the plate or, more likely, by their effects on the pituitary, have been implicated to explain the growth spurt at puberty and the plate closure that occurs at skeletal maturity.

As an organ system specifically concerned with the single function of longitudinal bone growth, the plate is sensitive to the biochemical, physiologic, and pathologic changes that occur in the body as a whole. It appears that the only stimuli to the growth zone in the plate are growth hormones and situations that produce hyperemia around the plate. Alterations of physiologic conditions or the application of other stimuli result in degenerative changes in the plate. Malnutrition, starvation, and severe chronic illness deprive the plate of adequate essential protein and other substances necessary for rapid growth. Longitudinal growth is retarded as a result of diminished cellular activity and matrix production in the growth zone. Normal growth processes resume promptly when an adequate diet or normal health is restored.

Abnormal pressure applied to the plate may also result in retardation of growth. Angulation of the shaft of a bone, asymmetrical pres-

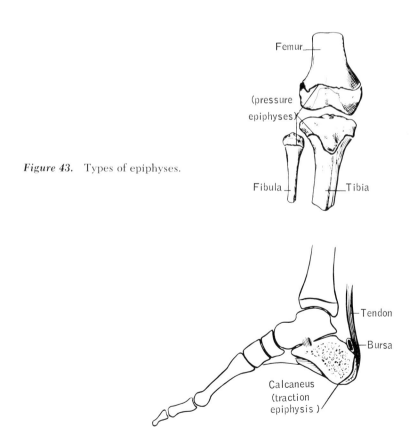

Figure 43. Types of epiphyses.

sures as a result of abnormal muscle pull or joint laxity, or the application of corrective braces or casts that produce angular forces may cause deformity by slowing growth on the side of compression.

The normal growth plate, as seen in standard histologic sections, is divided into four layers: the layer of germinal cells, the layer of proliferating cells, the layer of hypertrophied cells, and the layer of endochondral ossification (Fig. 44). The zone of growth consists of the germinal cell layer and the proliferating cell layer. The space between the cells is filled with cartilage matrix or intercellular substance. The intercellular substance, not the cells, provides the strength of the growth plate, particularly its resistance to shear. In the first two layers of the plate the matrix is abundant and the plate is strong. In the third layer the matrix is scanty and the plate is weak. Thus it is through this third layer that the plane of cleavage occurs in traumatic epiphyseal separations.

Growth is accomplished by proliferation of cartilage cells from the germinal layer (Fig. 45). Subsequent changes in the area are concerned

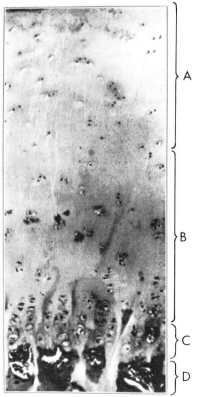

Figure 44. Normal human growth plate showing the various layers. *A*, resting cells. *B*, proliferating cells. *C*, hypertrophying cells. *D*, endochondral cells (metaphysis). (From Salter, R. B.: Injuries involving the epiphyseal plate. J. Bone and Joint Surg., *45-A*:587, 1963. By permission.)

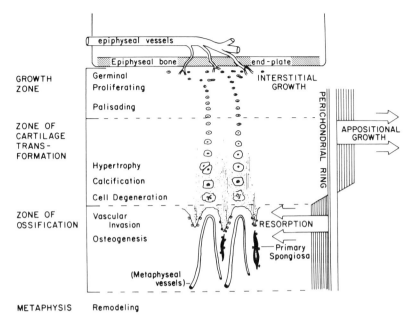

GROWTH
ZONE

ZONE OF
CARTILAGE
TRANS-
FORMATION

ZONE OF
OSSIFICATION

epiphyseal vessels

Epiphyseal bone   end-plate

Germinal   INTERSTITIAL
Proliferating   GROWTH

Palisading

Hypertrophy

Calcification

Cell Degeneration

Vascular
Invasion   RESORPTION

Osteogenesis

        Primary
        Spongiosa

(Metaphyseal
vessels)

PERICHONDRIAL RING

APPOSITIONAL
GROWTH

METAPHYSIS   Remodeling

Figure 45. Diagram of the growth plate of a long bone. The vascular supply to the germinal cells, which are concerned with chondrogenesis, enters through the epiphysis and penetrates the osseous end-plate. The vascular supply to the metaphysis plays no role in the nutrition of the plate but participates in the removal of the cellular and matrix end-products of chondrogenesis, in osteogenesis, and in remodeling. Actual longitudinal growth occurs only in the growth zone (interstitial growth) as a result of cell reproduction and elaboration of intercellular matrix. In the zone of cartilage transformation, complex physiological and biochemical processes are concerned with preparation of the cartilage matrix formed in the growth zone for later replacement by bone in the zone of ossification. Widening of the plate (appositional growth) and later external remodeling are the functions of the perichondrial ring. (From Siffert, R. S.: The growth plate and its affections. Am. Academy of Orthopaedic Surgeons Instructional Course Lectures, Vol. XVIII, J1, 1962–1969, p. 27. By permission.)

with preparation of the newly formed cartilage for replacement by bone. Complex physiologic mechanisms are involved in this preparation and are all geared toward rendering the matrix calcifiable. Conditions interfering with these basic physiologic mechanisms, or inborn errors of metabolism, may result in failure of the matrix to prepare for calcification or in lack of normal osteogenesis with consequent skeletal deformity. Similarly, nonavailability of the necessary bone salts, as in rickets, will interfere with orderly osteogenesis by making calcification impossible.

Blood is supplied to the epiphysis by two sets of vessels, those arising from the epiphysis and those arising from the metaphysis. The epiphyseal vessels arise as branches of the nutrient vessels to the ossification center of the epiphysis. The growth and survival of the epiphyseal cartilage and growth plate are dependent upon the blood supply from the epiphyseal side. Interference with the vascular supply to the germinal cells results in failure of chondrogenesis and complete failure of growth.

The possibility of restoring or providing increased length of a bone or an extremity through the transplantation of a growing epiphysis has intrigued clinicians and challenged researchers for years. The generally unfavorable experimental results reflect the difficulty researchers have encountered in developing techniques to maintain an intact epiphyseal circulation. It is this loss of blood supply that probably causes failure of epiphyseal transplants. Interference with the epiphyseal circulation is also thought to be the pathophysiologic basis of avascular necrosis of an epiphysis, a situation encountered clinically in Legg-Calvé Perthes disease (p. 85) and sometimes as a complication after a slipped capital femoral epiphysis (p. 344).

The metaphyseal vessels arise from the nutrient and periosteal vessels of the diaphysis. The rich and relatively abundant circulation on the metaphyseal side of the growth plate plays a much less vital role in the growth process. It can even be interrupted for short periods by such clinical problems as fracture or epiphyseal separation with only, at most, a temporary growth alteration. The metaphyseal blood supply is apparently involved in endochrondral ossification, a process of exchanging cartilage for bone.

CLINICAL CONSIDERATIONS

From the foregoing discussion it can easily be recognized that skeletal growth is a complex mechanism subject to the perfect operation of many variables. Disruption of one or more of the variables may have disastrous effects on human form and function. Developmental abnormalities of growth are assumed to be hereditary disorders of metabolism involving essential physiologic and biochemical complexes. Varying degrees of involvement, mixed disorders of chondrogenesis and matrix formation, and enzymatic errors can produce marked alteration in normal growth and unlimited variations in the clinical patterns of these diseases. Two developmental disorders in which specific defects have been identified are achondroplasia (p. 164) and osteogenesis imperfecta (p. 167).

Local conditions that exert some deleterious effect on the growth plate are seen fairly frequently in clinical practice. A force applied to a growing bone may cause the intact epiphysis to shear off at the growth plate, with a clinical result similar to a fracture of the bone. Of all injuries to the long bones during childhood, approximately 15 per cent involve the growth plate.

Disuse of an extremity can cause shortening by removal of the normal weight bearing stresses needed for orderly growth. Theoretically, this could be brought about by prolonged immobilization in a plaster cast or traction apparatus. Severe muscular paralysis following poliomyelitis or some cases of spina bifida deformity is frequently accompanied by retardation of bone growth with sometimes extreme shortening.

Growth disturbance secondary to abnormal pressure effects on the epiphysis may be seen with cerebral palsy or congenital dislocation of the hip. Pronation of the feet may exert abnormal pressure effects on the epiphyses at the knees, resulting in the development of a secondary knock knee deformity.

Infection can directly involve the epiphysis and cause its destruction, with resultant shortening of the bone. The growth plate, which forms an effective barrier to the spread of infection in older children, forms no such barrier in infants. In infants the cartilaginous growth plate itself is resistant to infection, but since the metaphyseal vessels penetrate it, the exudate can easily spread to the epiphysis from the metaphyseal focus. The epiphyseal center of ossification can therefore be destroyed by the actual infection, or the development of the epiphysis may be impaired by thrombosis or interruption of its blood supply. One condition characterized by this epiphyseal impairment is pyogenic arthritis of infancy (p. 136).

Since hyperemia in the region of the growth plate may act as a stimulus to growth, a pocket of infection localized in a bone shaft adjacent to an epiphysis could stimulate the epiphysis to overgrow and lengthen the bone.

TRAUMA

A shearing or avulsing force applied to a growing bone may cause the intact epiphysis to separate from the bone through the growth plate, with a clinical result similar to a fracture of the bone. The cartilaginous growth plate is weaker than the joint capsule or normal ligaments and tendons; thus, injuries that produce joint dislocation or major tendon rupture in the adult produce epiphyseal separation in the child. The epiphyses most commonly involved are distal radius, proximal radius, proximal humeral, and distal tibial. The child notes immediate pain and disability, and clinical deformity may be present. X-ray examination defines the problem as one involving the epiphysis.

Trauma to traction epiphyses may give rise only to locally painful conditions of limited significance, because these epiphyses do not contribute to longitudinal bone growth. The real orthopaedic problems involve disturbances to pressure epiphyses.

The three main types of injury sustained by a pressure epiphysis are separation of the epiphysis through its growth plate, fracture that crosses the growth plate, and crushing injury of the growth plate itself. Separation of the epiphysis is more common than the other two types of epiphyseal trauma (Fig. 46). The separation almost invariably occurs on the diaphyseal side of the growth plate through the area of hypertrophied cartilage cells, the area of greatest structural weakness. In the vast majority of instances, it is possible to replace the epiphysis into proper alignment by a gentle manipulative maneuver. In this type of injury the growth cells remain intact with the separated epiphysis, and the prognosis for renewed growth after replacement is good unless the injury simultaneously damages the nutrient vessels to the epiphysis. If that occurs, avascular necrosis may complicate the problem.

The other two types of epiphyseal injury carry with them a generally more serious prognosis with regard to growth disturbance. Fractures crossing the growth plate often result in gaps in the plate that fill

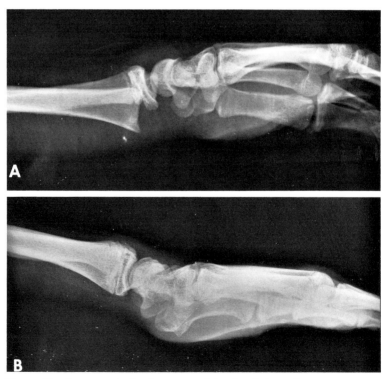

Figure 46. A, traumatic displacement of distal radial epiphysis at wrist. B, normal position of distal radial epiphysis on lateral x-ray view.

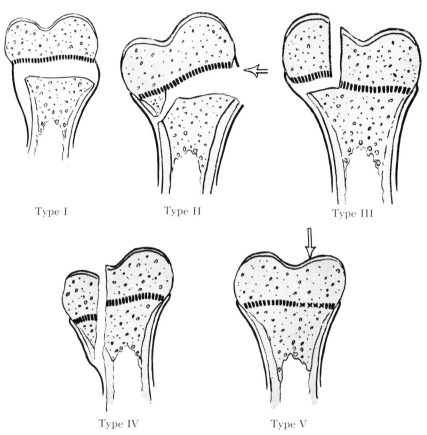

Type I   Type II   Type III

Type IV   Type V

Figure 47. A, Type I growth plate injury: separation of the epiphysis. B, Type II growth plate injury: fracture-separation of the epiphysis. C, Type III growth plate injury: fracture of part of the epiphysis. D, Type IV growth plate injury: fracture of the epiphysis and growth plate. E, Type V growth plate injury: crushing of the growth plate. (From Salter, R. B.: Injuries involving the epiphyseal plate. J. Bone and Joint Surg., 45-A:587, 1963. By permission.)

with bone if the integrity of the plate is not anatomically restored by either closed or open reduction. Crushing injuries carry the worst prognosis, since they invariably allow bony bars to grow across the growth plate, leading to premature closure.

Epiphyseal injuries have been classified by Salter and Harris into five types (Fig. 47). Injuries of Types I, II, and III carry a good prognosis for growth, provided the blood supply to the epiphysis is intact. Type IV injuries have a bad prognosis unless the growth plate is completely and accurately realigned. Type V injuries are associated with actual crushing of the growth plate and carry the worst prognosis (Fig. 48).

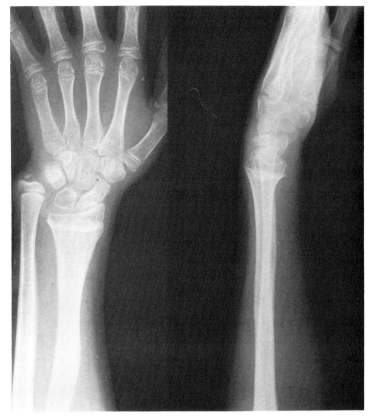

Figure 48.   Premature closure of distal radial epiphysis following crushing injury to growth plate (Salter Type V).

If the entire growth plate ceases to grow, the result is progressive shortening without angulation. However, if the involved bone is one of a parallel pair, such as tibia and fibula or radius and ulna, progressive shortening of the one bone will produce progressive deformity in the neighboring joint. If growth ceases in one part of the plate but continues in the rest, progressive angular deformity occurs (Fig. 49).

CORRECTION OF EPIPHYSEAL DISTURBANCES

Developmental abnormalities affecting the growth plate are puzzling conditions. In most instances, the specific defect remains obscure and definitive treatment is lacking. Occasionally local surgical treatment, such as osteotomy, may be required to improve the form or function of an extremity.

Except for the use of human growth hormone in children with hypopituitarism, no medical therapy is available that will reliably and safely add to the ultimate stature of short children or reduce the ultimate height of excessively tall ones. The orthopaedist is most frequently called upon for advice when local disturbances affect the growth plate.

After injury to a growth plate, local growth may either cease immediately or continue at a retarded rate for a period of time before stopping. In addition, the growth disturbance may involve either the entire growth plate or only part of it. The main types of clinical deformity that may develop are shortening of the bone, angulation of the bone, or a combination of the two. In any case, the resultant deformity is progressive until the end of the child's growth period. Because of the secondary tilting effect on the pelvis and spine, shortening of more than one inch becomes a problem when it involves the leg. Shortening of less than one inch can be accepted and adequately compensated for by the use of a heel lift in the shoe. Shortening of the upper

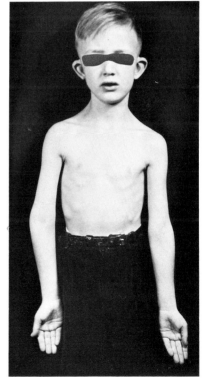

Figure 49. Carrying angle deformity of right elbow secondary to growth plate damage.

extremity may be cosmetically objectionable, but it usually causes no functional problem.

Unequal length of the extremities can also develop from causes other than epiphyseal damage. Fracture through the shaft of a long bone, when allowed to heal with the fragments in an overlapped position, can result in shortening. Injury or disease causing loss of bone substance can have the same effect. However, it is possible in many instances definitively to correct leg length inequality of more than one inch if certain criteria are met.

Progressive angulation of a bone at a joint is best treated by osteotomy of the bone, so that the growing potential of the undamaged portion of the growth plate may be preserved and some lengthening of the extremity may be gained. When progressive angulation exists in a very young child, it may be necessary to perform osteotomy more than once during the growth period.

The orthopaedist's most frequent challenge in this regard is progressive shortening of the lower extremity, which can give rise to significant leg length discrepancy if allowed to continue. There are, theoretically, five methods of obtaining leg length equalization:

1. *Stimulation of growth of the short leg.* Such stimulation may follow the hyperemia induced by a fracture, a surgical osteotomy, or surgical stripping of the periosteum. The effect operates for only a short period of time and the results are unpredictable. Attempts to stimulate growth artificially have either failed or proved impractical.

2. *Elongation of a short bone.* Bone lengthening operations should be restricted to older children and adolescents. A one-stage procedure is fraught with the danger of vascular and nerve complications. Gradual lengthening of the femur or tibia and fibula over a period of weeks, using a special frame and skeletal traction, is feasible and has been carried out successfully.

3. *Shortening of a long bone.* Bone shortening operations may be performed in the femur and tibia but should be reserved for patients who have completed or nearly completed their growth.

4. *Amputation and prosthetic replacement.* This is usually reserved for patients with the extreme shortening most frequently associated with congenital limb defects.

5. *Retardation of growth of the long leg,* which is the method most commonly employed.

To retard the growth of the long leg, the epiphyses of the normal leg must be operated upon so that its growth may be delayed and the short leg may have time to catch up in length. At the time of epiphyseal surgery on the longer leg, it is possible to permanently or temporarily inhibit its growth, depending upon which type of operative procedure is carried out.

To be a candidate for this type of surgery, the child must have enough growth potential left to make the procedure worthwhile. The surgery must be performed at just the right age in order to allow time for this "catching up" to occur. The proper time to perform epiphyseal surgery is decided after determining the patient's bone age and after consulting growth prediction charts. These charts indicate the amount of correction expected by arrest of each epiphysis at various ages. A long-term plan must include careful study of growth prediction charts, determination of bone age, and, if possible, a longitudinal study for several years prior to any growth retardation operation. The rate of growth should be graphed and projected into the future so that accurate determination of the desired shortening will be obtained. Since 70 per cent of the longitudinal growth of the leg comes from the epiphyses around the knee, the lower femoral and upper tibial and fibular epiphyses are the ones usually chosen for surgery.

Two types of growth retardation operations are in general use. The growth plate can be permanently arrested by a procedure called

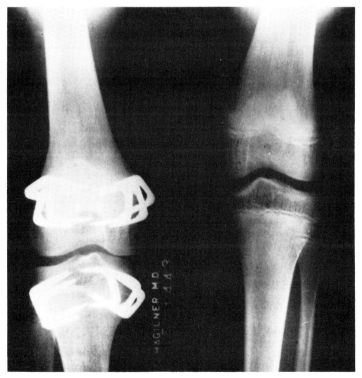

Figure 50. Temporary growth arrest obtained by stapling growth plates of lower femur and upper tibia at knee joint.

epiphysiodesis. The selected growth plates of the long leg are prematurely arrested by destroying the germinal cells by surgical curettage. The epiphysis is then prematurely fused to the shaft by the insertion of multiple small bone grafts across the destroyed growth plate. The epiphyses of the short leg continue to grow, and gradually the leg length inequality lessens. Growth of the shorter leg is the factor that corrects the discrepancy. This procedure is useful when maximum retardation must be obtained.

Temporary arrest of growth can be obtained by straddling each side of the growth plate with three metal staples (Fig. 50). If the staples are properly placed and if they do not loosen or break, this procedure can effectively inhibit the activity of a growth plate. Growth will resume after removal of the staples. Stapling causes a quantitative retardation of growth, retarding growth between 70 and 90 per cent of normal. The operation must be performed earlier than an epiphysiodesis to achieve the same retardation. If growth is to be resumed, the staples must be removed before growth of the epiphysis has ceased. The advantage and sole indication for epiphyseal stapling over the other form of arrest is reversibility.

THE OSTEOCHONDROSES

The term osteochondrosis refers to a curious self-limiting disorder affecting pressure epiphyses during the growth period. This disorder has been described in just about every pressure epiphysis in the body and, unfortunately, the describers' names have clung as identifying tags. The unwary might suppose that the terms Legg-Calvé-Perthes disease, Freiberg's disease, and Scheuermann's disease, for example, have little in common. The truth of the matter is that these terms all describe the same underlying pathologic process, the only difference being the functional importance of the involved pressure epiphysis. Legg-Calvé-Perthes disease, for instance, is an osteochondrosis of the capital femoral epiphysis; Kohler's disease involves the tarsal navicular bone; Freiberg's disease involves the head of the second metatarsal bone, while Scheuermann's disease is an osteochondrosis of the vertebral body epiphysis.

The pathologic process in an osteochondrosis is an avascular necrosis of the developing epiphysis produced by causes that are still unknown. Whatever the underlying cause, interference with the epiphyseal circulation occurs, resulting in avascular necrosis involving the epiphysis. The bone of an epiphysis so affected softens, dies, and is gradually absorbed. However, the cap of articular cartilage surrounding the epiphysis remains intact and unaffected, because its nutrition is derived from the synovial fluid. Because the bony tissue contained within the cartilage cap is soft and degenerating, the epiphysis may collapse and flatten under the pressure of the body weight. The body attempts to repair the damage almost immediately, and gradually the dead bone is replaced by new bone growing in from the adjacent viable bone. This process of repair is known as "creeping substitution."

Any pressure epiphysis so affected, then, undergoes an avascular necrosis but always heals spontaneously, with some permanent residual flattening or deformity. The factors producing the derangement of the epiphyseal circulation that causes the avascular necrosis remain unidentified, but trauma, infectious diseases, endocrine imbalance, faulty metabolism, and nutritional and hereditary predisposition have been mentioned as inciting factors.

LEGG-CALVÉ-PERTHES DISEASE

Osteochondrosis of the capital femoral epiphysis bears the name of the three physicians who described it, independently, about 1910. Also known as coxa plana (flat hip), it is one of the important causes of painful limp in childhood. The incongruity of the hip joint secondary to the residual flattening of the femoral head caused by this disorder may lead to a painful osteoarthritis of the hip during adult life (Fig. 52). For this reason it is the most important of the osteochondroses.

The underlying pathologic process in Legg-Calvé-Perthes disease, as in all of the osteochondroses, is an avascular necrosis resulting in massive necrosis of the bone of the capital femoral epiphysis, with the articular cartilage covering the femoral head remaining intact. Almost immediately bone repair begins, with new bone from the adjacent viable bone invading the necrotic epiphysis and gradually replacing the dead bone. This process of "creeping substitution," the method employed by bone tissue to heal an area of avascular necrosis, gives the self-limiting character to an osteochondrosis and accounts for the distinguishing x-ray changes. Complete healing will occur, but the contour of the epiphysis flattens and the shape and appearance of a completely normal epiphysis are never regained. It usually takes from 12 to 36 months for healing to be completed.

Clinical Features. Legg-Calvé-Perthes disease affects children between the ages of four and 10 years and is more common in boys. It is usually unilateral but may be bilateral. It frequently affects children of low birth weight who are not quite "up to par" physically as compared with their peers. It rarely occurs in the Negro. The attack rate is approximately one in 750 male children and one in 4000 female children. The disease has two striking characteristics: a clinical onset within a relatively narrow age range, usually between four and eight years, and a marked predilection for boys.

The initial complaint is usually vague discomfort in and about the affected extremity, with pain possibly referred to the thigh or knee. The child limps in an effort to avoid or lessen the pain (antalgic gait). Examination reveals restriction of hip motion on the involved side as compared with the unaffected side. Usually the first hip motion lost is that of rotation. Spasm of the adductor muscles may be present.

Serial x-ray films disclose the changes in the epiphysis brought about by necrosis and repair in the manner characteristic of this disorder (Fig. 51). Early the epiphysis appears to thin out or flatten. It then appears to break up or fragment. Dense areas, representing dead bone, appear in the head but later disappear as healing progresses. Neighboring bone is hypervascularized and therefore osteoporotic, particularly in the metaphysis. The diminished density of the osteoporotic bone causes, by contrast, an apparent increase in the density of the necrotic bone. The fragmented epiphysis tends to coalesce into a single mass of healing bone as repair proceeds. The femoral neck tends to shorten and broaden. The acetabulum tends to alter its shape to fit the contour of the femoral head. When healing is completed, there is almost always some residual deformity of the femoral head, varying from slight flattening to complete collapse with mushrooming of the head about the neck. The younger the patient at the onset the better will be the ultimate clinical and x-ray result. The amount of final shortening depends, to a great extent, on the amount of residual deformity.

Treatment. Once the diagnosis has been established, the child must be taken off his feet to remove the pressure of weight bearing from the epiphysis. Weight bearing will seriously and permanently deform the soft necrotic epiphysis. It has been well established that patients treated by complete and absolute recumbency during the active phase of the process heal with the least amount of deformity. For the few patients hospitalized in children's hospitals for treatment, it is usually possible to achieve such absolute recumbency. For the majority of patients treated at home, however, it is not possible to maintain complete recumbency for the many months required. Most of the children with this disease, therefore, are treated by a compromise form of ambulatory non-weight bearing.

The aim of treatment in Legg-Calvé-Perthes disease is the reduction of deformity during healing of the avascular necrosis of the capital femoral epiphysis. The efficacy of any form of treatment is judged by how near to normal the involved hip becomes. Usually, the earlier the age of onset, the better will be the final result.

The physician must impress both the patient and his family with

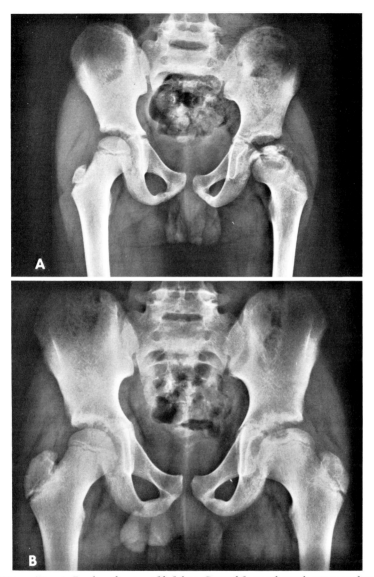

Figure 51. A, Perthes disease of left hip. Capital femoral epiphysis is undergoing necrosis and fragmentation. B, same hip, five years later, showing residual flattening of femoral head.

the absolute necessity of not bearing weight on the affected extremity until healing occurs. Initially, if there is a great deal of pain and muscle spasm, the child is put to bed until the spasm subsides. If necessary, the hip can be put to rest for several weeks in a plaster hip spica cast or in Buck's traction. When ambulation is allowed after the acute pain and muscle spasm have subsided, the hip must continue to be protected from weight bearing by the use of some protective device.

An ischial weight bearing caliper brace can be worn on the affected leg with an elevated shoe on the opposite foot. An older child may use crutches with the foot of the affected leg held off the ground by a shoulder sling. Some centers favor "containment" splints, which hold the leg in a flexed and abducted attitude and thus position the femoral head deeper into the acetabulum. The selected program is continued until x-ray examination discloses healing of the femoral head epiphysis. X-ray examination of the affected hip is made every several months to evaluate the progress of healing. The total healing process may take from 12 to 36 months.

There have been some attempts to treat Legg-Calvé-Perthes disease surgically. Theoretically, it was thought that surgical drilling of the growth plate would allow the metaphyseal vessels easy access to the epiphysis and hence materially shorten the necrotic phase. The clinical results, unfortunately, have generally been disappointing.

Arthrograms of hip joints affected with Legg-Calvé-Perthes disease made during the fragmentation and reparative stages have occasionally revealed enlargement of the femoral head not adequately demonstrated by plain x-ray films. This would indicate that a significant amount of the femoral head was not contained in the acetabulum and, therefore, could not be properly remodeled into a more normal contour. Many of these patients healed with severe femoral head deformity. It is the severe mechanical malalignment of the hip joint associated with significant femoral head deformity that can be expected to lead to secondary osteoarthritis of the joint in adult life (Fig. 52).

Two surgical procedures are possible to correct this situation and provide for better containment of the femoral head in the acetabulum. An osteotomy could be performed through the subtrochanteric area of the femur. This would permit deeper placement of the femoral head into the acetabulum. Or an innominate osteotomy (see p. 62) could be performed through the pelvic side of the joint. This would allow the roof of the acetabulum to be placed more squarely over the femoral head. Both procedures give the better relationship between femoral head and acetabulum so necessary for normal contouring. The results reported from both procedures have been quite promising.

Most patients with Legg-Calvé-Perthes disease, given adequate treatment, can be expected to heal with relatively minimal femoral head deformity. Long-term follow-up studies show that only the occasional patient with severe residual femoral head deformity develops secondary painful hip symptoms during adult life.

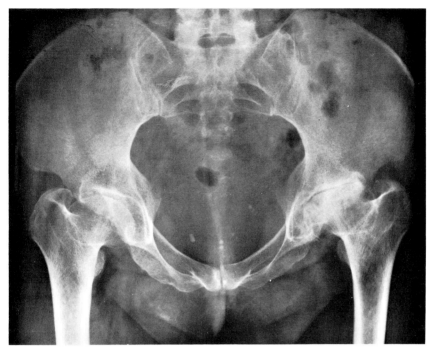

Figure 52. Osteoarthritis of the left hip, which has developed in a mechanically imperfect joint. Patient had Legg-Calvé-Perthes disease in both hips as a child.

SCHEUERMANN'S DISEASE

Osteochondrosis of vertebral body epiphyses is known as Scheuermann's disease. It has also been called vertebral epiphysitis and adolescent kyphosis or round back. The area of the spine most frequently involved is the thoracic segment. The pressure of weight bearing on an affected spinal segment will cause anterior wedging and some flattening of the softened vertebrae. If this is sufficiently severe, a kyphotic deformity or "hump" will appear in the thoracic segment of the spine. This disorder is the most common cause of "round back" deformity in children (see p. 297).

Symptoms usually appear between the ages of 10 and 16, with involvement being about twice as common in girls. The initial symptom is usually back pain or fatigue. This may be followed by the gradual appearance of the "round back" deformity. X-ray examination shows involvement of the vertebral epiphysis, with or without flattening of the body, depending on the stage of the avascular necrotic process. The affected vertebrae appear wedge-shaped, with undulating end plates.

Mild cases of Scheuermann's disease may be treated by hyperextension spinal muscle exercises to counteract the tendency to anterior vertebral body wedging and kyphosis. If any degree of deformation of the spine is present, the back should be first immobilized in a plaster body jacket and then supported by a long spinal brace with shoulder straps to hold the spine erect until healing occurs.

A section of the spine affected by Scheuermann's disease during the growth period may in adulthood develop degenerative changes secondary to the vertebral deformation. Pain in the thoracic segment of the spine during adult life not infrequently has its origin in adolescent Scheuermann's disease.

QUESTIONABLE OSTEOCHONDROSES

Two other painful conditions occurring in children, one involving the tibial tubercle and the other the os calcis, were in the past frequently classified with the osteochondroses. Authorities now question their right to belong in this category, since neither involves a pressure epiphysis and bone biopsy material has failed to disclose evidence of avascular necrosis. It is now considered that both conditions represent simply a tendinous attachment strain on a traction epiphysis.

OSGOOD-SCHLATTER DISEASE

This condition, characterized by a painfully tender and enlarged tibial tubercle, is seen most commonly in boys between 10 and 15 years of age. It is caused by a pull of the patellar tendon on the tibial tubercle epiphysis. Pain is accentuated by local pressure, such as kneeling, and by any activity that causes forceful contracture of the patellar tendon on the tubercle, such as running, stair climbing, or bicycle riding. The disease may occur bilaterally.

X-ray examination may reveal some fragmentation and separation of the tibial tubercle, but serial films will not show the gamut of changes characteristic of avascular necrosis and "creeping substitution."

The condition is self-limited and the ultimate prognosis is excellent. However, the knee pain suffered by the patient during the acute phase is often severe enough to require treatment. Mild cases may respond favorably to simple restriction of activities, such as prohibiting kneeling, running, and bicycling. In more severe cases it may be necessary to immobilize the extremity in a plaster walking cylinder for six weeks. Extreme local tenderness about the tubercle may respond to local injections of hydrocortisone. The local pain and tenderness disappear with time, but residual enlargement of the tibial tubercle may be permanent.

SEVER'S DISEASE

This condition causes painful heels, usually in boys between the ages of seven and 10. Also known as apophysitis of the os calcis, it is caused by pull of the Achilles tendon on this traction epiphysis. Pain is brought on by walking, especially on the toes, and causes a limp. The back of the heel is locally tender to palpation.

X-ray examination may be interpreted as showing a "dense fragmentation" of the epiphysis, but not too much significance has been ascribed to this interpretation. True avascular necrosis does not occur.

If the heel of the shoe is raised one-half inch on the affected side, painful pressure on the heel is usually relieved. Removal of the back counter of the heel portion of the shoe is also useful in relieving pressure. It is frequently beneficial to gouge out the heel of the shoe to form a foam rubber-filled saddle for the os calcis.

References

Anderson, M., Green, W. T., and Messner, M. B.: Growth and prediction of growth in the lower extremities. J. Bone and Joint Surg., *45-A* 1, 1963.

Catteral, A.: The natural history of perthes disease. J. Bone and Joint Surg., *43-B*:37, 1971.

Eaton, G. O.: Long term results of treatment in coxa plana. J. Bone and Joint Surg., *49-A*:1031, 1967.

Frantz, C. H.: Epiphyseal stapling: A comprehensive review. Clin. Orth. and Rel. Res., *77*:149, 1971.

Legg, A. P.: An obscure affection of the hip joint. Boston Med. and Surg. J., *1962* 202, 1910.

Ponseti, I. B.: Legg-Calvé-Perthes disease. Pathogenesis and evolution. J. Bone and Joint Surg., *43-A*:261, 1961.

Salter, R. B., and Harris, W. R.: Injuries involving the epiphyseal plate. J. Bone and Joint Surg., *45-A*:587, 1963.

Siffert, R. S.: The growth plate and its affections. J. Bone and Joint Surg., *48-A*:546, 1966.

Chapter Five

Disorders of Joints

INTRODUCTION

Normal joint cartilage is bathed with synovial fluid, a transudate of plasma derived from a moderately vascular synovium. This fluid supplies nutrients to the cartilage and functions as the perfect lubricant. Under normal conditions synovial fluid is viscous and serous in appearance, containing few polymorphonuclear leucocytes and no crystalline elements. The glucose levels of normal joint fluid and plasma are similar. Fluid aspirated from normal joints does not clot spontaneously. The precipitate formed by adding normal synovial fluid to dilute acetic acid is characteristically discrete and firm in appearance ("mucin" clot test). These characteristics of normal synovial fluid may be altered in various disease states of joints.

The classic pathologic response to a noxious stimulus affecting a joint is inflammation characterized by local heat, redness, swelling, and pain. The degree of the inflammatory response will depend greatly upon the type and extent of the offending stimulus, its location, and the state of the host tissue. By its nature the inflammatory response cannot involve the musculoskeletal system exclusively. The reticuloendothelial system, the cardiovascular system, and connective tissue are intimately concerned in this response. Consequently the inflammatory response frequently makes itself known as a systemic illness characterized by malaise, prostration, fever and, finally, localized pain.

Joint inflammation starts in the synovial membrane which, as a consequence of the irritation, may secrete large amounts of fluid into the joint cavity, together with numerous inflammatory cells. This resulting synovial effusion is usually painful and interferes with normal joint function. The inflammatory joint fluid is characterized by an

92

increased content of serum proteins, decreased viscosity, and a decreased content of hyaluronic acid. Cloudiness of the fluid results from increased numbers of white blood cells. Fluid obtained from inflamed joints clots because of the presence of fibrinogen, which enters an inflamed joint by means of increased vascular permeability. In most types of inflammatory joint disease, the "mucin" test shows a flocculation instead of a mucin clot.

The inflammatory joint response runs the gamut from a mild effusion to a severely destructive process causing permanent joint damage. Trauma to a joint frequently irritates the synovium to evoke an outpouring of synovial fluid and a joint effusion. Rheumatoid arthritis is characterized by chronic joint inflammation. Bacterial joint infection may be accompanied by joint cartilage destruction if the chondroid matrix is digested by proteolytic enzymes. The final result may be irreversible and permanent joint damage.

Emphasis must be placed upon identification of the cause of the inflammatory joint response at the earliest possible moment. Adequate and timely treatment can greatly modify the joint response and mitigate its harmful effects. The laboratory reflections of joint inflammation include an elevated serum uric acid in gout, leucocytosis in bacterial infection, and a persistent elevation of the erythrocyte sedimentation rate in the serum of the patient with rheumatoid arthritis. Additional diagnostic information may be obtained from an examination of the aspirated synovial fluid with reference to color and appearance, culture, cell count, sugar content, acid-phosphatase activity, and the presence or absence of crystals. Joint and synovial tissue biopsy may be required to establish a diagnosis.

ARTHRITIS

By definition, the term arthritis means simply "inflammation of a joint." Theoretically, any lesion or disorder associated with or causing inflammation of a joint may be said to produce a form of arthritis. Most cases seen clinically will fall within the following groups:

1. Rheumatoid arthritis (including juvenile rheumatoid arthritis and ankylosing spondylitis)
2. Arthritis due to rheumatic fever
3. Osteoarthritis (degenerative joint disease)
4. Arthritis due to infection (pyogenic arthritis, tuberculosis arthritis)
5. Traumatic arthritis
6. Metabolic disease affecting joints (gout)
7. Neuropathic joint disease (Charcot joint)

8. Monarthritis
9. Special forms
   a. Hemophilic arthritis
   b. Psychogenic rheumatism

In terms of total number of victims, arthritis leads all other diseases as a cause of crippling and economic loss to the community. It actually results in more lost work days than accidental injuries. The total number of people affected can be expected to increase as the life span lengthens, because osteoarthritis, the most frequently seen form of arthritis, is predominantly a disease of middle and old age.

RHEUMATOID ARTHRITIS

Rheumatoid arthritis, a chronic inflammatory disease of undetermined etiology and pathogenesis, is systemic in nature and is characterized by the manner in which it involves the synovial membrane of joints, tendons, or bursae.

The disease is seen most commonly in those between the ages of 25 and 50, but it may also be seen in children and in the aged. It shows a sex ratio of three women affected for each male. There is a slight tendency for the disease to be familial. Psychogenic factors are thought to be of some importance in the precipitation or exacerbation of the disease in many patients. This is the most feared form of arthritis because of the profound crippling that may result.

Pathologic Features. The major target organ for rheumatoid involvement is the synovial tissue. Inflammatory disease may be present wherever synovium is found. The disease is thus not limited to synovial joints, but may also occur in tendon sheaths and bursae.

Despite extensive study, the etiology of rheumatoid arthritis remains obscure. It is generally accepted, however, that immune mechanisms play an important role in the initiation and perpetuation of this disease. The articular changes, once started, become self-perpetuating because of mechanisms within the synovial membrane itself. Presumably an antigen-antibody reaction takes place directly within the synovial cavity, causing injury to and marked proliferation of the synovium. This diseased synovium, primarily by the release of proteolytic enzymes, damages the articular cartilage and adjacent tissues. These enzymes cause further injury to the synovium as well as perpetuating the disease process.

Joint involvement is heralded by synovial inflammation with effusion. The inflammatory changes may also involve the capsule and periarticular soft tissues, causing the swelling, tenderness, and painful motion seen in the joint clinically. There is regional atrophy of bone and muscle. Joint effusion is present in the active stage but disappears during remissions and in the chronic stage. Although the synovial tissues are densely infiltrated by mononuclear cells, the synovial fluid typically contains thousands of neutrophils, giving it a cloudy appearance. Hyaluronate is reduced in the fluid, and the "mucin" test shows a flocculation instead of a clot.

Since there is as yet no definitive treatment for rheumatoid arthritis, the initiating antigen persists and evokes a chronic state of inflammation. Round cells, particularly lymphocytes and plasma cells, become the predominant cell types in the synovium. The synovium proliferates extensively and becomes a permanently thickened, hyperemic, densely cellular membrane with enlarged erythematous villi. This thickened granulomatous tissue contributes to the formation of an eroding and invading membrane known as a *pannus*.

The excess joint fluid derived from the inflammatory synovium precipitates a layer of fibrin, which coats the synovial and articular surfaces. This fibrin layer gradually becomes organized into a highly vascular, spreading, granulation tissue membrane or pannus by the growth into it of cells and vessels from the synovium. The pannus gradually spreads over the joint surfaces, eroding and pitting the underlying cartilage and bone (Fig. 53). A reasonable hypothesis of

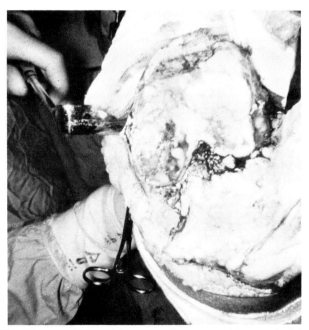

Figure 53.   Rheumatoid knee joint exposed at surgery. Note marked destruction of articular cartilage.

mechanism is that lysosomal enzymes, released from the proliferating rheumatoid synovium in contact with cartilage, gain access to the cartilage matrix and degrade it, thus preparing the way for the actual invasion of the cartilage by the pannus.

Pannus formation is a characteristic of rheumatoid pathology. The pannus destroys articular cartilage and may even erode subchondral bone, resulting in progressive and crippling joint deformity and permanent loss of motion. This destructive pathologic process renders the joint quite unstable, and muscle pull across the joint may cause flexion or extension contractures, subluxations, or even joint dislocation.

As the acute inflammatory process subsides, the granulation tissue may become converted to dense scar, causing fibrous ankylosis of the joint. If this fibrous scar is converted to bone, a true ankylosis results. The fibers of associated skeletal muscles undergo localized or diffuse degenerative changes, with the degenerated muscle being gradually replaced by fibrous tissue. The involved bones show osteoporosis or bone rarefaction.

Clinical Features.   Most often rheumatoid arthritis has an insidious onset. Joint involvement is usually symmetrically distributed, with the proximal interphalangeal joints of the fingers especially susceptible. Frequently one or just a few joints gradually become swollen and painful at the onset, with other joints becoming affected later. In many patients rheumatoid arthritis is relatively mild, and remission occurs before extensive joint damage has taken place. In advanced rheumatoid arthritis, chronic deformities including contractures, subluxation, ankylosis, and gross local distortion of joints may be found.

The painful swelling in and about the joint limits motion. The thickening of the periarticular tissues, combined with the muscle atrophy above and below, gives the joint a characteristic spindle-shaped appearance. The proliferating connective tissue tends to overgrow and erode the joint cartilage and invade the supporting cancellous bone, leading to severe disability and deformity, often with ankylosis of the joint. These changes are most likely to be seen in the hands, wrists, knees, hips, and feet, but almost every point in the body may be involved (Fig. 54).

As the disease progresses, the patient may experience fatigue, exhaustion, lassitude, vasomotor disturbances, paresthesias, generalized morning stiffness of one or several hours' duration, and general debility. Underweight frequently accompanies rheumatoid arthritis. Muscular weakness and atrophy are prominent. The skin of the extremities may become smooth, glossy, and atrophic. Constitutional manifestations may include elevated temperature, tachycardia, generalized lymphadenopathy, and malnutrition with bodily wasting.

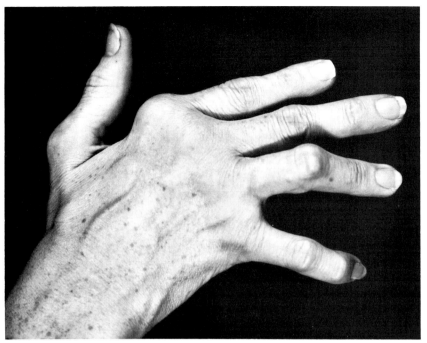

Figure 54. Typical changes in the hand caused by rheumatoid arthritis.

Subcutaneous nodules are found near the elbow in about 20 per cent of all patients. These are a characteristic pathologic feature of the disease and are thought to represent a reactive process of the reticuloendothelial system that leads to infarction and necrosis of the surrounding connective tissue.

Spontaneous subluxation of the cervical spine is a well-recognized and not uncommon complication of rheumatoid arthritis. It occurs most commonly at the atlantoaxial level but may also occur at lower levels in the cervical area. Although many of these patients are free from symptoms or complain only of increasing neck pain, cord pressure with tetraplegia can ensue.

X-ray Features. A single film of the hand and wrist is usually more useful diagnostically in peripheral rheumatoid arthritis than a view of any other part (Fig. 55). However, roentgen changes other than soft tissue swelling may not appear for several months after the onset of the disease.

The degree of x-ray change will vary with the stage of the disease and can be summarized as follows:

Early Stage
1. Soft tissue swelling

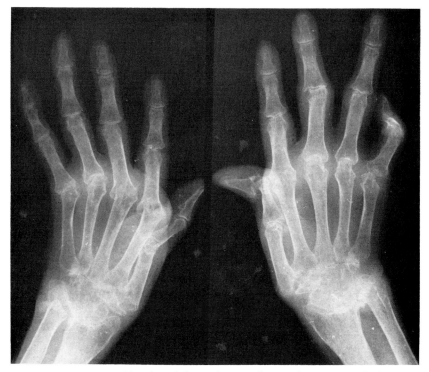

Figure 55. X-ray of hands, exhibiting bone and joint changes typical of rheumatoid arthritis.

2. Osteoporosis or bone rarefaction
3. Loss of joint space without alteration in contour
   Intermediate Stage
1. Bone erosion at the margins of the articular cortices
2. Subchondral cyst formation
3. Progressive osteoporosis
4. Progressive loss of joint space
5. Joint contracture deformities
   Late Stage
1. Severe osteoporosis
2. Complete destruction of the joint resulting in subluxation, dislocation, or ankylosis

Laboratory Features. There are no laboratory tests that are specifically diagnostic for rheumatoid arthritis. Aspirated joint fluid is often cloudy and of reduced viscosity. The "mucin" test of synovial fluid shows a flocculation instead of a clot. The joint fluid contains an increased number of polymorphonuclear leucocytes, but this finding is not pathognomonic. Most patients exhibit an elevated erythrocyte sedimentation rate, particularly during periods of disease activity. A secondary anemia with a normal white cell count is frequently found.

Serum from patients with rheumatoid arthritis contains a substance of unknown composition called the *rheumatoid factor*, produced by the plasma cells in the rheumatoid synovial membrane. Many authorities believe the rheumatoid factor represents a response to immunization to an unknown antigen in the joint, with the plasma cells throwing off rheumatoid factor as a byproduct of this process. Rheumatoid factor, in the presence of gamma globulin, is capable of agglutinating certain strains of streptococci, sensitized sheep cells, and latex particles. This reaction forms the basis for the latex flocculation test and the sheep cell agglutination test, both of which will ultimately be positive in a high percentage of patients with rheumatoid arthritis.

Management of the Patient. Most rheumatologists today will agree that the two major advances in the treatment of arthritic patients over the past decade have been the growing recognition of the need for a team approach in the rehabilitation of these patients and the increasing participation of the orthopaedic surgeon as a member of that team. It should be emphasized once again that rheumatoid arthritis is a systemic disease of unknown etiology, and no curative drug is known at the present time. Treatment is directed both at the general care of the whole patient and locally to the affected joints. The principal therapeutic objectives are control of the inflammatory process and preservation of joint function. Mechanical damage, muscular weakness, fluctuation of disease activity, and the psychological behavior of the patient all play relative roles in the assessment of functional disability. Ideally, the treating team should consist of a rheumatologist, a physiatrist, and an orthopaedist, bringing together, for the patient's benefit, the principles of medical care, rehabilitation, and orthopaedics. The orthopaedist's responsibility, as a member of the team, is to prevent or correct joint deformities.

Rest and the application of heat to the affected part are of great help in relieving joint and muscle pain and stiffness. A number of drugs may be helpful in controlling the inflammatory process. These include aspirin, gold salts, the antimalarial agents, chloroquine and primaquine, phenylbutazone, and corticosteroids, administered both systemically and by intra-articular injection. Most of these drugs have potentially serious side effects and must be given under close medical supervision.

Maintenance of joint function is of prime importance in the treatment of rheumatoid arthritis. Preservation of range of motion in affected joints must be emphasized during the treatment program. Active exercise must be part of the program in order to maintain muscle tone. Strengthening exercises may prevent disuse atrophy and restore wasted muscles. If muscle tone is very poor, the joint may have to be protected temporarily by bracing. Fixed flexion contractures about the joints may require traction, wedging casts, or open surgical release for their correction. Forced manipulation of joints under anesthesia is not favored because of the brittle nature of the bone.

The progressively destructive nature of rheumatoid arthritis frequently leads to permanent joint crippling or even complete invalidism for the patient. Early in the disease, a patient may voluntarily assume the "position of comfort" for a joint in order to relieve the pain caused by the joint inflammation. Usually this means a flexed position. If not constantly watched for and guarded against by the attending personnel, this "position of comfort" may become a permanent fixed flexion contracture. Every effort should be made to keep the joint in the "position of function," if necessary by resorting to traction, splints, casts, or braces.

Surgery may play an important role in the treatment and rehabilitation of the patient with rheumatoid arthritis who is not responding adequately to nonoperative measures. Surgical procedures on joints should be designed to reduce pain or deformity and thus lessen disability.

Since the major target organ for rheumatoid involvement is the synovial tissue, the operation of synovectomy, the surgical removal of the inflamed synovium, has a well-established place in the rehabilitation of patients with rheumatoid arthritis. The long-term results of joint synovectomy have not as yet been fully evaluated, but about 80 per cent of patients are reported to gain significant relief from pain. It is known, however, that a new synovium forms after operation, and recurrences of progressive disease in synovectomized joints are not rare. Yet despite recurrent synovitis, the relief of pain after synovectomy is maintained in many patients.

Recently there has been considerable interest in the use of synovectomy early in the course of the disease to prevent articular damage. Theoretically, with the joint cartilage intact, an early synovectomy should produce a better functional result than a late synovectomy If synovectomy can indeed prevent destruction of joints, it is clearly of great importance in the selected case and must be thought of as a conservative rather than radical measure. But although the short-term results are encouraging, no long-term results are yet available.

The joints that lend themselves most readily to surgical synovectomy are the knee, elbow, wrist, shoulder, ankle, and metacarpophalangeal joints of the hands. Attempts to perform medical synovectomy using cytotoxic drugs have generally failed.

Once joint destruction has occurred, synovectomy plays no useful part in treatment and more complicated operations are required. The joints most frequently requiring surgical attention because of destructive articular changes are the hip, knee, and joints of the forefoot (Fig. 56).

A stiff, painful, destroyed hip joint is best treated by an operation designed to restore motion to the joint. Cup arthroplasty or total hip replacement is the procedure of choice.

A stiff, painful, unstable, and severely affected knee also requires some type of replacement arthroplasty for its treatment. In recent years the availability of durable and inert plastics and metals has led to the development of tibial, femoral, and total knee prosthetic replacements.

Since rheumatoid arthritis is a polyarthritis with an almost unpredictable course even in the face of adequate medical management,

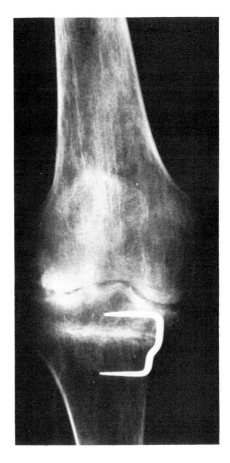

Figure 56. Severe destructive changes in knee joint due to rheumatoid arthritis. Staple is from previous surgery to correct angular deformity.

surgical fusion of a major joint is rarely performed. Present-day surgical emphasis is on attempting to restore relatively painless motion to the joint, provided joint stability can be maintained.

Rheumatoid arthritis frequently affects the forefoot with the development of stiff, painful feet. Typically, the forefoot broadens, the metatarsal heads are depressed into the sole of the foot, and a cock-up deformity of the toes develops (Fig. 57). Surgical removal of all the metatarsal heads relieves the forefoot pain and allows the toes to drop down into a more functional position.

JUVENILE RHEUMATOID ARTHRITIS

Juvenile rheumatoid arthritis is a chronic arthritis that may appear in different forms. It can begin as a fulminating systemic process known as *Still's disease.* Although the systemic aspects of the disease are usually more severe than in the adult form, the joints have the same appearance and there may be typical subcutaneous nodules. The streptococcus agglutination test is usually negative. Involvement of the cervical spine is common in this form of arthritis. The inflamma-

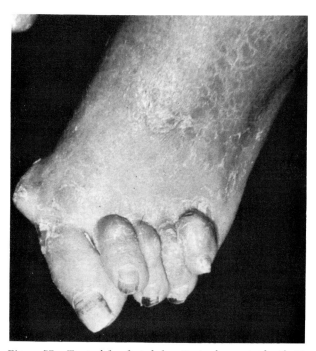

Figure 57. Typical forefoot deformity in rheumatoid arthritis.

tory reaction within the joints frequently destroys the growth cartilage, thus arresting longitudinal growth of bone.

Juvenile rheumatoid arthritis can have a polyarticular onset similar to that observed in adult arthritis, or it can present as a single joint disease that may or may not progress to polyarticular arthritis. The most valid criterion for diagnosing juvenile rheumatoid arthritis is the persistence of joint involvement for several months in a patient who has no other demonstrable disease. The laboratory tests for rheumatoid factor, useful in diagnosing adult rheumatoid arthritis, are not often positive in the juvenile form. It has been estimated that approximately 50 per cent of patients recover from juvenile rheumatoid arthritis without disability after receiving only nonsurgical treatment.

Synovectomy in children has not received universal approval, partly because of concern about interference with bone growth as a result of surgical trauma and partly because of isolated examples of severely restricted range of joint motion following operation. Recent studies, however, show that short-term results in children are no less favorable than those in adults. Indeed, the danger of abnormal bone growth as a result of rheumatoid inflammation is felt to be one of the indications for synovectomy by its proponents. This is felt to be especially true in a child with unilateral involvement of a knee. It is probable that the joint stiffness sometimes encountered after synovectomy derives from the difficulty of obtaining a young child's cooperation in postoperative exercises. If synovectomy is to be considered in a patient with juvenile rheumatoid arthritis, the question of timing is especially important in view of the fact that half or more of the patients recover from the disease with little or no residual disability.

MONARTHRITIS

Occasionally a patient, either child or adult, presents with signs of an inflammatory response confined to one joint, frequently the knee or ankle It is recognized that, although in some patients monarthritis is rheumatoid in nature and progresses to a typical polyarthritis, in many the diagnosis is not at all clear. In these patients arthrotomy and synovial biopsy should be performed. A lengthy period of observation is often necessary before a definitive diagnosis can be made, and in a substantial number of patients, the diagnosis is never made. In a few patients complete resolution of the monarthritis occurs.

ANKYLOSING SPONDYLITIS (MARIE-STRUMPELL DISEASE)

Ankylosing spondylitis is a chronic progressive polyarthritis characterized by involvement of the sacroiliac joints, the spinal apophyseal or synovial joints, and the adjacent soft tissues. Some patients may develop a peripheral joint involvement clinically indistinguishable from that seen in rheumatoid arthritis. Approximately 90 per cent of the patients are males between the ages of 20 and 40. The most frequent presenting complaint is back pain.

The cause of ankylosing spondylitis is unknown. It is not clear at the moment whether it is a variant of rheumatoid arthritis or exists as a totally different entity. Rheumatoid arthritis is seen about 15 times more frequently than ankylosing spondylitis. The essential pathologic joint changes, characterized by proliferative chronic synovitis, are indistinguishable in the two diseases, but the majority of patients with ankylosing spondylitis have a negative rheumatoid factor.

Inflammatory synovitis appears to begin in the sacroiliac joints and goes on to involve the apophyseal joints of the spine and the costo-vertebral joints, giving rise to the characteristic complaint of backache. As the disease progresses, cartilage and bone destruction results in fibrous and bone ankylosis of the spine. This causes the back stiffness or "poker spine" deformity which is the hallmark of this disease. One additional pathologic feature adds to the rigidity of the spine Calcification occurs beneath the anterior and posterior longitudinal spinal ligaments. As this process progresses, it may encase the entire vertebral column in a calcium shell, giving rise to the characteristic "bamboo spine" effect seen on x-ray (Fig. 58). The course of the

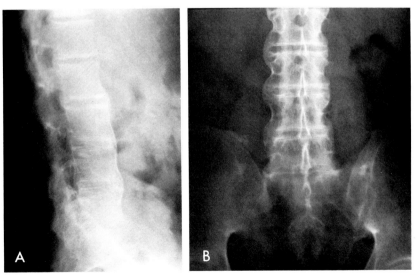

Figure 58. Ankylosing spondylitis of spine. Note bamboo effect on AP view and bony encasement of vertebral bodies on lateral view.

disease, measured by the progression of radiologic characteristics, is not modified by any available form of treatment. Mild or moderately severe disease with progressive ankylosis of the lumbar, thoracic, and cervical spine is the rule.

No treatment known at present will effectively check the progression of the arthritic process in ankylosing spondylitis. Treatment efforts are directed toward pain relief and keeping the spine erect. The overall prognosis for pain relief and maintenance of function is generally good. About three-quarters of the patients manage to work full-time in light occupations, supporting themselves and their families.

The main goal of treatment is to insure that the patient does not develop severe flexion contractures of the neck and back. Most patients tend to flex the spine voluntarily in order to relieve pain during the acute stages of the disease. If this tendency is not fought and corrected, the patient's spine may be permanently ankylosed in a flexed position. The patient must be instructed in the dangers of the flexed position and kept on a program of hyperextension spinal exercises. Brace support is occasionally indicated. Phenylbutazone orally and roentgen therapy are both effective in curtailing pain and making an exercise program more tolerable.

Occasionally a severe fixed flexion deformity of the spine can be corrected by a surgical osteotomy through the dorsolumbar junction. A few patients will develop significant peripheral joint involvement, particularly of the hip joints. Arthroplasty of the hip joint may be indicated for intractable hip pain with increasing joint stiffness and disability.

ARTHRITIS DUE TO RHEUMATIC FEVER

Rheumatic fever, an inflammatory disease occurring as a delayed sequel to infection with Group A streptococci, is an acute febrile illness affecting mostly children and frequently associated with a painful polyarthritis. Patients may have painful swollen joints due to synovial inflammation and effusion, but since the articular cartilage is not affected, no permanent joint damage is produced. Treatment of the underlying problem restores the joint to normal. Whatever permanent damage is associated with this disease is localized to the cardiac valves.

It is generally believed that the incidence of rheumatic fever, like that of streptococcal sore throat and scarlet fever, has been decreasing for several years, the rate of decrease presumably having been accelerated by the wide use of antimicrobial therapy. Rheumatic fever, however, remains a world-wide disease prevalent wherever poor economic conditions, overcrowding, and substandard housing prevail.

Osteoarthritis (Degenerative Joint Disease)

Osteoarthritis, also known as hypertrophic arthritis or degenerative joint disease, is a common progressive disorder, characterized pathologically by deterioration of articular cartilage and overgrowth of juxta-articular bone. It is a disease mainly of middle and old age and affects females more frequently than males. It strikes most weight bearing joints, particularly the cervical and lumbar spine, hip, and knee, giving rise to the clinical complaints of joint pain and stiffness. The distal interphalangeal joints of the fingers frequently show nodular thickenings known as *Heberden's nodes* (Fig. 59). Factors such as trauma, poor posture or body mechanics, obesity, and occupational strain may precipitate or aggravate symptoms.

The term osteoarthritis is actually somewhat of a misnomer, since it implies inflammation. At the present time, inflammation is not thought to play a significant role in the pathologic picture of osteoarthritis. The current concept of osteoarthritis implies degenera-

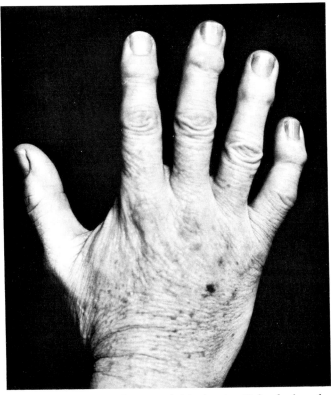

Figure 59. Patient with osteoarthritis showing Heberden's nodes.

tion in diarthrodial or synovium lined joints. Normally, degenerative changes found in joints are associated with the aging process. These changes, if solely related to age, are usually nonprogressive. They are quite distinct from the more severe and progressive process of cartilage degeneration and osteophyte formation characterizing osteoarthritis.

Osteoarthritis is said to be primary when it is inexplicable by at least current knowledge of predisposing factors. Osteoarthritis is defined as secondary when degeneration occurs in a previously abnormal joint, as in osteoarthritis secondary to hip dysplasia or dislocation.

Joints have a limited capacity to respond to trauma, inflammation, and biochemical challenge. The development of wear changes in the articular surfaces of joints is related in part to their ability to resist the compressive forces applied by activity. The capacity of a subchondral bone-articular cartilage system to withstand compressive dynamic forces is the joint's principal defense against these day-to-day pressures.

Most authorities believe that the first evidence of osteoarthritis is found in articular cartilage, where one of the earliest changes is diminution of chondroitin sulphate, an acid mucopolysaccharide, relative to the collagen of the matrix. This results in depletion of the ground substance and "unmasking" of the collagen, which, in itself, is probably stable. Normally the matrix dissipates stresses hydrostatically, but when the collagen is "unmasked," its fibers may rupture because they are subjected to excessive bending and torsional stress. This produces the characteristic lesions of early osteoarthritis: flaking, fibrillation, fissuring, and erosion of articular cartilage with loss of acid mucopolysaccharide staining. Subchondral bony sclerosis in the weight bearing areas, osteoporosis in the non-weight bearing areas, cysts, and marginal osteophyte formation are regarded as secondary phenomena produced by the loss of articular cartilage and the transmission of mechanical forces to the more labile bony tissues.

The way in which the articular cartilage is depleted of mucopolysaccharide is uncertain, but an enzymatic pathway is suspected. One such suggested pathway results from the presence of cathepsin-B, derived from the lysosomes of chondrocytes in human articular cartilage which can split chondroitin sulphate from the protein polysaccharide complex.

Pathologic Features. Both cartilage and bone are altered in osteoarthritis, but changes in other articular or periarticular structures are minimal. Degenerative change in the articular cartilage seems to be the primary pathologic lesion, with proliferation of bone at the joint margins and in areas of denuded bone occurring as a secondary effect.

Available data indicate that primary osteoarthritis of weight bearing joints is a focal disease demonstrating marked variation in histologic, biochemical, and metabolic parameters.

As we have seen, the earliest articular cartilage lesions show decreased concentration of chondroitin sulphate relative to the collagen of the matrix. The loss of polysaccharide from the cartilage matrix results initially in loss of elasticity, contributing to further breakdown of cartilage through physical stress. The normally smooth translucent cartilage becomes dull and opaque in appearance. Later, affected areas become roughened and soft. Fraying and fibrillation of the cartilage appear. Loss of cartilage substance progresses ultimately to denudation of underlying bone (Fig. 60).

Where the articular cartilage is thinned, the subchondral bone shows proliferation of fibroblasts and new bone formation, which appears on the x-ray film as subchondral bone sclerosis. Subcortical trabeculae also thicken. Subchondral cysts filled with fibrous tissue may appear (Fig. 61). Periosteal bone proliferation occurs at the joint margins and at the site of ligamentous and tendinous attachments, forming bony spurs or ridges called *osteophytes* (Fig. 62).

Synovial changes include villous proliferation with an increase in the number of surface cells and encroachment of synovia on the

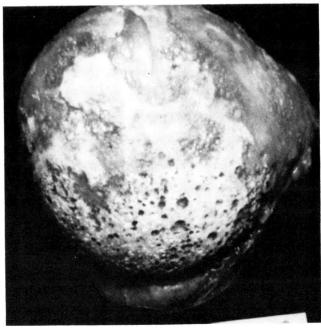

Figure 60. Femoral head specimen, showing cartilage denudation seen with osteoarthritis.

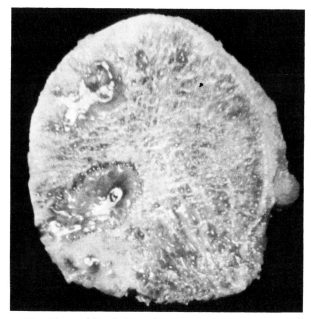

Figure 61. Femoral head slice, showing cysts seen in osteoarthritis.

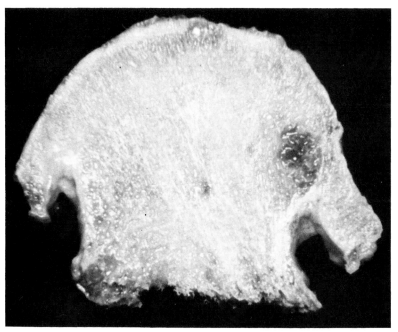

Figure 62. Femoral head slice, showing marginal osteophytes seen in osteoarthritis.

margins of the articular cartilage. The subsynovial areolar tissue is replaced by fibrous tissue, and chronic inflammatory cells may be evident throughout the synovium. With further progression, the capsule becomes markedly thickened by fibrous proliferation and adheres to adjacent structures. The joint space, as seen radiographically, is diminished, owing to loss of surface cartilage as well as to the advance of the subchondral bone into the deeper layers of existing cartilage.

It has long been held that the appearance of degenerative joint changes is commensurate with the aging process. However, there is presently sufficient evidence of focal, histologic, chemical, and metabolic changes, as well as of genetic and environmental influences, to permit the conclusion that degenerative joint changes, although correlated with age, are not necessarily an accompaniment of aging.

Clinical Features. Because articular hyaline cartilage is one of the first tissues to show degenerative changes with advancing age, over 80 per cent of people past 50 years of age will show some x-ray evidence of osteoarthritis, although only a small percentage will have annoying joint symptoms. In contrast to rheumatoid arthritis, osteoarthritis has no constitutional manifestations. The disease attacks principally weight bearing joints.

When present, the symptoms typically consist of pain, stiffness, and swelling in the affected joint. The pain tends to be of an achy nature and is definitely correlated with the stiffness. Characteristically, the pain and stiffness are brought on by immobility of the part and are relieved by mobility of the part, only to return with prolonged activity. This is why these patients feel worse after prolonged sitting and can relieve their stiffness, to some extent, by walking around. Where there is a large volume of synovial tissue, as in the knee joint, there may be a profuse effusion, causing increased pain through the mechanism of joint distension. With acute onset of the disease, the part may appear swollen, warm, and extremely tender.

The joints most frequently affected are the lumbar spine, knees, hips, and elbows. Around the shoulder area the glenohumeral joint is usually spared, but the acromioclavicular joint is frequently affected. In the hand the pattern of joint involvement is exactly opposite that of rheumatoid arthritis. In osteoarthritis the distal interphalangeal joints (Heberden's nodes) and the first carpometacarpal joints are primarily affected.

X-ray Features. The x-ray changes seen in most cases of osteoarthritis are quite striking and prove an invaluable aid to diagnosis. It is well to bear in mind, however, that in general there is no particular correlation between the severity of the x-ray findings and the degree of clinical distress. Frequently joints show striking changes on x-ray but few or no symptoms clinically.

The actual changes seen on x-ray result mainly from bony proliferation. Thus one sees subchondral sclerosis, which gives the bone its dense appearance on the x-ray film. This is usually associated with spur formation around the joint margins. Occasionally subchondral bone cysts are seen. The joint space becomes narrow and, to a certain extent, deformed. Unlike in rheumatoid arthritis, however, the general outlines of the joint are preserved and the bone texture remains normal (Fig. 63).

Management of the Patient. Even in the face of distressing symptoms and a frightening x-ray appearance, the joints in this condition generally retain a surprising degree of motion and do not go on to bony ankylosis as might occur in rheumatoid arthritis. This is basically because osteoarthritis is not associated with the formation of a pannus to eat away articular cartilage and the underlying subchondral bone. Flexion contractures may develop, however, particularly in the hip and knee.

Effective treatment of joints afflicted with osteoarthritis revolves around physical modalities (such as moist heat, exercise, splints, and

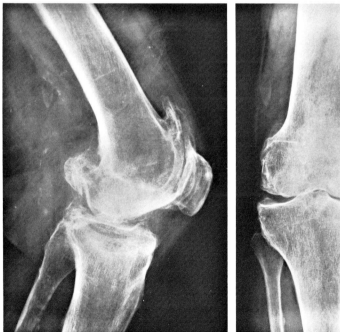
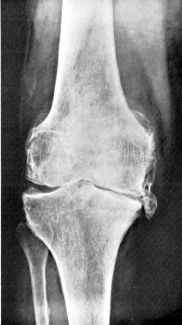

Figure 63. Severe osteoarthritis of knee joint.

occasionally brace support), medical treatment (particularly with the salicylates and anti-inflammatory drugs), and surgical procedures in carefully selected instances. The indicated surgical procedures are discussed more fully in the regional chapters.

The changes in the hands, although typical, usually do not progress to a functional deformity and rarely require specific treatment. A notable exception is involvement of the first carpometacarpal joint. Pain and stiffness in this joint can lessen the efficiency of the entire hand and may require intermittent immobilization, intra-articular hydrocortisone, or joint fusion for relief.

Involvement of the lumbar spine is heralded by pain and stiffness in this area (see p. 323). Since most of these patients are overweight, a weight reduction program is a necessary accompaniment of treatment. Exercise within toleration is helpful in maintaining muscle tone and joint mobility. Brace and corset support should be avoided if at all possible because of their tendency to increase the sensation of spinal stiffness. It will be remembered that these joints tend to stiffen with immobility and generally do better if kept flexible. Various physical therapeutic measures, such as diathermy and massage, are also helpful in allaying symptoms.

There are drugs available to aid in combatting the symptom of pain and the sensation of stiffness. Systemic treatment with salicylates is usually of benefit because of its analgesic effect. Butazolidin (phenylbutazone) has proven a very effective agent for controlling pain and stiffness in this condition, but patients receiving it must be closely watched and the medical contraindications observed (see p. 324). The systemic use of the corticosteroids has failed to help this condition consistently and their routine use is to be avoided.

As a rule surgery plays little part in the treatment of osteoarthritis of the lumbar spine. Spinal fusion is usually not feasible, since the process invariably involves several vertebrae and their associated joints. The one notable exception is the presence of nerve root compression secondary to an arthritic spur encroaching upon the intervertebral foramen. If the compression occurs in the lower lumbar segment, the patient will develop a distressing sciatica which may have to be relieved surgically by a nerve root decompression operation.

Involvement of the knee is signified by the complaint of pain and stiffness in the joint and frequently also in the thigh, calf, and popliteal area. A yellowish, clear, viscid effusion is often noted in the knee joint. Some decrease in the range of motion of the joint may be noted, but it is rarely as significant as that seen in the knee afflicted with rheumatoid arthritis. Subpatellar crepitus is frequently found. Fixed flexion contractures may be observed in joints in which the disease is

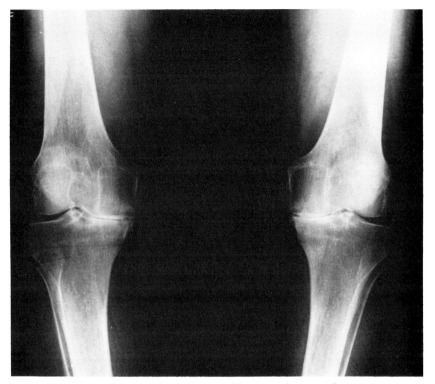

Figure 64. Angular deformity of knees with osteoarthritis.

long-standing. Angular deformities of the joint, either genu varum or genu valgum, may be seen (Fig. 64).

Medical treatment for a knee joint afflicted with osteoarthritis could include frequent periods of rest for the part, the use of local moist heat, or the use of intra-articular corticosteroids, injected after aspiration of the effusion. Local treatment to the joint could be combined, if necessary, with systemic salicylates or phenylbutazone. Fixed flexion contractures may have to be stretched in traction or plaster casts.

Surgery may be required for the knee joint that fails to respond to adequate medical management. Angular deformity at the knee can be corrected by an osteotomy performed through the proximal tibia. Various metal implants have been devised, such as tibial plateau prostheses, to replace part of the diseased joints. Various total knee replacement procedures are now in the development phase and show early promise. If all else fails, arthrodesis or surgical fusion of the joint could be carried out.

Involvement of the hip joint is probably the most serious complication from a strict orthopaedic viewpoint because of the crippling effect on the patient of a stiff, painful hip (p. 352). An osteoarthritic hip
may assume, in time, a flexed-adducted–externally rotated attitude,
which adds to the deformity and accentuates the painful limp. If the
hip joint is not damaged too severely, symptoms of pain and stiffness
can often be controlled by intra-articular corticosteroids and systemic
salicylates or phenylbutazone. If shortening is present, it should be
compensated for by a heel lift. The use of a cane in the opposite hand
as a walking aid is frequently of enormous help in relieving pain.

Surgical treatment is necessary more frequently in the hip joint
than in any other joint affected by osteoarthritis. Soft tissue procedures, such as flexion releases, adductor muscle release, section of the
iliopsoas tendon, and obturator neurectomy may have a temporizing
effect in the early stage of the disease. Many patients will ultimately
require a definitive surgical attack on the joint. The surgical procedures that have stood the test of time include displacement osteotomy,
arthroplasties of various types, total hip replacement, and arthrodesis.

Traumatic Arthritis

Any joint that has been previously damaged may later develop an
arthritis, confined to the involved joint, that is pathologically and
roentgenologically identical with osteoarthritis but is called traumatic
arthritis (Fig. 65). This term is somewhat unfortunate in that it con-
veys the suggestion that arthritis is caused by trauma. In reality it
means that osteoarthritis or degenerative arthritis may secondarily
implicate a joint whose hyaline articular cartilage has been damaged
or whose joint surface has been rendered incongruous by previous
trauma.

Articular cartilage, as previously noted, has almost no capacity to
regenerate once it is injured. The wear and tear of normal activity
leads to mechanical abrasion of the articular cartilage and damage to
the joint surface which is progressive as time passes. Damage is accelerated if the joint margins have been permanently distorted by the
trauma. The type of arthritis that may complicate such a traumatized
joint is pathologically and roentgenologically indistinguishable from
osteoarthritis, except for the fact that it will involve only the injured
joint.

The trauma may consist of small repetitive occupational stresses,
as frequently seen affecting the wrist, elbow, or acromioclavicular
joints. More often the arthritis follows major trauma to a joint, such as a

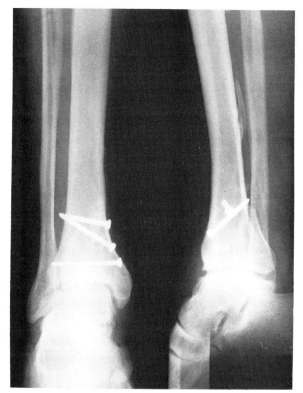

Figure 65. Traumatic arthritis in ankle joint nine years after reduction and internal fixation of ankle joint fracture.

displaced fracture or dislocation. It is particularly prone to develop following major trauma to weight bearing joints such as the ankle, knee, and hip, especially if a perfect anatomic reduction of the traumatic distortion has not been achieved. Another type of trauma is the wear and tear of normal activity on a joint that has been rendered incongruous by some congenital or developmental deformity. Thus osteoarthritis may develop later in life in a hip joint rendered imperfect from a prior congenital dislocation, Legg-Calvé-Perthes disease, or a slipped capital femoral epiphysis (Fig. 66).

Once an arthritic complication develops in the joint, the classic signs of pain, stiffness, and possibly swelling supervene. The x-ray findings are typical of osteoarthritis superimposed on some previously sustained traumatic deformity. The diagnosis is made from the history and x-ray evidence of involvement only in the traumatized joint.

Treatment is the same as that discussed under Osteoarthritis.

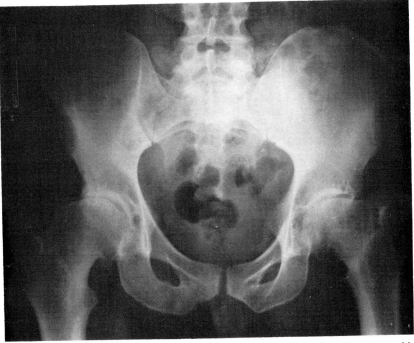

Figure 66. X-ray appearance of hip joints in a 32 year old male with untreated bilateral slipped capital femoral epiphysis.

GOUTY ARTHRITIS

Gout is a disorder of uric acid metabolism with hereditary predisposition and significant joint implications. The acute form of gouty arthritis is initiated by the deposition of sodium urate crystals within the joint space. The chronic form is characterized by the deposition of urate crystals in the subcutaneous tissue, cartilage, bone, and kidney. Uric acid precipitation within the renal collecting system leads to stones in many gouty patients.

Although there are other causes besides gout for hyperuricemia, all patients with gout have hyperuricemia resulting from overproduction of uric acid, defective excretion of uric acid, or both. Renal retention of uric acid is caused by the failure of renal tubules to secrete uric acid after it has been filtered at the glomerulus and reabsorbed. Regardless of whether hyperuricemia results from overproduction of uric acid or from renal retention, when the saturation point of a given serum is exceeded, crystallization may occur and the stage is set for gouty arthritis.

Ninety-five per cent of those affected are male and may be of any race, nationality, or social level. Acute gouty arthritis is typically a severe arthritis marked by an abrupt onset, involving one or more joints, and exhibiting natural periods of remission. The joints most often involved are peripheral. Gout should always be suspected in the presence of swollen, painful, and hot fingers, toes, wrists, or ankles. It is occasionally seen about the knees and elbows, infrequently in the shoulders, and rarely in the spine. In the classic description of gout, involvement of the great toe is cited. However, other areas of the foot, notably the fifth toe, tarsal, and ankle regions, can be involved (Fig. 67). In the hand the interphalangeal joints are most often affected, and the joint swelling is fusiform with exquisite tenderness.

If the diagnosis is not made early, urate salts may actually precipitate in a collection called a *tophus*, located in and about the joints and in other bony regions. Tophi occur commonly about the interphalangeal joints of the fingers, the wrists, and the toes, and in bursae such as the radiohumeral, olecranon, subdeltoid, prepatellar, trochanteric, and ischial. Many times this amorphous material in the soft tissues is mistakenly reported as "calcification" on the x-ray. It is thought that about 20 per cent of gallstones and renal calculi have their origin in gout. Deposits of urates may form bone tophi. These are seen as cystic areas in the bone near the joint margin.

An acute gouty arthritis can be precipitated in a patient with quiescent gout by surgery, trauma, or dietary indiscretion. Acute gouty arthritis may progress to the chronic type.

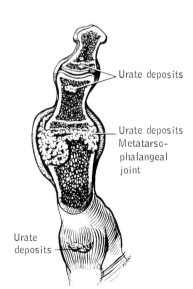

Figure 67. Urate deposits about the joints of the toe in gout.

X-ray Features.   If tophi are absent, the x-ray findings may be negative. If present, tophi may be seen in the soft tissues about the joints or in the bursae. Cystic areas may be noted in the bone at the articular margin.

Laboratory Features.   The most significant laboratory study to support the diagnosis of gouty arthritis is examination of the synovial fluid. Demonstration of sodium urate crystals in the fluid by the polarizing microscope confirms the diagnosis of gout. An elevated serum uric acid level and a diminished urate clearance in the absence of renal disease are suggestive but not confirmatory findings.

Management of the Patient.   The basic treatment for gout is medical and is well documented in standard texts. Two therapeutic approaches are used, the choice depending upon whether acute or chronic gouty arthritis is being treated. Acute attacks can be controlled by the use of anti-inflammatory drugs (colchicine, indomethacin, phenylbutazone, or corticosteroids). Chronic gout is best controlled by uricosuric agents that act to lower the serum uric acid level (ColBenemid, Benemid, allopurinol).

Specific orthopaedic care is reserved for those occasional patients requiring surgical excision of tophi.

NEUROPATHIC JOINT DISEASE (CHARCOT JOINT)

The term neuropathic joint disease, or Charcot joint, indicates a form of chronic progressive degenerative arthropathy affecting one or more peripheral or spinal joints. This represents a complication of various neurologic disorders, the common feature of which is a disturbance in sensation in the affected joints.

The underlying neurologic disorders that may give rise to Charcot joint include tabes dorsalis of syphilic origin, diabetic neuropathy, syringomyelia, myelomeningocele, spinal cord compression, peripheral nerve section, leprosy, and congenital absence of pain sensation. The main feature that these conditions have in common is absence or depression of pain sensation in the presence of continued physical activity. The patient loses the protective reactions in the joint to the minor traumata of everyday living, usually made worse by the underlying neurologic disorder. Being thus unprotected, the joint is subject to repeated sprains, hemarthroses, and fractures, leading to progressive joint destruction, debris formation, relaxation and stretching of supporting ligaments, and chronic instability of the joint (Fig. 68). If mechanical destruction outstrips the process of repair, the consequence is marked swelling, hemorrhage, debris formation, and local heat. Pain causes normal individuals to protect the area and prevent further trauma, with the result that healing takes place. In patients

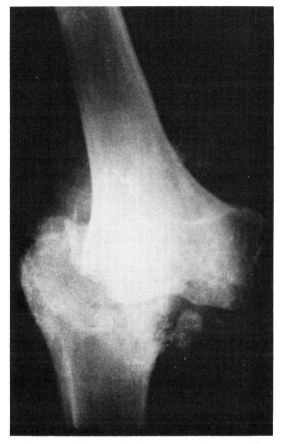

Figure 68. AP x-ray of knee, showing destruction secondary to neuropathic arthropathy (Charcot joint).

with neuroarthropathy, however, the vicious cycle may go on until the joint is totally destroyed.

Clinical Features. The outstanding orthopaedic feature of neuroarthropathy is the presence of an obviously abnormal joint that is clinically unstable. When the condition is related to tabes, the joints most often affected are the knee, hip, ankle, foot, shoulder, elbow, and spine. Involvement is frequently multiple. The typical patient is a male past 40 years of age. The affected joints are usually swollen and are typically unstable due to severe relaxation of the supporting structures. These joints are not always absolutely painless. Patients frequently complain of joint discomfort, particularly if swelling is present. However, the discomfort is disproportionately mild compared to the dramatic clinical and x-ray appearance of the joint. A careful neurologic examination will usually unearth evidence of the underlying neurologic disorder.

X-ray Features.   The changes seen in a Charcot joint are considered similar to those seen in exaggerated osteoarthritis: marked erosion of joint cartilage, destruction and fragmentation of subchondral bone, and large spurs at the joint margins. The spur formation may be flamboyant and bizarre in appearance. Compression fractures and free bodies in the joint cavity are frequent. The soft tissues are thickened and may contain scattered calcifications. Joint effusion is common.

Management of the Patient.   Careful clinical studies clearly indicate that inadequately protected fractures, sprains, and effusions of neuropathic joints are often the precursors of joint destruction. It has also been shown that these lesions, if adequately treated, generally heal without secondary joint damage. The key to proper treatment of neuroarthropathy, therefore, is the prevention of these injuries by early recognition of the problem and adequate protection of the joint, even to the extent of bracing.

Unfortunately, many patients are not seen until the damage has already been done. The outstanding orthopaedic feature in these patients is an obviously abnormal joint that is clinically unstable. Often sufficient stability can be obtained by the use of protective and supportive braces.

A Charcot joint exhibits a poor tolerance to surgery because of the difficulty of obtaining efficient postoperative immobilization. Operations on neuropathic bones are notorious for poor healing and nonunion. If a joint seems beyond salvage, fusion may be indicated, but it must be recognized that fusion is difficult to achieve and that nonunion is common. The main problem in a Charcot joint is instability, and for this reason arthroplasty operations, which tend by their very nature to cause instability, are never indicated. In selected instances amputation may be the treatment of choice.

SPECIAL FORMS OF ARTHRITIS

Hemophilic Arthritis.   In a patient afflicted with hemophilia, repeated joint hemorrhages lead to degenerative changes in the bone and cartilage associated with marked fibrous tissue contractures. The degree of degeneration and disability is directly proportional to the severity and frequency of the joint hemorrhages. It is not at all unusual to see severe arthritic changes at an early age in a hemophilic patient with severe bleeding tendencies.

Repeated joint bleeding leads to hemosiderosis of the synovial membrane and subsequently to shrinking and fibrosis of the joint capsule. The articular cartilage undergoes degenerative changes, with thinning and ultimately total or partial disappearance. The bone becomes atrophic and its structure becomes coarse. The articular surfaces are deformed by abnormal growth at the growth plate. Subchondral bone cysts, probably formed by the resolution of old hemorrhage, may be present.

The joints most frequently affected are the knees and elbows. The changes visible on x-ray resemble those of a type of secondary osteoarthritis, often with a superimposed osteoporosis.

Psoriatic Arthritis. Psoriasis occurs in about 3 per cent of patients with typical rheumatoid arthritis. Conversely, in certain instances of psoriasis, arthritic changes appear in the terminal interphalangeal joints of those fingers showing psoriatic nail lesions.

Psychogenic Rheumatism. This term refers to a common form of nonarticular rheumatism thought to represent the rheumatic manifestations of a psychoneurosis. Psychoneurotic patients in emotional conflict caused by psychic trauma, fear, anxiety, apprehension, or sorrow may experience arthralgia, muscle and tendon aches, stiffness, interference with joint motion, and other rheumatic symptoms that resemble some form of arthritis. The absence of true joint changes on clinical and x-ray examination and the concurrent evidence of psychoneurosis usually suffice to differentiate this condition from organic arthritis. Vague, nonspecific diagnoses, such as myositis, fibrositis, and neuritis, are frequently assigned to these patients.

BURSITIS

A bursa is a closed sac differentiated out of areolar tissue. Its delicate walls are normally separated from each other by a film of slippery fluid. Bursae exist as lubricating devices to diminish the friction of movement and are found beneath the skin, beneath tendons, and overlying joints. The international anatomical nomenclature (NA) lists 52 bursae in the body.

Inflammation of a bursa is a common clinical occurrence and its cause may be trauma, unusual use of the part, infection, gout, or rheumatoid arthritis. As a response to the stimulus of inflammation, the lining membrane may produce excess fluid, causing distension of the sac. In the case of trauma the fluid may be bloody, and in the case of gout urate crystals will be present. The symptoms produced by the inflammation are, in large measure, conditioned by the anatomic location of the bursa. Some of the more common are described.

Prepatellar Bursitis

The prepatellar bursa lies superficial to the distal pole of the patella and the upper half of the patellar tendon. It may become acutely inflamed and swollen from local trauma or may be chronically involved by repeated or prolonged kneeling. For that reason this condition has also been known as "housemaid's knee" or "nun's knee." Clinically a localized, well-circumscribed, fluctuant mass is seen lying over the anterior aspect of the knee. The knee joint proper is not involved.

Treatment consists of aspiration of the fluid, local instillation of corticosteroids, and a pressure dressing. If the cause of the inflammatory response is infection, incision and drainage with proper antibiotic coverage are indicated. Occasionally chronic recurrent enlargement justifies surgical excision of the bursal sac.

OLECRANON BURSITIS

Trauma to the point of the elbow frequently results in marked swelling of the olecranon bursa, giving rise to a large knob in this area (Fig. 69). Following acute trauma, the fluid in the bursal sac is frequently bloody and the bursal walls may become permanently thickened. Tender swelling of the olecranon bursa may also be seen with gout and rheumatoid arthritis. Repetitive minor trauma to the olecranon bursa, such as long periods of leaning on the elbows, may lead to chronic, relatively nontender enlargement of the bursa. Chronic enlargement has been known as "bartender's elbow."

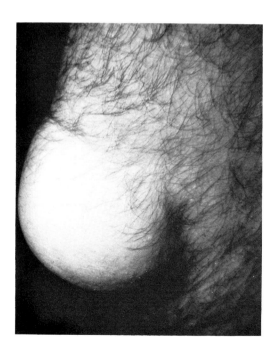

Figure 69. Distended olecranon bursa.

The treatment for olecranon bursitis is the same as that outlined for prepatellar bursitis.

TROCHANTERIC BURSITIS

Inflammation of the bursa overlying the greater trochanter of the femur is a frequent occurrence. It may appear as a primary entity, follow trauma, unusual use of the legs, or gout, or be associated with degenerative arthritis of the lumbar spine.

Typically, involvement of this bursa gives pain along the posterolateral hip and thigh area, particularly on direct palpation or when the hip abductors are tightened. The patient may find it painful to cross the involved leg over the opposite one or to lie on the involved area. Frequently the pain will run along the course of the tensor fascia lata to the knee, and will be described as a burning sensation.

Diagnosis is made by reproducing the pain by direct manual pressure over the greater trochanter in the absence of any physical findings referable to the hip joint proper. Trochanteric bursitis does not cause any restriction of passive motion of the hip joint. X-ray examination is usually negative, but occasionally small calcium deposits are seen adjacent to the trochanter.

Superficially, the pain caused by trochanteric bursitis could be mistaken for sciatica or for pain originating in the hip joint proper. Careful examination will clearly disclose the absence of any objective physical signs of sciatica and the presence of unrestricted hip motion.

Local injections of hydrocortisone into the bursa usually suffice to alleviate the condition. Moist heat to the painful area is beneficial. Rarely, the bursa may have to be excised.

BURSITIS OF THE HEEL

Several bursae are found in the region of the heel which may become painful when inflamed. One bursa lies subcutaneously between the skin and the Achilles tendon, and another lies between the Achilles tendon and the os calcis. Either can become inflamed, enlarged, and painful, particularly by irritation from a shoe or by excessive walking or running.

The patient usually obtains some relief by removing the counter of the shoe and using a heel pad to raise the painful area away from the back of the shoe. The inflamed bursa can be treated definitively by local injection of hydrocortisone or by surgical excision.

A third bursa is located on the plantar aspect of the heel, at the origin of the plantar aponeurosis and the short flexor muscles as they arise from the os calcis. Symptoms in this area are caused by direct pressure on the heel and the inflamed plantar bursa. This condition, seen most frequently in male adults, has been called "postman's heel" or "policeman's heel" and is the most common cause of adult heel pain. Occasionally on the x-ray a small bone spur may be seen arising from the plantar surface of the os calcis, but in these cases symptoms are more likely to be caused by an inflamed bursa than by the spur.

Treatment consists of local injections of corticosteroids into the inflamed bursa. A sponge rubber heel cushion, with a hole cut in the center, glued in the heel of the shoe frequently helps to relieve local pressure on the painful area.

Subdeltoid or Subacromial Bursitis

The physician will frequently hear a patient complain of "bursitis" of the shoulder. In this particular area, bursitis is too often used as an all-inclusive term to explain away all shoulder pain.

Although it is true that a primary subdeltoid or subacromial bursitis may occur, other causes of shoulder pain, often called bursitis by mistake, are far more frequent. These other causes of shoulder pain are covered in detail in the chapter on disorders of the shoulder joint.

References

Anderson, C. E.: The structure and function of cartilage. Am. Academy of Orthopaedic Surgeons Instructional Course Lectures. J. Bone and Joint Surg., 44-A:777, 1962.

Barnett, C. H., and Cobbold, A. F.: Lubrication within living joints. J. Bone and Joint Surg., 44-B:662, 1962.

Barnett, C. H., Davies, D. V., and MacConaill, M. A.: Synovial Joints. Springfield, Illinois: Charles C Thomas, 1961.

Bottlet, A. J.: An essay on the biology of osteoarthritis. Arthritis Rheum., 12:512, 1969.

Branernack, P. J., Eckholm, R., Goldie, R., and Lindstrom, J.: Synovectomy and rheumatoid arthritis, experimental biologic and clinical aspect. Acta. Rheumatol. Scand., 13:161, 1967.

Brower, T. D., and Hsu, Wan-Yi: Normal articular cartilage. Clin. Orth. and Rel. Res., 64:9, 1969.

Cathcart, E. S., and Cohen, A. S.: Synovial fluid and synovial membrane abnormalities in arthritis of the knee joint. Am. Academy of Orthopaedic Surgeons Instructional Course Lectures, Vol. XX:231. St. Louis: C. V. Mosby Co., 1971.

Chrisman, O. D.: Biochemical aspects of degenerative joint disease. Clin. Orth. and Rel. Res., 64:77, 1969.

Curtiss, P. H., Jr.: Changes produced in the synovial membrane and synovial fluid by disease. J. Bone and Joint Surg., 46-A:873, 1964.

Eising, L.: Dietary intake in patients with arthritis and other chronic diseases. J. Bone and Joint Surg., 45-A:69, 1963.

Gardner, E.: Nerve supply of joints. Am. Academy of Orthopaedic Surgeons Instructional Course Lectures. Vol. IX:155. Ann Arbor: J. W. Edwards, 1952.

Gardner, E.: Physiological mechanisms in movable joints. Am. Academy of Orthopaedic Surgeons Instructional Course Lectures, Vol. X:251. Ann Arbor: J. W. Edwards, 1953.

Gardner, E.: Synovial tissue and synovial fluid. Am. Academy of Orthopaedic Surgeons Instructional Course Lectures, Vol. IX:162. Ann Arbor: J. W. Edwards, 1952.

Gutman, A. B.: View on the pathogenesis and management of primary gout, 1971. J. Bone and Joint Surg., 55-A:357, 1972.

Hammerman, D., Rosenberg, L. C., and Schubert, M.: Diarthrodial joints revisited. Review article, J. Bone and Joint Surg., 52-A:725, 1970.

Hollander, J. L. (Ed.): Arthritis and Allied Conditions, 7th Edition. Philadelphia: Lee and Febiger, 1966.

Linscheid, R. L.: Surgery for rheumatoid arthritis — Timing and techniques: The upper extremity. J. Bone and Joint Surg., 50-A:587, 1968.

Luck, J. V.: Traumatic arthrofibrosis — A comparison of the etiology, pathogenesis and treatment of the traumatic arthritides. Am. Academy of Orthopaedic Surgeons Instructional Course Lectures, Vol. X:57. Ann Arbor: J. W. Edwards, 1953.

Mankin, H. J.: The articular cartilages — A review. Am. Academy of Orthopaedic Surgeons Instructional Course Lectures, Vol. XIX. St. Louis: C. V. Mosby, 1970.

McFarland, G., and Sherman, N. D.: The synovial reactions of rheumatoid arthritis. Clin. Orthop., 36:10, 1964.

Peterson, L. F. A.: Surgery for rheumatoid arthritis — Timing and techniques: The lower extremity. J. Bone and Joint Surg., 50-A:587, 1968.

Rodnan, G. P., Lewis, J. H., Warren, J. E., and Brower, T. D.: Hemophilic arthritis. Bull. Rheum. Dis., 8:137, 1957.

Sharp, J.: Differential diagnosis of ankylosing spondylitis. Bull. Rheum. Dis., 7:125, 1957.

Sokoloff, L.: The Biology of Degenerative Joint Disease. Chicago: University of Chicago Press, 1969.

Smyth, C. J.: Gout. Clin. Orth. and Rel. Res., 57:69, 1968.

Talbott, J. H. (Ed.): Surgical treatment in rheumatology. Seminars in Arthritis and Rheumatism, Vol. I, No. 1. New York: Henry M. Stratton, Inc., May, 1971.

White, R. K.: The clinical application of the rheology of synovial fluid. Clin. Orthop., 29:213, 1963.

Chapter Six

Skeletal Infection

INTRODUCTION

Bone tissue infections and joint infections present special problems, depending on the type of organism involved and the anatomy of the area invaded.

The most common infection is that caused by a pyogenic organism. If the infection is localized to the structure of the bone, the condition is called *osteomyelitis*. If the infection is confined to a joint, it is termed *pyogenic arthritis*. Even when the invading organism is the same, the two conditions produced are different and are dissimilar in clinical course, prognosis, and management. Under some circumstances the use of antimicrobial agents to combat bone or joint infection is curative, while under other circumstances such use is supportive to judicious surgery, undertaken chiefly to prevent septicemia and fulminating local sepsis.

The tubercle bacillus may attack bones and joints, which are the locus of about 3 per cent of all tuberculous infections. Bone can also be infected with *Treponema pallidum*, resulting in congenital and acquired bone syphilis. Although less common, fungus infections, particularly actinomycosis, can occur in bone.

PYOGENIC INFECTIONS

The most common bacterial invaders of the musculoskeletal system are *Staphylococcus aureus, Proteus, Pseudomonas, Aerobacter,* colon bacillus, *Salmonella,* and *Streptococcus,* with occasional infections caused by pneumococcus, meningococcus, gonococcus, and influenza bacillus. Infection of a part of the skeletal system with a

126

pyogenic organism is more common in infants and young children than in adults. The acute form of the disease is usually blood-borne and has a predilection for the rapidly growing child.

Infection of bones and joints was expected to fade into comparative insignificance with the coming of the antibiotic era, but this surmise proved false. Although the mortality associated with severe bone infections has been dramatically reduced by antibiotic treatment, reported studies have shown a steadily increasing rise in the incidence of bone and joint infections over the past two decades. Two factors have been identified as contributing to the increased incidence. One is the masking of the early signs of infection by the indiscriminate use of antibiotic therapy and the other is the emergence of antibiotic resistant strains of organisms. Since *Staphylococcus aureus* can be implicated as the causative agent in 65 to 70 per cent of bone and joint infections, the incidence of strains of penicillin resistant staphylococci is of serious concern. It has been found in clinical situations that when staphylococci are resistant to penicillin, they are invariably penicillinase producers. More recently, concern has also been expressed about the relative increase in gram-negative infections.

ACUTE OSTEOMYELITIS

When pyogenic organisms directly invade the substance of a bone, the condition is called osteomyelitis. This inoculation may be the result of erosion from a neighboring infection, or the organisms may be introduced directly into the bone by contamination accompanying open fractures or war wounds. By far the most frequent form of osteomyelitis, however, is the acute hematogenous form, in which the infection is spread by the blood stream to the bone from a distant focus such as infected tonsils, boils, abscessed teeth, or upper respiratory infections. The disease, therefore, is a systemic infection or bacteremia, of which the bone involvement is only a local manifestation.

Acute osteomyelitis is usually a blood-borne disease and is most frequently seen in the rapidly growing child. Boys are affected more frequently than girls. The bones most often involved are the tibia, femur, humerus, and radius. A history of trauma is frequently obtained, and there is reason to suspect that local injury influences the site of infection by creating an area of lowered resistance to an already present systemic infection.

Staphylococcus aureus is the infecting microorganism in 70 to 80 per cent of patients. *Salmonella osteomyelitis* is frequent in patients with sickle-cell disease. Less frequently found organisms are *Streptococcus* and pneumococcus. The organism enters the bone through the nutrient or metaphyseal vessels and localizes in the venous sinusoids of the metaphysis. Once established in a bone, infection may spread throughout the bone in an adult. In children infection does not gain direct transport across the growth plate because the epiphyseal cartilage blocks anastomosis between blood vessels in the shaft and those in the epiphysis. If any of the metaphyseal area lies within the capsule, such as in the hip joint, for example, infection can burrow around the growth plate to involve the joint (Fig. 70).

Pathology.   Initially there is acute exudative inflammation with increased vascularity, edema, and polymorphonuclear leukocytes. Within two to three days, thrombosis and obliteration of the vessels through increased intramedullary pressure produce ischemia and bone necrosis. An intramedullary abscess forms, and edema fluid and purulent exudate are forced through the haversian and Volkmann's canals, stripping periosteum from the bone. This isolates the cortical bone from its blood supply and produces more dead bone. The pus, following the line of least resistance, may re-enter the medullary canal through the cortex at another point, may form subperiosteal abscesses, may perforate the periosteum and enter soft tissues, or may extend

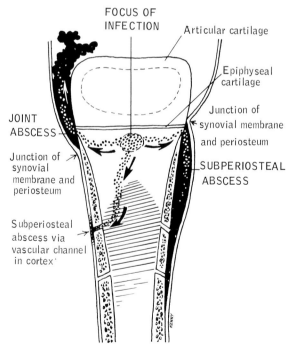

FOCUS OF INFECTION

Articular cartilage

Epiphyseal cartilage

Junction of synovial membrane and periosteum

SUBPERIOSTEAL ABSCESS

JOINT ABSCESS

Junction of synovial membrane and periosteum

Subperiosteal abscess via vascular channel in cortex

Figure 70.   The possible routes infection may take as it spreads from a focus in the metaphysis. (Redrawn from Shands: Handbook of Orthopaedic Surgery [After Hart]. St. Louis: C. V. Mosby Co., 1971.)

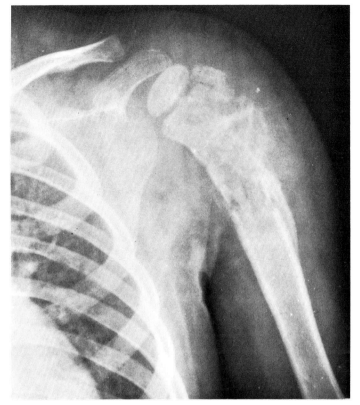

Figure 71. Acute osteomyelitis of proximal humeral shaft in young child.

into the neighboring joint. The admixture of dead and viable bone tissue explains the irregular decalcification seen on the x-ray film during the course of acute osteomyelitis (Fig. 71).

Elevation of the periosteum and vascular thrombosis both contribute to bone necrosis and portions of the bone die. The body tries to extrude the dead bone by forming granulation tissue beneath it, lifting it out of its bed in the bone. This separated dead bone is called a *sequestrum.* Small sequestra may revascularize after the infection is controlled, but large ones will persist. The presence of retained sequestra is the chief reason for continued drainage in osteomyelitis.

The elevated periosteum retains its osteogenic capability and starts to lay down new live bone as one of the first steps in the reparative process. This new live enveloping bone is called the *involucrum,* and it is laid down over and around the granulation tissue separating the sequestrum. The involucrum may be pitted with sinuses called *cloacae,* which permit the escape of pus. If an early diagnosis is made and if adequate and efficient treatment is carried out, infected bone tissue possesses the capability of reverting to a normal structure and appearance.

Clinical Picture.   The patient with acute hematogenous osteomyelitis may develop general and local symptoms. The general symptoms are those of an acute toxic illness with fever. There may be vomiting with subsequent dehydration. Locally the involved area may be swollen, warm, and exquisitely tender to touch. The most valid clinical sign is the presence of localized bone tenderness in a patient exhibiting a febrile course. Since there is pus under pressure in the bone, the patient may complain of severe, constant pulsating pain in the part, usually aggravated by motion. The adjacent joints may be held in a flexed position in an effort to splint the painful part.

For the first week or two, the x-ray examination may be negative except for soft tissue swelling. Roentgenographic evidence of bone destruction does not appear before the tenth to fourteenth day. As bone tissue dies, the x-ray film will reflect spotty irregular areas of decalcification, usually in the metaphyseal area of the bone. This type of change may gradually extend to involve the entire shaft. Periosteal new bone formation becomes visible. As sequestra form, they may appear as pieces of dead separated bone. Still later, involucrum formation becomes evident.

In the acute stage of the disease, study of the patient's blood may reveal an elevated leukocyte count and sedimentation rate. The blood culture is usually positive.

In a child, the presence of infection near a growth plate may trigger an abnormal growth response (Fig. 72). The result might be shortening, lengthening, or a directional change in growth of the bone.

Differential diagnosis should include cellulitis, Ewing's tumor, acute rheumatic fever, pyogenic arthritis, and blood dyscrasias, such as leukemia. The diagnosis of acute osteomyelitis ideally requires the identification of the organism from the pus or from blood culture.

Treatment.   A successful clinical outcome is completely dependent upon establishing an early clinical and bacteriologic diagnosis. Adequate treatment must be started early. There is usually a two to three day delay from the onset of symptoms to hospitalization. Blood cultures may require an additional two to three days. As soon as the diagnosis is suspected clinically, at least two blood specimens from different sites should be drawn for culture and antibiotic sensitivity studies. On examination of the patient, a source of infection may be found in the skin, middle ear, throat, lungs, or urinary tract. Appropriate cultures from these areas may be helpful.

Treatment should be begun as soon as the culture specimens are taken so that valuable time is not lost while waiting for the bacteriol-

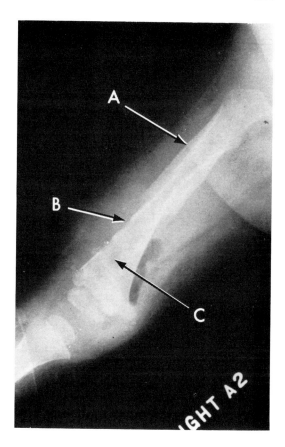

Figure 72. Acute osteo-myelitis of the femur in young child. A, reactive periosteal bone. B, multiple cortical defects. C, area of bone destruction. (Courtesy Dr. Roshen Irani, Thomas Jefferson University Hospital, Philadelphia, Pa.)

ogic results. Large doses of penicillin and methicillin are started immediately. Crystalline penicillin G in the range of 12 to 20 million units daily and 1 to 8 grams of methicillin daily, depending on the patient's age, are given in divided doses at three hour intervals, either intravenously or intramuscularly. Appropriate adjustments in the antibiotic program can be made when the results of the culture and sensitivity studies are known. As the disease is controlled, a corresponding reduction in dosage should follow. It appears that once acute hematogenous staphylococcal osteomyelitis is controlled with parenteral therapy, oral therapy should suffice. It is important not to give oral antibiotics with food, because this markedly reduces absorption from the gastrointestinal tract and seriously diminishes the drug level in the blood. Antibiotics should be continued for three to four weeks after the patient becomes afebrile.

The body's resistance is supported by the use of small blood transfusions and intravenous fluids to maintain electrolyte balance. Local treatment contists of plaster immobilization of the affected part.

The availability of effective antibiotic therapy has relegated surgery to a secondary position in the treatment of acute hematogenous osteomyelitis. Operative intervention is not necessary if effective medical treatment is instituted within 72 hours after onset of the disease. Bone is a highly vascular tissue and thus, until the infection progresses to the state of producing vascular thrombosis and pus with increased marrow pressure, antibiotic treatment will be effective.

Surgical intervention is reserved mainly for the drainage of subperiosteal abscesses and the removal of sequestra. Early surgical decompression of the bone is indicated if antibiotic treatment had not been instituted within 72 hours of onset or if it fails to control the infection completely.

With early diagnosis and effective treatment, a good result can usually be expected, with the infection eradicated and the bone substance returned to a normal state. A breakdown in either diagnosis or treatment may lead to chronic osteomyelitis or to a localized bone infection known as *Brodie's abscess*.

CHRONIC OSTEOMYELITIS

The progression from acute to chronic osteomyelitis is graded and is characterized by the accumulation of pus under pressure, causing bone ischemia and forcing bacteria into the vascular channels and bone lacunae. As the chronic infection continues, proliferative granulation tissue, once highly vascular, turns to dense scar. This avascular scar forms an impenetrable barrier around the infected area. New bone may be laid down adjacent to the old bone spicules and may further isolate dead infected bone. Chronic osteomyelitis, therefore, is a disease of ischemia more than of infection. Organisms thrive in avascular bone, and scar tissue acts as an impenetrable membrane to antibiotic therapy.

Clinical Picture.   The patient with chronic osteomyelitis may present in one of two clinical situations:

1. The infection may remain persistent and active and may be characterized by recurring sequestration of bone and continuous drainage of pus from sinuses (Fig. 73). Chronic drainage over a long period of time may lead to nephritis, amyloid disease, or squamous cell carcinoma in sinus tracts.

2. The process may seemingly quiet down and the sinuses close. However, residual infection may lurk within the bone substance, ready to flare up intermittently. When this occurs, the part becomes painful, swollen, and inflamed. The closed sinus tracts may open to discharge pus and occasionally pieces of dead bone. A pocket of infec-

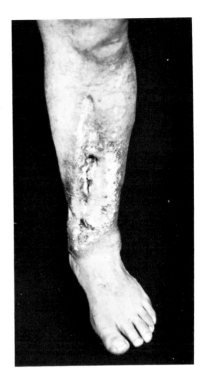

Figure 73. Chronic osteomyelitis of the tibia. Leg exhibits marked scarring of the skin and draining sinuses.

tion may be present within the bone and give no indication of its presence for years.

On x-ray examination, chronic osteomyelitis is characterized by an enlarged, irregular, and dense bone structure with involucrum formation. Cavities and sequestra within the bone substance are frequently noted (Fig. 74).

Treatment. Effective treatment of chronic osteomyelitis depends, first and foremost, on radical surgical debridement of the bone with excision of all sinuses, dead bone, scar, and grossly necrotic tissue. The role of antibiotics at this stage is more supportive than curative: they aid in preventing septicemia and fulminating local infection. Culture specimens are taken preoperatively from the depth of the wound or sinus, and the appropriate antibiotic is started 24 to 72 hours before surgery to ensure an adequate level of antibiotic in any small hematoma that might form postoperatively. Fresh culture material should also be taken from the depth of the wound at the time of operation. A large bolus of antibiotic should be given intravenously during the operative procedure to aid in sterilizing the hematoma. The wound should be closed, if possible, with stainless steel wire,

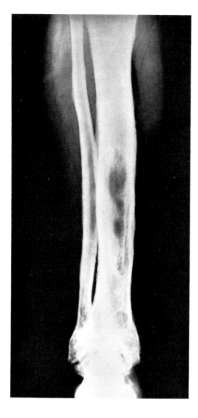

Figure 74. Chronic osteomyelitis of the tibia in an adult.

and as much dead space as possible eliminated by tight closure. A closed system of irrigation and suction should be incorporated into the wound at the time of closure.

The technique of primary closure, with irrigation and suction providing a constant antibiotic bath to the raw bone surfaces, has considerably reduced patient disability and has almost eliminated the incidence of secondary bacterial infection. In this method of treatment, a pair of multiperforated polyethylene tubes is placed in the cavity created by surgery, and the nonperforated ends are brought out through normal tissue as far away from the wound edges as possible. The outlet tube is connected by tubing to some type of electrically driven suction machine and adjusted to the least possible suction to maintain outflow. A prepared solution of physiologic saline containing penicillin or methicillin, an appropriate wide-spectrum antibiotic, or both, and either Varidase or a detergent, such as aerosol wash or Alevaire, is run through the inflow tube at the rate of about 2 to 3 liters during each 24 hours, depending on the results from the cultures obtained at operation. Appropriate antibiotics are given orally or intramuscularly during the period of closed irrigation. The material coming through the suction tube is cultured daily. When three successive negative cultures have been obtained, the system can be gradually discontinued and removed. An oral antibiotic is usually given for 4 to 6 weeks after removing the irrigation tubes in an attempt to reduce the incidence of recurrent infection.

In an occasional patient it may be impossible to obtain closure of the soft tissues. In this instance it would be preferable to pack the wound open with vaselinized gauze, allowing it to granulate from within outward.

Successful treatment of chronic osteomyelitis requires good viable skin and soft tissue coverage. For this reason the overlying skin frequently has to be replaced with skin grafts before or after definitive surgical intervention.

Regional perfusion of infected areas with antibiotic solutions for refractory infections of bones and joints has been described. Regional body perfusion is not without complications and, at present, should be regarded as a promising method of investigative surgery. The technique involves completely isolating the vascular tree of an area from the general body circulation and pumping artificially oxygenated blood through it. Appropriate antibiotic solutions can be added to the system to obtain a highly concentrated perfusion without fear of injury to parenchymatous tissue.

BRODIE'S ABSCESS

Brodie's abscess is a chronic localized form of osteomyelitis due, frequently, to a staphylococcus of low virulence. The infection causes localized bone destruction that becomes sealed off by fibrous tissue and sclerotic bone formation, resulting in a sharply demarcated lytic lesion in the bone. This localized bone abscess is frequently found at the lower end of the tibia.

The patient complains of bone pain of gradual onset, which is frequently worse at night. There may be tenderness to palpation over the site of the abscess.

X-ray examination reveals a well-circumscribed lytic lesion surrounded by an area of dense sclerotic bone (Fig. 75). Differential diagnosis includes unicameral bone cyst, osteoid osteoma, fibrous dysplasia, and eosinophilic granuloma.

Treatment consists of draining the abscess at operation and scraping the inside of the bone cavity clean. Occasionally it is possible to expedite healing by filling the empty cavity with bone chip grafts taken from the ilium.

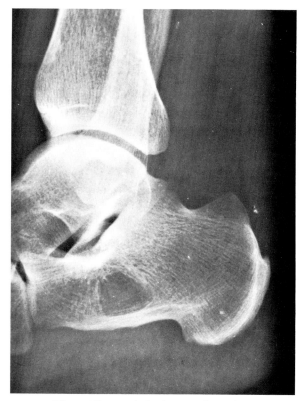

Figure 75.   Brodie's abscess of os calcis.

Pyogenic Arthritis

Infection of a joint with pus forming organisms is called pyogenic arthritis, infectious arthritis, or septic arthritis. It is more common in infants and children than in adults and has an affinity for the hip and knee joints. *Staphylococcus aureus* is the infecting agent in 40 to 60 per cent of these patients, with *Streptococcus* next in frequency. Pyogenic arthritis may be the result of metastatic infection arising from a primary infection source, such as pneumonia, gonorrhea, meningitis, upper respiratory infection, otitis media, furuncle, infected abrasion, or umbilical vein infection. Osteomyelitis localized in a bone may spread to involve an adjacent joint, or direct inoculation of a joint with organisms may follow trauma, penetrating wounds, or joint aspiration.

Regardless of how the organisms find their way into a joint, pyogenic arthritis, once established, is a grave problem in any age group and requires immediate recognition and vigorous treatment for its control. Militant attention to every suspected joint infection is demanded to prevent irreparable joint damage. Articular hyaline cartilage is digested by pyogenic exudates, and if this occurs, the joint will be damaged beyond repair. A nonvascular tissue such as articular cartilage is defenseless in the face of microorganism invasion. It has been shown experimentally that under certain conditions hyaline cartilage can be completely digested within 24 hours by action of the proteolytic enzymes in the pyogenic exudate.

Pathologic Features.　The organisms gain entrance to the joint by several routes. They may be blood-borne from some distant focus of infection. This is the usual mechanism in the infant or when pyogenic arthritis complicates an infectious disease such as gonorrhea. They may erode into the joint from an adjacent focus of osteomyelitis, or they may be inserted directly into the joint from outside. The pathologic changes in the joint, once microorganisms have gained entrance, are those changes initiated by infection. The inflammatory response begins in the synovial membrane, which becomes swollen, reddened, and hyperemic. The joint distends with cloudy fluid which, in a few days, becomes frank pus. If the pus is allowed to remain in the joint, it will destroy the articular cartilage through chondrolysis. This destruction occurs first and most extensively at points of joint contact. The process allows raw bone surfaces to be bathed by infection, potentially leading to fibrous or bony ankylosis of the joint or, if the infection has invaded the substance of the bone, to the development of osteomyelitis as a complication of the pyogenic arthritis.

Clinical Picture.　The acute onset of painful and hot joint swelling, associated with the systemic signs of infection, particularly after trauma or during the treatment of some primary source of infection, should immediately signal the possibility of pyogenic arthritis. The patient is sick, febrile, and irritable and shows a marked unwillingness to move the affected joint or bear weight on it because of pain. He will keep the joint in a flexed position, which is the position of comfort. If the joint involved can be palpated, it usually feels hot and is exquisitely tender to touch.

Laboratory studies reveal an increased leukocytosis and an elevated erythrocyte sedimentation rate. Except for signs of capsular swelling and widening of the joint space, the x-ray examination should be negative. If bone destruction is seen on the x-ray film, it means that osteomyelitis has already complicated the problem.

The diagnosis is made by inserting a needle into the joint and withdrawing pus. This immediately differentiates pyogenic arthritis from hemarthrosis, rheumatoid arthritis, joint tuberculosis, and any other condition causing joint symptoms.

HIP JOINT INVOLVEMENT.   Involvement of the hip joint, particularly in the infant, can easily be overlooked because the joint is deeply placed, causing the local signs of infection to be less readily apparent. The patient holds the leg in a flexed position at the hip and resists all efforts to move the joint either actively or passively. There may be swelling over the hip and trochanteric area. In children, a mechanical complication of pyogenic arthritis of the hip may be pathologic dislocation of the joint. This has been reported to occur in as many 40 per cent of children with pyogenic arthritis of the hip.

KNEE JOINT INVOLVEMENT.   Involvement of the knee joint is more obvious because of its exposed position in the body. The joint and suprapatellar pouch may distend with fluid, and the joint is usually held in a flexed position by hamstring muscle tightness and spasm. The joint will feel hot, and the overlying tissues will appear red and inflamed. The joint will be markedly tender to palpation, and the patient will resist movement of the joint. Because of the severe penalties attached to delay, there should never be any hesitation about aspirating a joint for verification if suppuration is suspected.

Treatment.   Treatment must be immediate and vigorous, considering the time limitations imposed by the defenselessness of the articular cartilage.

Accurate bacteriologic diagnosis is essential, since antibacterial agents and adequate surgical drainage complement each other in the treatment of pyogenic arthritis. Direct smear of the articular fluid frequently will give immediate valuable information concerning the involved microorganism. Organisms cannot always be cultured, even from purulent articular fluid, but often a presumptive etiologic diagnosis can be made by culture from other sources, such as blood, spinal fluid, and throat.

Due to its relative depth, the hip joint should be surgically drained and irrigated as soon as the diagnosis is made. Perforated polyethylene tubes are introduced into the joint, and solutions of methicillin and ampicillin are instilled four times daily. An alternative treatment method is a constant antibiotic bath with the irrigation and suction system previously described for the treatment of chronic osteomyelitis.

Other joints, since they are superficially placed in the body, may be aspirated with a large bore needle and then irrigated thoroughly with solutions of normal saline or Ringers lactate. One gram each of methicillin and ampicillin is instilled into the joint. Infected joints should be protected by traction or splinting. Methicillin and ampicillin are given parenterally until the results of the culture are known. The appropriate bactericidal antibiotic is continued for two to three weeks after the patient becomes afebrile and joint effusion ceases.

The joint is aspirated and irrigated, and the antibiotic is instilled as often as effusion recurs. Failure of the infection to begin to subside promptly indicates the presence of walled-off collections of pus, and surgical drainage of the joint should be performed without delay. The joint should be closed by the suction-irrigation technique previously described.

All treating physicians are not agreed on the need or even the desirability of repeated intra-articular drug injections or of constant joint irrigation with antibiotic solutions, even though it has been demonstrated experimentally that intra-articular instillation of appropriate antibiotics produces sterility of the joint more rapidly than does intramuscular administration. Opponents of intra-articular instillation point to present evidence that penicillin and other anti-infective agents may diffuse across inflamed synovial membranes to reach levels in the joint fluid approximating the level in the blood, provided they are given systemically in large enough doses. Antibiotics of large molecular size do not cross the synovial membrane with the same rapidity as those of smaller molecular size, although all presently known antibiotics do cross the synovial membrane in therapeutic concentrations. Until this divergence of opinion is better illuminated by more extensive clinical trials, most experienced clinicians will continue to favor joint aspiration and local instillation of an antibiotic, combined with its systemic use.

Prognosis. With early diagnosis and rapid effective treatment, the prognosis for joint function is good. Delay in diagnosis will lead to joint damage and, possibly, fibrous or bony ankylosis of the joint. If minimal or moderate damage is sustained in childhood, progressive joint deformity in adult life is possible, with the subsequent development of degenerative arthritis. Pathologic dislocation of the hip, occurring as a complication of the sepsis, may seriously impair the future function of the joint. With delay in diagnosis or ineffective treatment, the infection will progress in some patients to osteomyelitis.

TUBERCULOUS INFECTION

Tuberculosis is a constitutional infection caused by the tubercle bacillus and resulting in focal lesions in the respiratory or alimentary organs, with involvement of the regional lymph nodes. The infection produces metastatic lesions in other tissues and organs, notably the urogenital and skeletal systems, by means of lymphatic spread and arteriolar infarction. In the involved tissue or organ, the characteristic granulation tissue and spreading avascularity lead to necrosis, caseation, and abscess formation. The abscesses may spread along tissue planes, particularly along neurovascular pathways, for great distances.

INCIDENCE

During the early years of the present century, skeletal tuberculosis constituted the most common single cause of childhood crippling. Today skeletal tuberculosis is relatively uncommon except in underdeveloped countries. This dramatic change has been produced by rigid inspection of dairy herds, pasteurization of milk, efficient public health measures, and effective chemotherapeutic agents. In the countries where these measures are enforced, human contact is the most common form of transmission. Bovine tuberculosis is seen in those countries where the practice of drinking raw milk is allowed. Although tuberculosis is now a relatively rare disease in Europe, North America, and Australia, its continued manifestation in many parts of the world, notably Asia and Africa, should be a reminder that it is never far away. At any time tuberculosis might return with increased virulence and resistance to antibiotic treatment.

Although it is difficult to be certain of this, skeletal tuberculosis is thought to constitute about 3 per cent of total tuberculous infection. It is believed that most bone and joint lesions appear within two years of the onset of the primary lesion. Because their immunity is less developed than that of adults, about 85 per cent of patients with skeletal tuberculosis are children, the peak incidence occurring at about five years of age. Skeletal tuberculosis affects the spine, hip joint, or knee joint in about 90 per cent of patients. The joints of the upper extremity are affected relatively more frequently in adults than in children.

GENERAL CONSIDERATIONS

Since tuberculosis is a constitutional infection of which the skeletal focus is but a metastatic manifestation, a search must be made for the primary focus. If the focus is located, it must be determined if it is healed, quiescent, or active.

The pathologic response of bone tissue to the tubercle bacillus is rather characteristic, although influenced to a certain extent by the anatomy of the area involved. The infection causes local death of bone, with caseation necrosis and destruction of bone structure. Endarteritis occurs with further necrosis, and the ever-widening circle of destruction continues. The necrotic caseous material may burst through joint capsules and tissue planes and present under the skin as an abscess. This type of abscess, filled with necrotic debris, is called a "cold" abscess, in contrast to a "hot" abscess, which is filled with pyogenic pus. A "cold" abscess may burst through the skin to become a draining tuberculous sinus.

Unlike bone tissue involved with pyogenic organisms, bone tissue infected with tuberculosis makes little or no attempt to defend or protect itself and, as a consequence, no new bone formation is usually noted on the x-ray film. It is the presence of bone destruction associated with the absence of bone repair that is characteristic of the tuberculous skeletal lesion as seen on the x-ray film (Fig. 76).

When tuberculosis invades a joint, the synovial membrane becomes thickened, secretes excessive fluid, and becomes sprinkled with tubercles. A pannus of tuberculous granulation tissue slowly covers the articular hyaline cartilage, gradually destroying it and the underlying subchondral bone.

The x-ray picture reflects the pathologic changes brought about by tuberculosis. The presence of bone destruction and the absence of new bone formation are noted. Gradual destruction of the joint cartilage leads to joint narrowing. Continued weight bearing results in collapse of the involved joint.

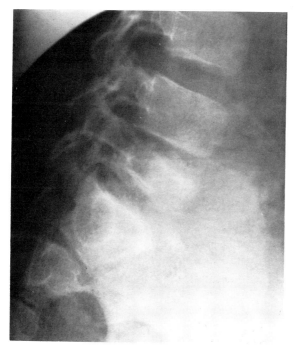

Figure 76. Tuberculosis involving body of fifth lumbar vertebra. Note narrowing of intervertebral disc space, destruction and collapse of vertebral body, and absence of a bony reparative process.

The symptoms of tuberculous involvement of the musculoskeletal system may be general and local. The general symptoms can include malaise, loss of appetite, loss of weight, and intermittent fever. The local presenting symptoms can include pain, swelling, limitation of motion, and possibly deformity of the affected part.

Even though the clinical picture presented by the patient and the changes noted on the x-ray film may seem typical of skeletal tuberculosis, experience has shown that dependence on these alone will lead to a wrong diagnosis in about 25 per cent of patients. Laboratory substantiation of the diagnosis must be obtained.

The tuberculin test is of value when negative, but it gives no specific information when positive. Unfortunately, culture of aspirated material and guinea pig inoculation give a negative result in a large number of patients who actually have tuberculosis. Synovial biopsy may prove to be the important diagnostic test in many patients.

For many years it was recognized that the cornerstone of treatment of tuberculosis was rest of the involved part. When the skeleton was involved, this treatment was carried out by prolonged plaster immobilization in a tuberculosis sanitarium, in association with nourishing food and exposure to sunlight. In 1911 Hibbs performed the first spinal fusion for tuberculosis and introduced the concept of total and complete rest to a joint by arthrodesis.

The next major advance in the treatment of skeletal tuberculosis came with the introduction of the chemotherapeutic drugs: streptomycin, para-aminosalicylic acid (PAS), and isonicotinic acid hydrazide (I.N.H.). The use of these agents has resulted in a reduction of the primary mortality in bone and joint tuberculosis. Because of these drugs, normal function has been restored to many joints that formerly would have gone on to destruction and ultimate fusion. These agents have also made it possible to gain adequate control over abscesses and sinus tracts. With adequate blood drug levels it is now possible to operate on skeletal tuberculosis without fear of hematogenous spreading of the disease or postoperative abscess or sinus formation, as was formerly the case.

TUBERCULOSIS OF THE SPINE

Tuberculous infection of the spine, by far the most common form of skeletal tuberculosis, is known as *Pott's disease* (Sir Percival Pott, 1779). It commonly affects the segment from the tenth thoracic to the first lumbar vertebra, called the thoracolumbar junction, since this is the segment possessing the greatest mobility. Although spinal tuberculosis may strike any age group, about half the patients are between three and five years of age at the time of onset. In general, spinal lesions can be much more serious than those in peripheral joints because of the possibility of implicating the spinal cord. Other factors that might add to the seriousness of the problem are the presence of multiple lesions, the degree of activity of the primary focus, the extreme youth or old age of the patient, and associated debilitating conditions, such as diabetes, nephritis, and anemia.

Pathology. The skeletal focus begins in the vertebral body, usually along the anterior aspect of the bone. In a way this is fortunate, for it is infection in the posterior aspect of the vertebra that is most likely to cause compression of the spinal cord. The disease causes destruction of bone, which leads to collapse of the vertebral body. As the vertebral body collapses, caseous necrotic material may be squeezed out into the soft tissues to form paravertebral abscesses. Infection may spread beneath the anterior longitudinal spinal ligament to involve several vertebrae.

Compression of the spinal cord may occur at any level from the foramen magnum to the upper lumbar region, but it is most common in the thoracic spine area. Here the spinal canal is narrow and the cord occupies most of the space, so that even a small abscess or bone sequestrum may produce cord pressure and paraplegia. In the cervical region, infected material can track sideways along the fascial planes and, in the lumbar region, along the psoas muscle sheath to the groin. In the thoracic region, pus tends to collect beneath the anterior and posterior longitudinal ligaments under tension, possibly spreading upward and downward to form a paravertebral abscess.

Clinical Picture. The patient complains of back pain that restricts spinal movement. Characteristically, a patient will squat rather than bend to retrieve an object from the floor. Because of pain, all spinal movements are guarded and the patient tends to walk with a protective gait. With marked anterior collapse of several vertebral bodies in the thoracic spine region, the patient may develop a sharp angular deformity of the spine called a *gibbus.* In the days when spinal tuberculosis was common, this was one of the chief causes of "hunchback" deformity.

The earliest sign on the x-ray film of tuberculous infection of the spine is deossification of the vertebral bodies, associated with thinning of the involved disc space. As the disease progresses, bone destruction leads to progressive anterior wedging of the vertebral bodies and ultimate vertebral collapse (Fig. 77). The psoas muscle shadow may appear enlarged on the x-ray film because of the presence of a paravertebral abscess. The x-ray film is then said to show the presence of a "psoas abscess."

Complications. The chief complications of spinal tuberculosis are psoas abscess, paraplegia, and tuberculous meningitis.

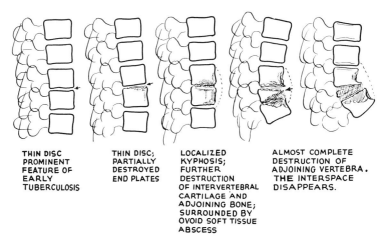

| THIN DISC PROMINENT FEATURE OF EARLY TUBERCULOSIS | THIN DISC; PARTIALLY DESTROYED END PLATES | LOCALIZED KYPHOSIS; FURTHER DESTRUCTION OF INTERVERTEBRAL CARTILAGE AND ADJOINING BONE; SURROUNDED BY OVOID SOFT TISSUE ABSCESS | ALMOST COMPLETE DESTRUCTION OF ADJOINING VERTEBRA. THE INTERSPACE DISAPPEARS. |

Figure 77.   The sequence of bone changes noted by x-ray in tuberculosis of the spine. (From Meschan, I.: Analysis of Roentgen Signs in General Radiology, Vol. 3. Philadelphia: W. B. Saunders Co., 1973.)

A psoas abscess is a paravertebral abscess composed of necrotic debris that pushes out against the psoas muscle, causing its shadow to appear enlarged on the x-ray film. This abscess may spread down tissue planes, point in the thigh, or spread backward through the lumbar triangle to form a lumbar abscess. If these abscesses drain out to the skin surface, tuberculous sinuses are formed.

Paraplegia is one of the most disabling and distressing complications of spinal tuberculosis. The type of paraplegia seen with tuberculous cord compression may vary from a slightly spastic gait to complete paralysis, and is encountered in about 10 per cent of patients with spinal tuberculosis. Partial or complete paralysis of the legs results from spinal cord compression secondary to pressure from abscess, tuberculous granulation tissue, a tuberculoma, or extreme gibbus formation. This complication is more common with involvement of the posterior aspect of the vertebral body, laminae, pedicles, or transverse processes, because of the close proximity of the spinal cord.

If a patient with spinal tuberculosis shows any evidence of incipient or actual paralysis, total and complete bed rest with adequate antibiotic coverage should be ordered. When indicated, abscesses are drained surgically and diseased tissue is removed as early and as thoroughly as possible.

Tuberculous meningitis is an extremely grave complication resulting from the rupture of a tuberculous abscess through the dura.

Before antituberculosis drugs were available for treatment, tuberculous meningitis frequently had a fatal outcome.

Treatment. Although all treating physicians are agreed on the value of immobilization and chemotherapy for the treatment of spinal tuberculosis, no standard treatment exists throughout the world. In many American and European centers, immobilization of the spine by bed rest, plaster cast, or spinal brace, coupled with prolonged chemotherapy, is considered adequate treatment for most patients. In other centers of the same countries, posterior spinal fusion of the involved segment is carried out to obtain complete immobilization of the joint.

The disease appears to be more destructive in Asia and Africa, and physicians in those areas believe surgery is needed much earlier than formerly was thought desirable. Most of these physicians favor a direct attack on the lesion through an anterior approach. This allows removal of diseased tissue by extensive vertebral body curettage. Bone grafts are used to fill the large intervertebral defect created by the removal of diseased tissue. This gives spinal stabilization by anterior spinal fusion.

Regardless of whether or not surgery is used, all are agreed that the introduction of chemotherapy has led to better results in all forms of treatment.

TUBERCULOSIS OF THE HIP JOINT

The second most common skeletal area for tuberculous infection is the hip joint. Here again the majority of patients are young children.

The disease may begin in the synovial membrane, in the metaphyseal portion of the bone adjacent to the capital femoral epiphysis, or in the acetabulum, but it eventually progresses to involve the entire joint. The disease usually does not spread across the growth plate to involve the capital epiphysis, and early in the process, this may differentiate the x-ray film from x-rays showing evidence of Legg-Calvé-Perthes disease. Tuberculous granulation tissue spreads over the articular cartilage of the joint like a pannus, ultimately destroying the cartilage and subchondral bone. Gradual collapse of the joint occurs with weight bearing. Abscesses formed within the joint space may eventually rupture through the joint capsule to cause draining sinuses.

A painful limp is often the first sign produced by tuberculous infection of the hip joint. The pain may radiate to the knee area. Examination usually discloses obvious muscle atrophy of the leg and limitation of hip joint motion. There may be a flexion-adduction contracture of the leg at the hip joint.

X-ray examination may show demineralization of the bone structure, with joint narrowing and some local bone destruction. There may be capsular swelling. As the disease progresses, gross destruction of the bones and collapse of the joint may be seen on the x-ray film.

Treatment.   The patient is put to bed and traction is used in the early stages to combat muscle spasm and pain. If the diagnosis is made early in the course of the disease before joint destruction occurs, immobilization and chemotherapy may induce healing and preserve joint mobility.

If there is irreparable joint destruction, operative fusion of the hip joint will be required for control of the infection and relief of pain. In this instance the joint is surgically cleaned of all tuberculous tissue and articular cartilage, and the denuded cancellous bones of the femoral head and acetabulum are placed in contact. An iliac bone graft is usually placed between ilium and femur to promote osteogenesis. Immobilization is obtained in a plaster hip spica cast.

In the event the hip joint is the site of abscess formation, or if draining skin sinuses exist about the hip joint, fusion can be obtained by bypassing the hip joint proper and running an iliac graft from the trochanteric area of the femur to the ischium. This is called an *extra-articular fusion.*

TUBERCULOSIS OF THE KNEE JOINT

The third most common locus for skeletal tuberculosis is the knee joint. The distinguishing characteristic of this form of tuberculosis is that the major involvement is initially in the synovia. The synovial membrane responds to tuberculous infection by villous hypertrophy and an effusion, with resultant distension of the joint capsule. Small tubercles may be seen on the inflamed synovial surface. Early diagnosis is necessary to save the joint from destruction and eventual fusion.

The patient with a tuberculous infection of the knee joint may develop a painful swollen boggy knee. The suprapatellar pouch may be filled with fluid and a thickened synovial membrane. There may be a flexion contracture of the knee joint and marked quadriceps muscle atrophy of the thigh.

Immobilization and chemotherapy, if started before bone destruction appears, often arrest the process and preserve a well functioning joint. Some authorities recommend surgical excision of the synovial membrane (synovectomy) and others do not. If bone destruction is severe, joint fusion will be necessary to control the infection and provide pain relief.

References

Bulmer, J. H.: Septic arthritis of the hip in adults. J. Bone and Joint Surg., *48-B*:289, 1966.

Clawson, D. K., and Dunn, A. W.: Management of common bacterial infections of bones and joints. J. Bone and Joint Surg., *49-A*:164, 1967.

Compere, E. L., Metzger, W. I., and Mitria, R. N.: Treatment of pyogenic bone and joint infections by closed irrigation with a non-toxic detergent and one or more antibiotics. J. Bone and Joint Surg., *49-A*:614, 1967.

Curtis, P. H., Jr., and Klein, L.: Destruction of articular cartilage in septic arthritis. J. Bone and Joint Surg., *45-A*:797, 1963.

Drutz, D. J., Schaffner, W., Hillman, J. W., and Koenig, W. G.: Penetration of penicillin and other antimicrobials into joint fluid. Three case reports with the reappraisal of the literature. J. Bone and Joint Surg., *49-A*:1416, 1967.

Friedman, B.: Chemotherapy of tuberculosis of the spine. J. Bone and Joint Surg., *48-A*:451, 1966.

Hibbs, R. A.: An operation for progressive spinal deformities. A preliminary report of three cases from the service of the orthopaedic hospital. N.Y. Med. J., *93*:1013, 1911.

Kagan, B. M. (Ed.): Antimicrobial Therapy. Philadelphia: W. B. Saunders Co., 1970.

Kelly, P. J., Martin, W. J., and Coventry, M. B.: Bacterial (suppurative) arthritis in the adult. J. Bone and Joint Surg., *52-A*:1595, 1970.

Miller, J. E. (Ed.): Bone infections. Clin. Orth. and Rel. Res., *No. 96*, 1973.

Obletz, B. E.: Acute suppurative arthritis of the hip in the neonatal period. J. Bone and Joint Surg., *42-A*:23, 1960.

Pott, P.: Remarks on the Kind of Palsy of the Lower Limbs which is Frequently Found to Accompany Curvature of the Spine. London: Johnson, 1779. Also in: Medical Classics, *1*:218, 1936.

Tuberculosis of the spine and paraplegia (Editorial). J. Bone and Joint Surg., *49-B*:605, 1967.

Waldvogel, F. A., Medoff, G., Swartz, M. N.: Osteomyelitis, a review of clinical features, therapeutic considerations, and unusual aspects. Part I. N. Engl. J. Med., *282*:198, January 22, 1970.

Waldvogel, F. A., Medoff, G., and Swartz, M. N.: Osteomyelitis, a review of clinical features, therapeutic considerations, and unusual aspects. Part II. N. Engl. J. Med., *282*:260, January 29, 1970.

Waldvogel, F. A., Medoff, G., and Swartz, M. N.: Osteomyelitis, a review of clinical features, therapeutic considerations, and unusual aspects. Part III. N. Engl. J. Med., *282*:316, Febuary 5, 1970.

Chapter Seven

Neuromuscular Disorders

Pathologic conditions may affect the neuromuscular system to produce disorders of orthopaedic interest. Some of these disease states have congenital, infectious, metabolic, or traumatic causes. In others the cause is totally unknown. In general the symptoms and signs produced by a disorder of this type will depend upon the level of involvement within the neuromuscular system. This involvement may be at the brain, spinal cord, nerve root, or peripheral nerve level, producing a set of findings characteristic of either an upper or lower motor neuron lesion.

An upper motor neuron lesion is characterized by muscular spasticity and increased muscular tone, increased tendon reflexes, diminished or absent superficial reflexes, and the appearance of pathologic reflexes, such as the Babinski. An example of upper motor neuron lesion is *cerebral palsy.*

A lower motor neuron lesion is associated with injury or disease of the anterior horn cells, the anterior roots, the peripheral nerves, the nerve plexuses, or the cauda equina. It is characterized by muscular flaccidity and loss of muscular tone, absent tendon reflexes, muscle atrophy, and the reaction of degeneration. Examples of lower motor neuron lesion are *paralytic poliomyelitis* and the *nerve root compression syndromes.*

Failure of muscular function, on the other hand, may have no neurologic basis, but rather may represent a disease state primary in the muscle tissue. This state, which is referred to as *myopathy,* takes the form of an intrinsic degenerative or inflammatory disease of

148

muscle, the innervation of which is intact. An example of this state is *progressive muscular dystrophy.*

Finally, there may be no abnormality of the neural or muscular elements but only an interference with the transmission of the impulses from the neuron to the muscle across the myoneural junction. An example of this is *myasthenia gravis.*

INVOLVEMENT AT BRAIN LEVEL

CEREBRAL PALSY (LITTLE'S DISEASE)

The term cerebral palsy refers to a nonprogressive state of muscular dysfunction caused by damage or defect of the upper motor neuron either in the brain stem or brain, resulting in interference with voluntary motor function. The clinical state produced is characterized by muscular incoordination, lack of balance, speech difficulties, convulsions, and in many instances, mental deficiency.

The causes of cerebral palsy are multiple and may arise before, during, or after birth of the child. In some instances congenital defective development of the brain stem is responsible for the condition. In other instances certain pathologic conditions in the mother may pass the placental barrier to cause fetal insult. Incompatability of maternal and fetal blood types (Rh factor) may result in destruction of fetal blood cells with resulting anoxic damage to the brain of the developing embryo. At birth, trauma to the head, resulting in cerebral hemorrhage or anoxia, may cause cerebral palsy. After birth, whooping cough, encephalitis, and trauma are possible causes. The causative brain lesion in cerebral palsy is irreparable but not progressive.

Incidence. With the incidence of skeletal tuberculosis and poliomyelitis shrunken by effective public health measures, cerebral palsy and congenital deformities now rank as the most frequent causes of childhood crippling. It has been estimated that seven new patients with cerebral palsy are discovered in every 100,000 births. Statistics show that of these seven patients, one usually dies during infancy, two have severe mental deficiency requiring institutional care, one is so severely handicapped that treatment is ineffective, and one is so mildly affected that treatment is not needed. The two remaining patients are moderately handicapped and are the ones upon whom treatment efforts are concentrated.

Clinical Types. The clinical type of cerebral palsy depends upon the location of the damage in the brain or brain stem.

The *spastic* form of cerebral palsy is caused by lesions in the cerebral cortex, which tend to eliminate the motor control system and allow reception of excessive impulses from the lower motor neurons. These children, forming about 70 per cent of the entire group, exhibit spastic muscles which undergo involuntary contraction when suddenly stretched. Since the flexor muscle groups are stronger than the extensor muscle groups, the spasticity tends to pull the limbs into flexion deformities. Hyper-reflexia is present.

The typical positional deformity of the upper extremity in this condition is a flexed elbow, pronated forearm, palmar flexed wrist with the hand in ulnar deviation, and flexed fingers with the thumb adducted. The typical positional deformity of the lower extremity is an adducted, flexed, and internally rotated position of the hip joint, with a flexed knee, equinus deformity of the foot, and a dorsiflexed large toe. If both lower extremities are affected, the patient may walk with a type of mincing gait known as a scissors gait, which is caused by a spasticity of the adductor muscles (Fig. 78).

The *athetoid* form of cerebral palsy is produced by lesions in the basal ganglia area. These children, forming about 20 per cent of the entire group, exhibit purposeless involuntary muscular movements,

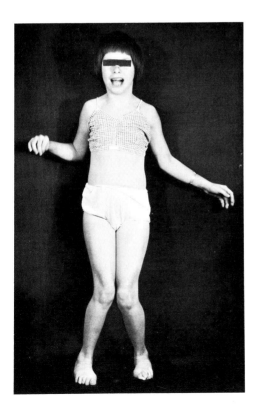

Figure 78. Spastic form of cerebral palsy, illustrating the typical positional deformities of the upper and lower extremities. (Courtesy Dr. John Dowling, Lankenau Hospital, Philadelphia, Pa.)

which are characteristically exaggerated by excitement or by attempts to perform purposeful activities, such as walking or speaking. Some children in this group exhibit muscular tremor or muscular rigidity.

The *ataxic* form of cerebral palsy is produced by lesions in the cerebellum. These children, forming about 10 per cent of the entire group, exhibit a disturbed sense of balance and equilibrium that greatly lessens their muscular efficiency.

In many children the pathologic changes involve more than one area of the brain or brain stem, resulting in mixed types of cerebral palsy.

These patients may also be classified according to the extent of regional involvement: *monoplegia* refers to involvement of a single extremity; *diplegia* refers to involvement of both upper extremities; *hemiplegia* refers to involvement of an upper extremity and a lower extremity on the same side of the body; *paraplegia* refers to involvement of both lower extremities; and *quadriplegia* refers to involvement of all four extremities. It has been estimated that about 60 per cent of patients with cerebral palsy are quadriplegic.

Treatment. The treatment of cerebral palsy is a major rehabilitation effort and is best carried out in special clinics or treatment centers where a trained team is available to manage the problem. The goal of treatment is to make the patient as independent as possible. Unfortunately, some patients never progress beyond the sitting stage, although others are improved to such a degree that they become able to compete with normal individuals in earning their own living.

Treatment of cerebral palsy takes many directions, all aimed at ultimate improvement for the child. Attention is directed toward improving speech difficulties and mental defects as far as it is possible. The child is taught balance, posture, and muscular relaxation. The most important facet of this program, however, is the re-education of muscles.

Muscular re-education in cerebral palsy is carried out over a long unhurried treatment period by making use of exercises with the guidance of trained therapists. Passive stretching exercises are used by the therapists to correct or prevent joint contractures. Bracing is a useful adjunct to help the patient accomplish a specific activity, such as walking.

Drugs such as Prostigmin (neostigmine) and Dilantin (diphenylhydantoin) may have a temporary relaxing effect on muscle spasm and tension and are occasionally used as adjuncts to treatment, particularly if epilepsy accompanies cerebral palsy.

Occasionally operations are performed on patients with cerebral palsy as an aid to muscular re-education. The greatest benefit from surgery is gained by the spastic group. Surgery is contraindicated in patients with the athetoid form of cerebral palsy and in those with severe mental defects.

The goals of operative treatment in cerebral palsy and the surgical measures for attaining those goals are:

1. To diminish muscle spasm by operations upon motor nerves, such as neurectomy.

2. To correct joint contractures by cutting tight joint capsules, tendons, and other soft tissues.

3. To restore muscle balance by equalizing the power of opposing muscles by tendon transplantation.

4. To stabilize poorly controlled joints by surgical fusion.

ADULT SPASTIC PARALYSIS

Spastic hemiplegia in the adult may follow cerebral vascular disorders, such as hemorrhage, thrombosis, or embolus formation. As in cerebral palsy, treatment involves muscular re-education through therapy and exercise, and the use of splints or braces if necessary. Nerve blocks may be used to relieve spasticity. Surgical correction of joint contractures or tendon transfer operations may be useful to restore muscle balance and improve function.

INVOLVEMENT AT SPINAL CORD LEVEL

ANTERIOR POLIOMYELITIS (INFANTILE PARALYSIS)

Until recently, anterior poliomyelitis ranked as the most frequent cause of childhood crippling in this country, supplying large numbers of paralytic problems to orthopaedic services for rehabilitation and reconstruction. The incidence of the disease has been sharply curtailed since the mid-1950's by the use of prophylactic poliomyelitis vaccine. However, sporadic cases requiring orthopaedic care will undoubtedly continue to appear.

Etiology. Anterior poliomyelitis is an acute infectious disease caused by a filtrable virus of the enterovirus group, of which there are three principal strains. The chief pathway for entrance of the virus is thought to be the alimentary tract, since organisms have been isolated from the feces and oral secretions of patients. The disease characteristically appears both sporadically and in epidemic form during midsummer and early fall, which is known as the "polio" season.

Pathology. The virus inflicts its principal damage on the anterior horn cells of the spinal cord and brain stem, which may be damaged or destroyed, with resulting flaccid paralysis in the muscles innervated by the affected motor cells.

The possibility of recovery of any paralyzed muscle is dependent upon the condition of the anterior horn cells that innervate the muscles. Destroyed cells can never be repaired or replaced. If all the neurons that innervate a particular muscle are destroyed, that muscle will exhibit complete and permanent flaccid paralysis.

Cells that have been damaged but not destroyed may recover their physiologic function. Under these circumstances there will be partial or complete return of muscle power, depending on the relative number of motor cells that recover.

Clinical Picture.   Although poliomyelitis is essentially a disease of childhood, adults are not infrequently affected.

Studies of past epidemics show that only a small percentage of patients contracting anterior poliomyelitis actually develop muscle paralysis. Those who do, however, are the ones who come to the attention of the orthopaedic surgeon.

Two clinical forms of the disease are distinguished: (1) the more common *spinal* form, in which involvement of the anterior horn cells in the spinal cord may result in flaccid paralysis of the muscles of the trunk or extremities, and (2) the *bulbar* form, in which damage to the brain stem and upper cord may result in respiratory and circulatory collapse with an attendant high mortality rate.

Three stages of the disease are recognized:

1. The *acute* stage is characterized by the onset of flaccid muscular paralysis, which may be patchy in distribution, combined with painful muscle spasm in the antagonist muscles. This stage may last from one to four weeks.

2. The stage of *convalescence and recovery* is the period during which spontaneous recovery of motor power may occur. Some authorities believe that maximum muscle recovery occurs during the first six months following onset, while others extend the period to two years.

3. The *residual* stage is the final stage of the disease and begins at the end of the spontaneous recovery period. No further spontaneous improvement in motor power occurs, and any remaining paralysis will be permanent. The orthopaedic surgeon is most concerned with this stage.

Treatment.   ACUTE STAGE.   Treatment during the acute stage consists of symptomatic and supportive medical care of an acutely ill febrile patient needing rest and quiet. Respiratory difficulties may require a respirator or tracheostomy. Hot moist packs applied to the body relieve painful muscle spasm.

Orthopaedic interest during this stage centers upon the prevention of joint contractures. Muscles in spasm, unopposed by the paralyzed ones, tend to pull joints into contracted positions. Unless this pulling is prevented by splinting, shortened muscles may develop fixed contractures.

CONVALESCENT STAGE. By the time the convalescent stage is reached, the period of painful muscle spasm is over and definitive exercise therapy to muscles can be given. Trained therapists, under orthopaedic supervision, give passive exercises to preserve joint motion and prevent contractures. Active exercises are used to develop strength and function in weak muscles.

The orthopaedic surgeon adds crutches and braces to the program as they may be needed by the patient for support and ambulation. Splints and casts may be used to prevent joint deformities.

It has been estimated that with good supportive care, 75 to 85 per cent of patients with paralysis will show marked spontaneous improvement or complete recovery of muscle function.

RESIDUAL STAGE. Any muscular paralysis remaining at this time will be permanent. The crippling effects of motor paralysis can be ameliorated in many patients by definitive orthopaedic surgical procedures designed to correct deformities and improve function. The orthopaedic surgical procedures most frequently used to accomplish these goals are joint fusion and tendon transplantation, either singly or in combination, as illustrated in the following examples:

1. If the muscles motivating a joint (e.g., hip or ankle) are paralyzed, the joint will be flail and unstable and the patient greatly incapacitated. If the joint is stabilized by arthrodesis, the functional efficiency of the patient will be markedly increased.

2. The motion lost when a particular muscle becomes paralyzed may be regained by transplanting the tendon of a normal muscle to perform the job of the paralyzed muscle. Thus the motion of thumb opposition, lost with paralysis of the opponens pollicis muscle, may be regained by transplanting a normal flexor sublimis tendon from the fourth finger to the base of the thumb.

3. A "foot drop" deformity resulting from paralysis of the anterior tibial muscle may be corrected by a combination of both operative procedures. Surgical fusion of the subtalar joints eliminates the motions of eversion and inversion of the foot, which are normally performed by the posterior tibial and peroneal muscles. These tendons, no longer having motions to perform, may be transplanted to the front of the foot, where they then act to dorsiflex the ankle.

Severe muscular paralysis involving a child's leg may be accompanied by considerable shortening of the extremity due to retardation of epiphyseal growth. Operations on the epiphyses may be required to correct the leg length inequality (see p. 80).

Friedreich's Ataxia

Friedreich's ataxia or hereditary spinal ataxia is a heredofamilial disorder exhibiting both dominant and recessive inheritance patterns and involving chiefly the posterior columns of the spinal cord. The disease manifests itself somewhere between five and 20 years of age, with the highest incidence at puberty. The course of the disease is generally slow, with frequent periods of remission. Affected patients develop a lurching ataxic gait which may progress to a severe disability. Intention tremors and scanning speech are noted with progression of the disease. As a result of muscle weakness and deformity, the patient is often unable to walk by the fourth decade, and death from intercurrent disease frequently supervenes by the age of 40.

This disease is of orthopaedic interest because the resulting muscle imbalance may allow the development of a particular foot deformity known as a cavus or "claw foot," characterized by a high curved longitudinal arch, prominence of the metatarsal heads, and

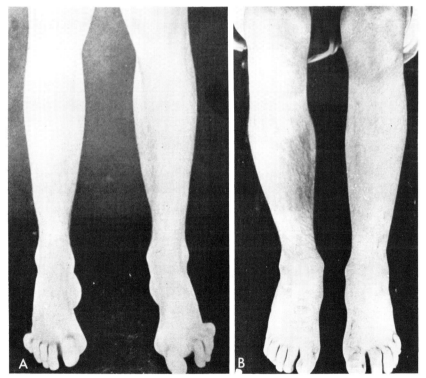

Figure 79. A, positional foot deformity in Friedreich's ataxia. B, appearance after surgical correction.

clawing of the toes (Fig. 79). "Claw foot" is frequently a painful deformity because of malalignment of the weight bearing surface of the foot.

In many patients progress of the neurologic disease is slow, and operative correction of the deformity is indicated to bring about a more functional alignment of the weight bearing surface of the foot.

CHARCOT-MARIE-TOOTH DISEASE

Charcot-Marie-Tooth disease or progressive muscular atrophy of the peroneal type is a heredofamilial disease transmitted either as an autosomal dominant, X-linked recessive, or autosomal recessive trait. The disease, affecting males more often than females, is associated with degenerative changes in the posterior columns of the spinal cord, the spinal roots, and the peripheral nerves.

When dominant, the disease manifests itself at about 30 years of age and tends to run a prolonged course with only moderate atrophy. The X-linked variety is usually manifested during the second decade of life and tends to run a more severe course with marked disability by about 30 years of age. The most severe form, the autosomal recessive, has its onset at about eight years of age and usually produces profound weakness by the second decade.

Orthopaedic attention focuses upon the peripheral deformity brought about by the neurologic changes. The characteristic changes seen in the upper extremity are intrinsic atrophy and weakness of the radially innervated forearm muscles. Paralysis of the peroneal and toe extensor muscles in the lower extremity may allow the foot to assume a club foot appearance resulting from overpull of the unaffected foot muscles (Fig. 80).

Deformity in the lower extremity may be lessened by supporting the foot in a brace. If the disease is not rapidly progressive, operative correction of the foot deformity by removal of bone wedges followed by triple arthrodesis will provide a better functioning extremity for the patient.

SYRINGOMYELIA

Syringomyelia is a chronic, slowly progressive disease of the cervical portion of the spinal cord, characterized by cavity formation within the substance of the spinal cord tissue. The disease chiefly affects young people and causes a variety of motor, sensory, and trophic disturbances.

Orthopaedic interest in this neurologic disease centers about the appearance of a Charcot joint deformity in the upper extremity. Syr-

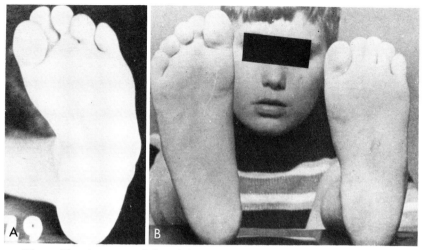

Figure 80. A, positional foot deformity in Charcot-Marie-Tooth disease. B, appearance after surgical correction.

ingomyelia usually results in a segmental loss of pain and temperature sensation, and a loss of position and vibration senses. In 10 to 40 per cent of patients, these sensory and trophic disturbances will allow the formation of a neurotrophic or Charcot joint deformity, frequently affecting the shoulder joint.

Traumatic Paraplegia and Quadriplegia

Severe injuries to the spine, such as fracture-dislocations and gunshot wounds, may damage the spinal cord and result in traumatic paraplegia or quadriplegia. Injuries below the level of the first thoracic vertebra produce a paralysis of both lower limbs (paraplegia); those above this level produce a paralysis of all four limbs (quadriplegia). Complete transection of the spinal cord results in permanent paralysis of all muscles supplied by motor neurons below the level of the lesion and permanent loss of skin sensation in all areas supplied by sensory neurons below the lesion.

Initially after injury, the patient exhibits a state of spinal shock characterized by flaccid paralysis and complete loss of skin sensation. After a few weeks the affected muscles develop permanent spasticity and the skin sensibility may drop to a slightly lower permanent level. Among the serious complications of spinal cord injury are paralytic incontinence of the bladder and rectum, urinary tract infections, and decubitus ulcers.

Surgical decompression of the spinal cord may be indicated if the paraplegia is incomplete at the beginning or if there is evidence of progression in the neurologic deficit. If the paraplegia is complete from the beginning, there is no value in surgical decompression. If an unstable fracture-dislocation of the spine is present, operative reduction and stabilization by fusion facilitate nursing care and enable the patient to get up with safety and comfort at an early stage in the rehabilitation period.

As soon as the patient's condition will permit, transfer to a spinal paraplegic center or a center for long-term care and rehabilitation should be effected. The overall management of paraplegic patients requires the combined skills of a large team. With wheelchair transfer, long leg braces, crutches, and gait training, the strongly motivated paraplegic whose cord lesion is not at too high a level may return to walking and may become self-supporting.

INVOLVEMENT AT NERVE ROOT LEVEL

OBSTETRICAL PALSY

Obstetrical palsy is the name given to a traction injury of the infant's brachial plexus caused by pulling on the arm during a difficult delivery. Injury to the nerve roots contributing to the brachial plexus may cause a muscular paralysis involving either the entire arm, the upper arm and shoulder only, or just the lower arm and hand. The most common injury involves the fifth and sixth cervical nerve roots and is associated with paralysis of the upper arm and shoulder region (*Erb's palsy*).

Following traction injury to the fifth and sixth cervical nerve roots, paralysis involves mainly the abductors and external rotators of the upper arm and shoulder. As a result the infant will be noticed to lie with the shoulder and arm in adduction and internal rotation and the forearm pronated. If the limb is allowed to remain in this position, the deformities will become fixed because of contracture of the unopposed normal muscles (Fig. 81). If this occurs, the child will be unable to abduct the arm well or to elevate it beyond the shoulder level.

The majority of patients suffering traction injuries to the brachial plexus recover spontaneously. During this time all joints of the involved limb must be put through a full range of motion in an attempt to prevent contractures. The affected upper extremity may be supported in a brace, with the arm held in a position opposite to that assumed by the deformity. The brace supports the weakened musculature while it regains strength, and also helps prevent the formation of joint contractures.

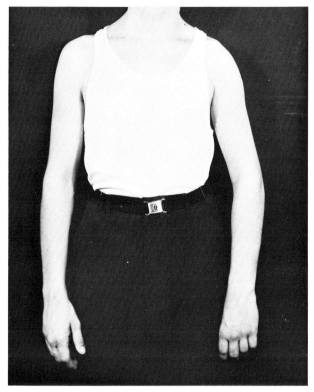

Figure 81.   Internal rotation contracture of left upper extremity in adolescent boy with untreated obstetrical palsy.

Operative treatment may be indicated in older children in whom complete spontaneous recovery has not occurred. Cutting through contracted tendons and muscles may allow better positioning of the arm. Transplantation of normal muscles to replace the paralyzed ones may effectively increase the muscular strength and function of the arm and shoulder. In some patients osteotomy through the shaft of the humerus is performed to allow rotation of the deformed upper extremity into a more functional position.

NERVE ROOT COMPRESSION

Abnormal conditions arising in the spine may be associated with mechanical compression of the adjacent spinal nerve roots. Herniated intervertebral disc, bony compression of the intervertebral foramen, tumor, or an osteoarthritic spur projecting posteriorly into the nerve root may give rise to rather characteristic signs and symptoms that would indicate compression at the nerve root level.

Abnormalities associated with nerve root compression occur most frequently in the cervical and lumbar segments of the spine.

The cervical nerve root compression syndrome is discussed on page 285. The lumbosacral nerve root compression syndrome is discussed on page 312.

INVOLVEMENT AT PERIPHERAL NERVE LEVEL

POLYNEURITIS

The term polyneuritis may be applied to any condition associated with irritation of multiple peripheral nerves. In general the condition is characterized by pain and tenderness along the affected nerve trunks and associated musculature. Paresthesias are common. Examination may disclose decreased or absent tendon reflexes along with motor and sensory disturbances.

Polyneuritis commonly has a nutritional, metabolic, or infectious basis.

Nutritional polyneuritis may be seen in the alcoholic and is thought to be due largely to avitaminosis. Polyneuritis may also be seen in the true vitamin deficiency diseases, such as beriberi and pellagra, and in leprosy.

Diabetes is the most frequent metabolic cause of polyneuritis. Polyneuritis is more likely to affect those patients whose diabetes is not under adequate control. It has been estimated that it occurs at one time or another in about 5 per cent of all patients with diabetes.

Infectious polyneuritis *(Guillain-Barré syndrome)* is an acute process characterized by an ascending progressive, symmetrical paralysis. The onset of this disorder frequently follows an upper respiratory infection. There is usually no associated sensory change. The process is differentiated from anterior poliomyelitis by the fact that the patient is afebrile and by the presence of an abnormally elevated spinal fluid protein content. Most patients make a spontaneous recovery following symptomatic and supportive treatment.

TRAUMA TO PERIPHERAL NERVES

Certain specific orthopaedic lesions carry with them the potential for damage to adjacent peripheral nerves. The examiner must be aware of this possibility so that the status of the peripheral nerve can be determined at the time of the initial examination. The radial, median, ulnar, and sciatic nerves are injured more frequently than other peripheral nerves in the body.

Radial Nerve. The radial nerve may be damaged in association with fractures through the mid-shaft of the humerus (see p. 238).

Trauma to the radial nerve at this level may result in a "wrist drop" deformity, in which the patient loses the ability actively to raise the wrist and the thumb and the metacarpophalangeal joints of the hand. Improper use of crutches, taking weight through the axilla rather than on the hand, may also in time produce a radial palsy with "wrist drop."

Median Nerve. The median nerve may be damaged by dislocation of the lunate bone at the wrist and may be implicated in the carpal tunnel syndrome (see p. 260). Trauma to the median nerve at this level may result in paralysis of the opponens pollicis muscle. If this occurs, the patient loses the ability actively to oppose the thumb to the remaining fingers.

Ulnar Nerve. The ulnar nerve may be damaged by trauma or fracture involving the medial epicondyle of the humerus at the elbow (see p. 250). Trauma to the ulnar nerve may result in paralysis of intrinsic hand muscles, and the patient may lose the power to spread and bring together all the fingers. Clawing of the fourth and fifth fingers may develop.

Sciatic Nerve. The sciatic nerve may be damaged in association with a fracture through the mid-shaft of the femur (see p. 359), or it may be damaged by the femoral head following traumatic posterior dislocation of the hip joint (see p. 351). Trauma to the sciatic nerve may result in complete paralysis of all the muscles of the lower leg and foot and partial paralysis of the thigh muscles.

Axillary Nerve. The axillary nerve may be damaged in association with anterior dislocation of the shoulder joint. Trauma to the axillary nerve may result in paralysis of the deltoid muscle, and the patient may lose the ability actively to abduct the arm at the shoulder joints.

Common Peroneal Nerve. The common peroneal nerve may be damaged by excessive pressure or injury to the head and neck region of the fibula. The most frequent orthopaedic cause of this involvement is a tight or inadequately padded plaster leg cast. Trauma to the common peroneal nerve may result in paralysis of the long toe extensor muscles, the anterior tibial muscle, and the peroneals. The patient may note a "foot drop," with loss of the ability actively to dorsiflex or evert the foot.

INVOLVEMENT AT MUSCLE LEVEL

PROGRESSIVE MUSCULAR DYSTROPHY

Progressive muscular dystrophy is a genetically determined, primary degenerative disease of muscle tissue transmitted as a sex-linked recessive character to male children predominantly. Although several types have been described, the *Duchenne* type of muscular dystrophy (pseudohypertrophic muscular dystrophy) is the commonest and most disabling form.

The disease usually has its onset during the first three years of life, primarily affecting the musculature of the pelvic girdle and shoulder girdle. In general, the muscles and segments of muscles formed first in the embryo are the first to be involved in the dystrophic process. Often the calf muscles appear thickened and enlarged but are actually quite weak in strength. The patient usually stands with an increased lumbar lordosis and walks with a waddling gait, with the trunk lurching from side to side with each step. The disease tends to be progressive, and the patient may ultimately lose all power over the hip, knee, ankle, shoulder, and elbow joints. Positional deformities with joint contractures may develop. Frequently, the disease terminates fatally during the second or third decade of life.

Laboratory investigation reveals an elevation of certain cellular enzymes which probably arise from affected muscles. These enzymes include creatine kinase, aldolase, and alanine transaminase. Electromyography is helpful in differentiating neurogenic muscular weakness from myogenic weakness. Muscle biopsy may assist in determining the exact type of muscular dystrophy. In pseudohypertrophic muscular dystrophy, the increased bulk of the muscle is due to excessive fibrous tissue and fat, rather than to muscular hypertrophy.

There is no known treatment. Orthopaedic care is supportive only. Lightweight braces are often helpful.

INVOLVEMENT AT MYONEURAL JUNCTION LEVEL

MYASTHENIA GRAVIS

Myasthenia gravis is a disease characterized by excessive fatigability of voluntary muscles. The disease is thought to be due to an abnormality at the myoneural junction and may affect a single muscle, a group of muscles, or all the muscles. Characteristically, muscle fatigue and weakness are aggravated by exertion and are typically worse toward the end of the day. A degree of muscle strength can usually be restored by rest.

The disease affects adult females most commonly. Most patients note facial symptoms due to fatigue of ocular, facial, jaw, and tongue muscles. Symptoms due to weakness of the upper and lower extremity muscles may also be noted. The muscles of the abdomen and the back may be affected. As a rule, myasthenia gravis is not progressive and may be characterized by long periods of remission.

Muscles fatigued as a result of myasthenia gravis show a dramatic return of strength following the administration of neostigmine bromide, which is a parasympathetic stimulant. Treatment of this disorder consists of a properly adjusted dose of neostigmine bromide, usually given in three oral doses of 15 mg. each, or the use of other indicated parasympathomimetic drugs.

References

Banker, B. Q.: Neuromuscular diseases. Med. Sci., 8:575, 1960.

Bechtol, C. O.: Muscle physiology. Am. Academy of Orthopaedic Surgeons Instructional Course Lectures, Vol. V:181. Ann Arbor: J. W. Edwards, 1948.

Bechtol, C. O.: Surgical application of muscle physiology. Am. Academy of Orthopaedic Surgeons Instructional Course Lectures, Vol. XII:161. Ann Arbor: J. W. Edwards, 1955.

Curtis, B. H.: Orthopaedic management of muscular dystrophy and related disorders. Am. Academy of Orthopaedic Surgeons Instructional Course Lectures, Vol. XIX. St. Louis: C. V. Mosby Co., 1970.

Denhoff, E., and Robinault, I. T.: Cerebral Palsy and Related Disorders. New York: McGraw-Hill, 1960.

Eggers, G. W., and Evans, E. B.: Surgery in cerebral palsy. J. Bone and Joint Surg., 45-A:1275, 1963.

Engels, W. K. (Ed.): Review of current concepts of myopathies. Clin. Orth. and Rel. Res., No. 39, 1965.

Holdsworth, Sir F.: Fractures, dislocations and fracture-dislocations of the spine. J. Bone and Joint Surg., 52-A:1534, 1970.

Last, R. J.: On the form and structure of muscles. J. Bone and Joint Surg., 34-B:195, 1952.

Levitt, R. L., Canale, S. T., Cooke, A. J., Jr., and Gartland, J. J.: The role of foot surgery in progressive neuromuscular disorders in children. J. Bone and Joint Surg., 55-A:1396, 1973.

Mommaerts, W. F. H. M.: Fundamental aspects of muscle function. J. Bone and Joint Surg., 41-A:1315, 1959.

Patterson, R. L., Jr., and Adler, J. B.: Erb's palsy: Long term results of treatment in 88 cases. J. Bone and Joint Surg., 49-A:1052, 1967.

Phelps, W. M.: Description and differentiation of types of cerebral palsy. Nerv. Child., 8:107, 1949.

Spencer, G. E., Jr.: Orthopaedic care of progressive muscular dystrophy. J. Bone and Joint Surg., 49-A:1201, 1967.

Vignos, P. J., Jr.: Diagnosis of progressive muscular dystrophy. J. Bone and Joint Surg., 49-A:1212, 1967.

Vignos, P. J., Jr., Spencer, G. E., Jr., and Archibald, K. C.: Management of progressive muscular dystrophy of childhood. JAMA, 184:89, 1963.

Chapter Eight

Disturbances in Skeletal Development

INTRODUCTION

In this chapter are described the relatively rare but frequently bizarre orthopaedic conditions brought about by abnormal influences on bone tissue. These abnormal influences are of a generalized character and include errors in calcium metabolism, errors in tissue metabolism, dietary or nutritional errors, endocrine dysfunction, and congenital errors in bone tissue development.

Constitutional diseases of bone with a known pathogenesis include chromosomal aberrations, metabolic abnormalities, and the mucopolysaccharidoses. Constitutional diseases of bone with an unknown pathogenesis include abnormalities of cartilage or bone growth and development; disorganized development of cartilage and fibrous components of the skeleton; malformation of individual bones, singly or in combination; and abnormalities of density of cortical diaphyseal structure, of metaphyseal modeling, or of both. Bone abnormalities may also arise secondary to a disturbance in an extraskeletal system, as in the endocrine, hematologic, neurologic, renal, gastrointestinal, or cardiopulmonary systems.

CONDITIONS ASSOCIATED WITH GENETIC ABNORMALITIES

ACHONDROPLASIA

Achondroplasia is congenital dwarfism resulting from a developmental error of enchondral ossification in which there is failure of nor-

164

mal ossification of the long bones but not of the flat bones. Skeletal changes are usually noticeable at birth, which is frequently premature. Subsequent growth results in the formation of a dwarf with short limbs and a relatively large head (Fig. 82). Epiphyseal closure usually occurs at the normal time. The adult height of an achondroplastic dwarf is seldom more than 4 feet. As a rule, mental and sexual development are normal.

The deformity is transmitted by an autosomal dominant gene. The underlying defect is a failure of longitudinal growth in the cartilage of the growth plate. The exact nature of this error of localized cartilage growth is unknown.

Orthopaedic treatment is sometimes required for associated skeletal deformities. The achondroplastic dwarf may have marked lumbar lordosis with low back pain. Bowleg deformity, deformities about the hip, and deformities about the elbow may require corrective treatment.

MULTIPLE EXOSTOSES (DIAPHYSEAL ACLASIS)

Multiple exostoses is the result of a developmental error that restricts metaphyseal remodeling during longitudinal growth. Multiple outgrowths of bony exostoses or spurs capped with cartilage gradually develop from the abnormally broad metaphyseal region of long bones.

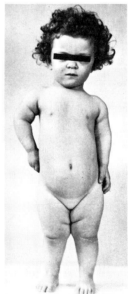

Figure 82. Achondroplastic dwarf. (Courtesy Dr. Beckett Howorth, Greenwich, Conn.

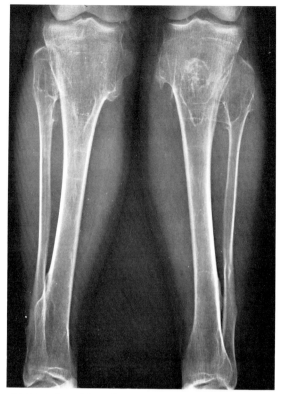

Figure 83. Multiple broad-based exostoses projecting from both the proximal and distal ends of the tibia and fibula.

These exostoses always point away from the adjacent epiphysis (Fig. 83).

The deformity is transmitted by an autosomal dominant gene. The underlying defect is believed to be an absence of the normal osteoclastic activity in the process of remodeling the metaphysis during longitudinal growth. This not only results in the formation of the exostoses but also may cause shortening and bowing of some long bones.

The patient may exhibit many exostoses of varying size, usually found at the ends of long bones at the knee, wrist, or shoulder, or at both ends of the fibula. These changes are infrequent in the bones of the hands and feet. As a rule the exostoses stop growing and their cartilage caps ossify after skeletal bone growth ceases.

X-ray examination reveals the presence of multiple broad-based exostoses projecting from the shafts of the affected bones. The parent long bones are frequently thickened and distorted in shape.

Most exostoses produce no symptoms and do not require surgical removal. Some are associated with pain, caused by local pressure against tendons, nerves, or other sensitive tissues. Those exostoses causing pain should be excised. The development of chondrosarcoma in an exostosis has been reported in adults, but it is quite rare.

This condition must not be confused with the presence of a single solitary osteochondroma, which is considered a benign tumor of bone (see p. 196).

Osteogenesis Imperfecta (Fragilitas Ossium)

Osteogenesis imperfecta is a crippling condition associated with weakness and fragility of all bones of the body. As a result the bones are soft and fragile, and multiple fractures are the rule.

The disease is transmitted by an autosomal dominant gene. The underlying defect is believed to involve bone matrix and to be associated with an impaired maturation of collagen fibers, or possibly with the synthesis of an abnormal collagen. Some evidence suggests a qualitative defect in the osteoblasts, resulting in excessive osteoclasis.

Osteogenesis imperfecta may be apparent at birth or may appear shortly thereafter. Many infants survive only a few weeks. In many patients with this condition a very definite China blue coloration of the sclerae may be noted.

X-ray examination reveals slender, frequently deformed osteoporotic bones with very thin cortices.

Surviving patients may sustain multiple fractures, which usually heal surprisingly well following immobilization. Prolonged immobilization must be avoided, however, since it adds the problem of disuse atrophy to the already weak bones.

The skeletal deformity that results from bone softening and multiple fractures may cause dwarfism and structural abnormalities of the extremities, spine, and pelvis. Severe bowing of long bones can be corrected by performing multiple segmental osteotomies through the bone and using intramedullary metal rod fixation as internal support until bone healing occurs.

Osteopetrosis (Albers-Schönberg Disease, Marble Bones)

Osteopetrosis is a rare condition characterized by the formation of extremely hard dense bones throughout the skeleton. The formation of abnormally dense bone continues until skeletal growth ceases. The markedly increased bone density gives rise to the synonym marble bone disease.

The disease is transmitted by an autosomal recessive gene. The essential pathologic defect is believed to be failure of osteoclastic resorption of bone.

X-ray examination reveals the excessive density of all the affected bones.

The dense sclerotic bone may compromise the marrow cavity, causing an aplastic anemia that may be fatal. Optic atrophy may be noted. Pathologic fracture through these bones may occur. Healing of this type of bone tissue may be slow, and delayed union of the fracture is relatively common.

Neurofibromatosis (Von Recklinghausen's Disease)

Neurofibromatosis is a bizarre developmental anomaly characterized by multiple light brown pigmented spots on the skin (café au lait spots), multiple fibrous pedunculated tumors in the skin and soft tissue, and multiple neurofibromata of the peripheral nerves, cranial nerves, or spinal nerves.

The abnormality is transmitted by an autosomal dominant gene. It may appear at any age and affects males more frequently than females. It is also known as Von Recklinghausen's disease, but the reader should be aware that occasionally hyperparathyroidism is known as Von Recklinghausen's disease as well.

Orthopaedic interest is focused upon the skeletal complications of neurofibromatosis which develop in about one-half of the afflicted patients. Severe scoliosis is frequently an associated deformity. Fibromatous lesions may cause local erosion defects in bone, and occasionally actual cysts may be found within the bone substance. Neurofibromatosis has been suspected as a cause of congenital pseudarthrosis of the tibia. Occasionally, gross enlargement or gigantism of all or part of an extremity is seen. Symptoms and signs resulting from peripheral nerve involvement vary according to the particular nerve affected. The tumors possess a definite tendency to undergo secondary sarcomatous change with an ultimately fatal outcome.

The Mucopolysaccharidoses

In 1919 Gertrude Hurler, a German pediatrician, described two children suffering from a disease characterized by mental retardation, skeletal dysplasia, and a gibbus. Hurler's syndrome, which is autosomal recessive, and the X-linked form described by Hunter became the prototypes of the mucopolysaccharidoses, a group of related heritable disorders of connective tissue with skeletal manifestations of varying severity. A defect in connective tissue metabolism results in widespread deposition of specific mucopolysaccharides in the tissues and their excessive excretion in the urine.

These patients are usually normal at birth with the stigmata of their disease frequently not appearing until after the first year of life. A striking feature in the history is the progressive nature of these diseases. As a result of the biochemical abnormality, these patients develop varying and progressive degrees of mental retardation and severe skeletal disorders. Hurler's syndrome usually terminates fatally at a young age.

To date, six distinct syndromes have been described and the specific mucopolysaccharide identified.

TYPE	MUCOPOLYSACCHARIDE
Hurler's syndrome	Heparan sulphate and dermatan sulphate
Hunter's syndrome	Heparan sulphate and dermatan sulphate
Sanfilippo's syndrome	Heparan sulphate and chondroitin sulphate
Morquio's syndrome	Chondroitin sulphate and keratan sulphate
Scheie's syndrome	Heparan sulphate and dermatan sulphate
Maroteaux-Lamy syndrome	Dermatan sulphate

The diagnosis of mucopolysaccharidosis is made by the characteristic historical, clinical, and biochemical findings. Biochemical analysis to determine the specific mucopolysaccharide excreted in excess in the urine aids in early diagnosis. Fibroblast cultures are also helpful for diagnosis and genetic counseling. These studies take advantage of the tendency of the intracellular mucopolysaccharides to stain pink with toluidine blue dye. Clinically normal-appearing carriers also show a high incidence of pink-staining fibroblasts. This information is useful in genetic counseling.

Various skeletal abnormalities may be encountered. Skeletal dysplasia is present in all mucopolysaccharidoses but varies markedly in severity, being mild in Sanfillippo's syndrome and severe in patients with Hurler's and Morquio's syndromes. Spine deformities may be a problem in patients with Morquio's and Maroteaux-Lamy syndromes. Odontoid dysplasia and cord compression have been seen in these patients. Occasionally a patient with Morquio's syndrome may develop progressive quadriparesis or die suddenly while sleeping or during the induction of anesthesia.

Bowleg deformity is seen mostly in patients with Morquio's syndrome. This deformity can be corrected by osteotomy. Flexion contractures are found in all the mucopolysaccharidoses except Morquio's syndrome, in which patients tend to be loose jointed. Carpal tunnel syndrome and cavus feet have been reported in patients with Scheie's syndrome.

GAUCHER'S DISEASE

Gaucher's disease is a rare reticuloendothelial disease due to an inborn error of lipid metabolism. In this disease, proliferating reticuloendothelial cells in the spleen, liver, lymphoid tissue, and bone marrow are filled with the lipid kerasin. The kerasin filled cells are called Gaucher's cells. The disease is characterized by a relatively slow course, enormous enlargement of the spleen, anemia with leukopenia, hemorrhagic tendencies, and bone lesions. The more severe forms of Gaucher's disease, seen in early childhood, have a worse prognosis than the forms encountered later in life.

Gaucher's cells infiltrate the bone marrow and cause localized osteolytic lesions of bone. Some lesions may be complicated by avascular necrosis, particularly in the femoral head. Gaucher's disease is usually associated with a mottled-appearing enlargement or expansion of the lower end of the femur. It is said that when viewed on the x-ray film, the lower end of the femur in Gaucher's disease resembles an Erlenmeyer flask.

Diagnosis is made by demonstrating Gaucher's cells in bone marrow obtained by marrow aspiration.

No specific curative treatment exists, although x-ray therapy is usually effective in decreasing the size of the bone lesions.

CONDITIONS ASSOCIATED WITH DIETARY OR METABOLIC ABNORMALITIES

CALCIUM DEFICIENCY DISEASES

The bony skeleton of vertebrates serves two principal functions. It gives a rigid structural protection for the soft tissues of the body, and it provides a calcium reservoir for maintaining calcium homeostasis in the living organism. Normally the body's major source of calcium is the diet. Calcium, however, is poorly absorbed from the gut, and vitamin D is required to increase the rate of calcium absorption from this area. The actual rate of calcium absorption from the intestine is regulated by calcium ion concentration of the extracellular fluids. A type of feedback control system operates constantly to maintain a normal calcium ion concentration. The agent maintaining this feedback system is thought to be parathyroid hormone.

The metabolism of vitamin D and its mechanism of action are quite complicated and not yet completely understood. Vitamin D in the human is derived from the diet and from the skin. It appears that 7-dihydrocholesterol is synthesized from steroids in the body and converted at an unknown anatomic site in the skin to cholecalciferol (vitamin D3). Cholecalciferol is then metabolized in the liver to 25-hydroxycholecalciferol (25-HCC). This is the circulating, biologically active form of vitamin D carried in the blood stream on an alpha globulin.

Recently a further metabolite, apparently produced in renal tissue, has been identified as 1,25-dihydroxycholecalciferol (1,25-DHCC). This substance functions as a hormone and is active in the serosa of the intestine, the bone cell nucleus, and kidney tubular cells. The level of 1,25-dihydroxycholecalciferol is controlled by a negative feedback mechanism through dietary and serum calcium. The action of 1,25-DHCC is thought to be stimulation of messenger RNA production in the cell nucleus, leading to an increased production of calcium-binding protein. This in turn increases pickup of calcium ions at the brush border of the serosal cell and transport of calcium ions into the cell and eventually into the serum.

Bone tissue, because of its calcified collagenous intercellular substance, serves an important bodily function by acting as a storage depot for calcium. As a result of physiologic demands, bone tissue may release some of its stored calcium to meet the immediate needs of the patient for this ion and to maintain a normal calcium ion concentration in the extracellular fluids.

The body will readily sacrifice structural integrity of the skeleton to maintain serum calcium levels. When the physiologic demands become abnormal, serum calcium homeostasis is maintained at the expense of intact skeletal development, and calcium deficiency diseases may appear.

The calcium deficiency disease of infants and children is called rickets. The same disease appearing in the adult is called osteomalacia. Both rickets and osteomalacia can be found in association with renal disease, in addition to appearing independently.

Rickets.   Rickets, the calcium deficiency disease of infants and children, is caused by vitamin D deficiency or dietary lack of calcium and phosphorus. Improved infant nutrition has now made nutritional rickets a medical curiosity except in the underdeveloped areas of the world. However, malabsorption may cause a nutritional rickets in spite of adequate dietary intake of vitamin D by preventing the intestinal mucosa from absorbing the available vitamin D. Gluten sensitive enteropathy or celiac disease, liver disease, such as congenital biliary atresia, and fibrocystic disease with pancreatitis are among the disorders predisposing to malabsorption. The calcium deficiency allows the infant's bones to soften and become deformed.

This physiologic abnormality causes a relative increase throughout the body of osteoid tissue, which is the protein base in which the calcium and phosphorus have failed to deposit. This results in cranio-tabes, or frontal and parietal bossing of the skull; epiphyseal thicken-ing, noted particularly about the wrist, ankle, and knee; enlargement of the cartilage of the costochondral junctions, giving a beading effect known as the rachitic rosary; generalized weakness and lethargy; and delayed milestones of sitting, standing, and walking.

The pull of the diaphragm produces a horizontal depression on the thorax called "Harrison's groove." The thorax may become flat-tened laterally, producing a pigeon breast deformity, and in severe cases the thoracic deformities may seriously compromise pulmonary ventilation. Once sitting commences, a kyphoscoliosis may develop. Once walking commences, deformities in the long bones may occur with the stress of weight bearing. Knock knee, bowleg, and coxa vara deformity are not uncommon (Fig. 84). Greenstick fractures of long bones may occur. Because of the involvement of epiphyseal cartilage, rickets may affect longitudinal bone growth.

The x-ray findings in rickets are distinctive. There is a general-ized osteoporosis and a thinning of the cortices and bone trabeculae. Affected epiphyses may appear irregular and fuzzy, with widening of the growth plate. The metaphyses may appear frayed, widened, and

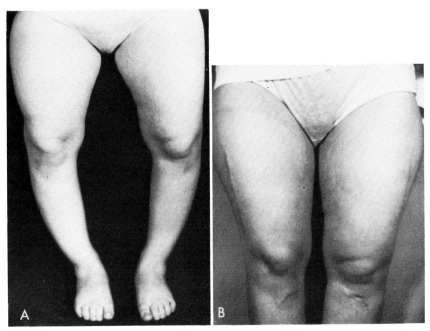

Figure 84. A, severe bowleg deformity in patient with hypophosphatemic rickets. B, same patient after correction of deformity by femoral and tibial osteotomies.

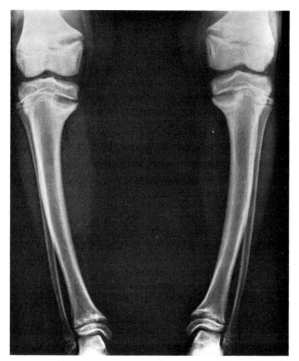

Figure 85. X-ray of lower extremities of patient with hypophosphatemic rickets. Note the irregular, fuzzy, and broadened growth plates at the knee and ankle joints and the typical bowing of the tibiae.

occasionally cup-shaped (Fig. 85). The areas of most rapid bone growth show the greatest involvement. These areas include distal radius and ulna, distal femur, proximal tibia, proximal humerus, and the costochondral junctions.

Laboratory examination usually reveals a low serum phosphorus and a high serum alkaline phosphatase. Although rickets is a calcium deficiency disease, the serum calcium is usually maintained at a normal level through withdrawals of calcium from the skeletal storage depot by parathyroid hormone.

Treatment of active rickets includes the use of a high calcium diet, large doses of vitamin D, and exposure to sunlight or ultraviolet rays. Many of the skeletal deformities spontaneously regress with correction of the physiologic defect. Some orthopaedic deformities may be corrected by the use of braces. Persisting deformities of the long bones frequently require surgical correction by osteotomy.

Osteomalacia. Osteomalacia (the term means "softening of the bone") is the adult form of rickets. The main difference is that in osteomalacia epiphyseal cartilage and longitudinal bone growth are unaffected because onset of the disease occurs after closure of the growth plates. Osteomalacia may be caused by dietary calcium deficiency, chronic diarrhea, excessive calcium demands of pregnancy and lactation, longstanding lack of sunshine, or renal acidosis.

Renal Disease (Renal Rickets, Renal Osteodystrophy). In recent years a definite physiologic relationship has been established between chronic renal insufficiency and the appearance of abnormal skeletal changes. Although several different clinical states exist, the general relationship was, in the past, described by the loose term renal rickets. Severe renal insufficiency is associated with a renal acidosis. All available calcium is used by the body to neutralize the renal acidosis. When this supply proves insufficient, a compensatory parathyroid hyperplasia occurs to increase the amount of circulating parathyroid hormone. This hormone releases calcium from the skeletal storage depot. The skeleton, thus deprived of calcium, undergoes abnormal changes. If this process occurs in children, rickets results. If it occurs in adults, osteomalacia is produced. In addition to the changes of rickets or osteomalacia, the secondary parathyroid hyperplasia may promote osteoclastic resorption and fibrosis of bone, with the production of cystic changes and bone destruction resembling the changes seen with osteitis fibrosa cystica (see p. 179).

Skeletal changes are now known to occur with two broad categories of renal disease. The term renal rickets is being abandoned in favor of more specific nomenclature.

The first category consists of renal diseases associated with impaired glomerular filtration. The primary cause may be chronic glomerulonephritis, chronic pyelonephritis, congenital anomaly of the kidney, obstructive uropathy, or heavy metal poisoning. These patients present with chronic renal failure and uremia. The skeletal disturbance accompanying this state has been referred to as *renal osteodystrophy.*

The second category consists of renal diseases associated with defective function of the renal tubules. At least seven different clinical states have been determined to fit this second category. The commonest is hypophosphatemic rickets, inherited as a sex-linked dominant trait. This was formerly known as vitamin D resistant rickets. These patients are usually not sick but present with the physical signs and x-ray findings of rickets or osteomalacia. They exhibit a low serum phosphate due to phosphaturia and tubular inability to absorb phosphate.

Fanconi's syndrome is a less common clinical state associated with renal tubular defects and skeletal changes. In this condition there is failure to resorb phosphates, glucose, and amino acids normally, and acidosis is frequently present. Serum calcium is normal or low; phosphorus is low; and alkaline phosphatase is increased. Dwarfism and skeletal deformity may be severe.

VITAMIN INFLUENCES ON BONE TISSUE

Vitamin A. Vitamin overdosage may result in chronic vitamin A intoxication which, in children, may cause disturbances of bone growth because of this vitamin's specific effect on osteoblasts, osteoclasts, and epiphyseal chondroblasts of growing bone. Short thick bones result from cortical thickening and premature epiphyseal closure. Prognosis for normal development is excellent after correction of the vitamin overdosage.

Vitamin C (Scurvy). Scurvy is a nutritional disease caused by a lack of vitamin C in the diet. Vitamin C is an important factor in regulating the formation of intercellular substances such as osteoid, collagen, and ground substance. Deficiency of this essential vitamin causes an abnormality of the intercellular matrix, particularly of cells and tissues of mesodermal origin. The disease is characterized by hemorrhagic tendencies, particularly beneath mucous membranes and the periosteum. Wound healing is poor in those with scurvy.

Subperiosteal hemorrhages are the characteristic orthopaedic phenomena of scurvy and involve the knee and shoulder areas most frequently. The growth plate may weaken, sometimes allowing affected epiphyses to displace from their normal position. The effects of scurvy may cause a delay in osteogenesis, with a resulting decrease in the density of the bone tissue. Pathologic fractures may occur.

Treatment consists of the addition of citrus fruits, fruit juices, and ascorbic acid to the diet. Specific orthopaedic treatment is rarely required for skeletal complaints.

Vitamin D. The human organism requires vitamin D to influence the rate of absorption of ingested calcium from the gastrointestinal tract. This is absolutely essential to maintain normal calcium and phosphorus levels in the blood without making abnormal physiologic demands on the skeletal system. As previously discussed, deficiency of vitamin D causes rickets and osteomalacia.

OSTEOPOROSIS

Osteoporosis is a type of metabolic bone atrophy with an unknown mechanism of causation. The bone tissue is qualitatively normal, but there is too little of it as a result of a deficiency in protein matrix formation, caused by decreased osteoblastic activity combined with increased osteoclastic resorption of bone. This results in a marked decrease in the total amount of bone in the skeleton.

Osteoporosis is the commonest metabolic affection of bone tissue and involves mostly the vertebral bodies, the pelvis, and areas containing large amounts of cancellous bone. It has been estimated to be radiologically detectable in 50 per cent of all persons over 65 years of age. It is believed that approximately 20 per cent of elderly persons develop symptoms attributable to osteoporosis because bone tissue that is lost by normal catabolism is not replaced in equal measure by new bone.

Calcium and phosphorus metabolism are unaffected in osteoporosis. The bony trabeculae become thin and sparse, with the result that compact bone is transformed into spongy bone with more open texture. Thus bone mineral content is normal but matrix is insufficient. The most important clinical implication of osteoporosis, of course, is that affected bones are prone to fracture.

There are many causes of osteoporosis: disuse of a part, prolonged immobilization, protein deficiency states, hormone deficiency (including postmenopausal) states, conditions associated with negative calcium balance, and prolonged corticosteroid therapy. The most frequently encountered cause of osteoporosis, however, is senility. The condition is seen more than twice as often in women as in men and is frequently manifested as an impairment of the bony strength of the spine.

Spinal osteoporosis, the result of the decreased osteoblastic activity that may accompany senility and postmenopausal states, may lead to pain and deformity. Compression fractures in the thoracolumbar segment are common. Progressive loss of height of the vertebral bodies due to compression of the softened bone may produce kyphosis or round back deformity or actual shortening of the patient's stature.

On x-ray examination the vertebral bodies appear translucent, and there is loss of the normal trabecular pattern (Fig. 86). The thoracic vertebrae become wedge-shaped, and the bodies of the lumbar vertebrae appear biconcave as a result of pressure of the intervertebral discs on the softened bone. Often spontaneous compression fractures are seen in the thoracic and lumbar spine.

Treatment is empiric and generally unsatisfactory because the mechanism of causation is not understood. Brace support for the spine may be necessary in the presence of painful compression fractures. A diet high in protein, calcium, and phosphorus, with vitamin D supplement, helps obtain a positive calcium balance. The administration of estrogens and androgens, alone or in combination, is thought to be indicated because of the anabolic effect of these hormones on bone tissue. Their use is helpful in relieving pain but does not demonstrably result in increased bone production. Currently, there is clinical inter-

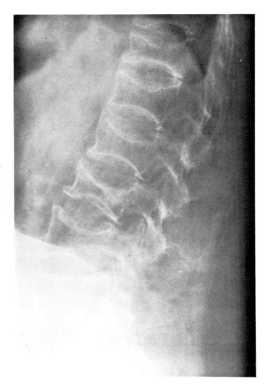

Figure 86. Lateral x-ray of lumbar spine, illustrating the biconcave appearance and compression of vertebral bodies in senile osteoporosis.

est in using fluoride to treat osteoporosis because of its supposed ability to strengthen the apatite crystal of bone. No convincing long-term therapeutic results have yet appeared.

CONDITIONS ASSOCIATED WITH ENDOCRINE DYSFUNCTION

Dysfunction of certain endocrine glands may have far-reaching orthopaedic implications because of the effect of the imbalance on skeletal tissue. The specific effect exerted on the skeleton will depend largely on the age of the patient at the time the particular endocrine dysfunction arises. As a rule, the younger the patient at the time of onset, the more profound will be the effect on skeletal tissue.

Pituitary, thyroid, and parathyroid gland problems are generally associated with the greatest changes in skeletal tissue. Hypersecretion of growth hormone by the anterior lobe of the pituitary may cause acceleration of bone growth, resulting in overgrowth and increased stature. On the other hand, decrease in secretion of either growth hormone or thyroid hormone may have the opposite effect on bone growth, resulting in undergrowth and dwarfism. Oversecretion of parathyroid hormone gives rise to a curious medical disease called *generalized osteitis fibrosa cystica,* which is characterized by diffuse skeletal osteoporosis, cystic changes in bone, and certain abnormalities in blood chemistry. Thyroid hormone has an effect on the maturation of bone tissue in children.

HYPERPITUITARISM

Hypersecretion of growth hormone is caused by an eosinophilic adenoma of the anterior lobe of the pituitary gland. If this tumor appears during childhood, the excess of growth hormone stimulates the growth plate to a remarkable degree to cause bone overgrowth and gigantism. Growth hormone exerts no particular delaying effect on the growth plate, so epiphyseal closure usually occurs at the normal time. Children so affected often show subnormal sexual development. The condition may be complicated by slipping of the capital femoral epiphysis (see p. 344).

Excess of growth hormone in the adult cannot affect longitudinal bone growth but does affect circumferential bone growth, resulting in thicker bones. If hypersecretion of growth hormone occurs in the adult, a condition known as *acromegaly* results. The bones of the skull, face, and jaw and those in the hands and feet become thick and enlarged. Enlargement and thickening of the soft tissues of the face, hands, feet, and viscera contribute to the physical deformity that characterizes an acromegalic patient.

HYPOPITUITARISM

Hyposecretion of growth hormone may be caused by a tumor or suprasellar cyst compressing the anterior lobe of the pituitary gland. Deficiency of growth hormone causes marked undergrowth of skeletal tissue and dwarfism. The dwarfism may be present at birth or may appear during the first few years of life.

Some patients with hypopituitarism may exhibit dwarfism associated with normal body proportions and normal mental development (*Lorain* type of dwarfism). Other patients may exhibit relatively normal growth associated with obesity, subnormal sexual development, and a predilection to develop slipping of the capital femoral epiphysis (*dystrophia-adiposo-genitalis, Fröhlich's syndrome*).

HYPOTHYROIDISM

Congenital hypothyroidism in children results in a condition known as *cretinism.* The cretin typically has a dull, sleepy facial expression, thick lips, a thick, protruding tongue, and mental and sexual retardation.

Deficiency of thyroid hormone delays ossification of skeletal tissue and retards longitudinal growth of bone. The epiphyses appear later than normal and may remain open for many years past regular closure time, but they do not make a significant contribution to longitudinal bone growth. For this reason, a cretin may be a dwarf. If this condition is diagnosed early and treated by thyroid extract for life, significant improvement can be anticipated.

Hypothyroidism in the adult produces a condition called *myxedema*. There are usually no specific associated skeletal abnormalities in the adult.

HYPERPARATHYROIDISM

Tumors of the parathyroid gland, usually occurring in adults, may result in excessive secretion of parathyroid hormone, which can exert profound metabolic effects on skeletal tissue to produce a relatively rare clinical condition known as *generalized osteitis fibrosa cystica* or primary hyperparathyroidism. Excess of parathyroid hormone causes excessive osteoclastic resorption of bone with marrow fibrosis, upsets calcium and phosphorus metabolism, and results in a generalized osteoporosis and decrease in bone density. Fibrous lined cysts of irregular size and distribution may appear in any bone but are most frequently seen in the bones of the extremities and pelvis. Growths resembling giant cell tumors may be found at the ends of long bones. The bones are softened by the osteoporosis, decreased density, and cystic changes. Actual bone absorption may be noted on the x-ray film (Fig. 87).

The patient with primary hyperparathyroidism may complain of severe skeletal pain. The bone softening may result in skeletal deformities and pathologic fracture. Between 50 and 75 per cent of patients may have associated renal complications, including hematuria, kidney stones, and renal failure with uremia.

Laboratory examination reveals elevation of the serum calcium and alkaline phosphatase levels but decrease in the serum phosphorus level.

Primary hyperparathyroidism with skeletal changes must be differentiated from osteoporosis, osteomalacia, polyostotic fibrous dysplasia, Paget's disease, multiple myeloma, and metastatic carcinoma.

Secondary hyperparathyroidism may be seen in patients with chronic renal insufficiency. Severe renal insufficiency is associated with a renal acidosis. All available calcium is used by the body to neutralize the renal acidosis. When this supply proves insufficient, a

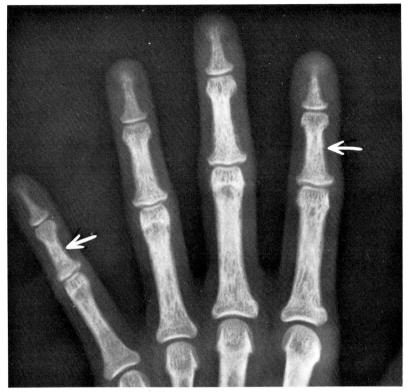

Figure 87. Hyperparathyroidism. Note subperiosteal absorption of bone. This is seen only with hyperparathyroidism.

compensatory parathyroid hyperplasia occurs to increase the amount of circulating parathyroid hormone so that extra calcium can be released from the skeletal storage depot. The skeleton, thus deprived of calcium, undergoes abnormal changes (see p. 174).

CONDITIONS CAUSED BY UNKNOWN FACTORS

RETICULOENDOTHELIOSIS (HISTIOCYTOSIS X)

Under the heading of Reticuloendotheliosis are listed a group of unusual granulomatous conditions implicating the skeletal system. Although clinically these conditions differ considerably, they are thought to be related because of fundamental pathologic similarities. Proliferation of reticuloendothelial cells within bone may produce disseminated granulomatous lesions throughout the skeleton, characterized histologically by the presence of histiocytes.

1. EOSINOPHILIC GRANULOMA

Eosinophilic granuloma is a localized benign form of reticuloendotheliosis, developing as a granulomatous lesion in bone. The lesion is composed of histiocytes and an overabundance of eosinophils. These lesions most frequently affect children and young adults and usually involve ribs, flat bones, vertebrae, and shafts of long bones.

Although it is most common to see a single lesion, multiple lesions and involvement of several bones have been described. The growth of this granulomatous tissue within the bone substance may cause pain and local tenderness. Pathologic fracture may occur through the lesion, but healing of the fracture always follows.

On x-ray examination the lesion of the eosinophilic granuloma resembles an oval or circular cyst within the medullary area of the bone, showing clear-cut margins and no surrounding reactive bone formation (Fig. 88). These lesions may be mistaken for osteomyelitis, osteoid osteoma, Ewing's sarcoma, osteogenic sarcoma, multiple myeloma, bone cyst, and giant cell tumor.

The natural history of these lesions seems to indicate gradual spontaneous healing. Frequently biopsy is carried out to rule out the other conditions often confused with eosinophilic granuloma. Exci-

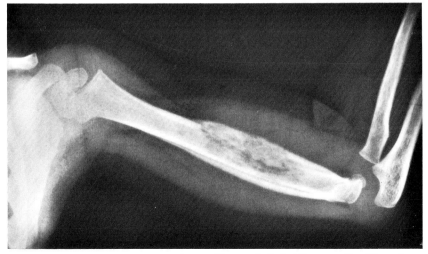

Figure 88.   Eosinophilic granuloma of humeral shaft. (Courtesy Dr. Albert Berg, Staten Island, N.Y.).

sion or curettage of the lesion induces healing. Radiotherapy may also be curative when surgical treatment cannot be carried out.

2. HAND-SCHÜLLER-CHRISTIAN DISEASE

This is a relatively rare chronic granulomatous type of reticuloendotheliosis with an onset during early childhood. It is characterized by multiple destructive lesions in the skull, spine, pelvis, and long bones. In addition, the patient may have exophthalmos and diabetes insipidus.

Histologically, granulomatous material from a Hand-Schüller-Christian disease lesion contains histiocytes laden with cholesterol.

X-ray therapy may induce healing of the skeletal lesions, but a fatal outcome is often the result in a patient with extensive involvement.

3. LETTERER-SIWE DISEASE

This is a very rare generalized form of reticuloendotheliosis of infancy which some authorities regard as an acute form of Hand-Schüller-Christian disease. The disease is characterized by an acute onset, typically short course, and invariably fatal outcome. The patient usually succumbs to the disease before significant bone lesions develop.

ENCHONDROMATOSIS (DYSCHONDROPLASIA, OLLIER'S DISEASE)

Enchondromatosis is a rare condition resulting from an unknown developmental error affecting cartilage cells at many growth plates. Masses or nests of cartilage cells in varying stages of development become displaced into the metaphyses of the affected bones instead of being calcified and ossified in the normal manner.

Curiously, the lesions caused by this developmental error tend to involve one side of the body more then the opposite side. These cartilage filled spaces in abnormal skeletal locations may cause shortening, deformity, or pathologic fracture of the affected bone. Malignant degeneration of the abnormal cartilage may occur.

The lesions of enchondromatosis are most often found in the hands and feet and at the growing ends of the long bones. Disturbances of development at the growth plate may result in a knock knee or bowleg deformity, clubhand deformity, or cubitus varus deformity at the elbow (see pp. 377–378, 66, 240).

X-ray examination reveals mottled cystic spaces of irregular size

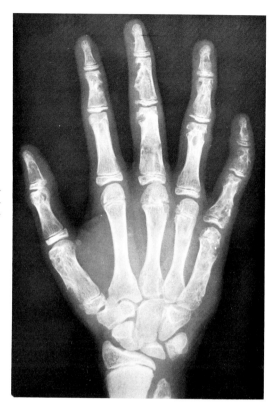

Figure 89. Multiple irregular cyst formation and bone deformity typical of enchondromatosis.

and shape in the metaphyses of affected bones (Fig. 89). Enchondromatosis should not be confused with benign enchondroma, which is a single enchondroma in bone and is classified as a benign bone tumor.

There is no specific treatment for enchondromatosis. Leg length equalization operations or osteotomy to correct angular deformities may be indicated occasionally.

FIBROUS DYSPLASIA

Fibrous dysplasia is a peculiar skeletal anomaly brought about by a disturbance in the normal physiologic rhythm between bone formation and bone replacement in mature bone tissue. Normally, bone tissue is constantly dying and being replaced by new bone. Fibrous dysplasia arises when some bone tissue is instead replaced by an irregular mass of tissue containing spicules of bone and masses of cartilage embedded in a fibrous tissue matrix. This abnormal tissue is thought to develop during the growth period of bone and to stop producing with the cessation of bone growth. The etiology of the disorder is unknown, but most authorities consider it to be a noninherited dysplasia of developmental origin.

Clinically, fibrous dysplasia may be seen in one of three forms. It may be confined entirely to one bone, in which case it is called *monostotic* fibrous dysplasia. If more than one bone is involved, it is referred to as *polyostotic* fibrous dysplasia. *Albright's syndrome* is a relatively rare triad seen mostly in girls, which consists of polyostotic fibrous dysplasia, irregular patches of café au lait pigmentation on the skin, and precocious puberty.

The lesions of fibrous dysplasia grow slowly, frequently deforming bone and causing premature closure of epiphyses. The disorder may affect any bone, but involvement of long bones is most common. The clinical effects may be pain, enlargement or deformity of bone, or pathologic fracture. The fractures usually heal well, except those of the upper third of the femur. Severe femoral deformation is the rule after multiple fractures in this area, causing some of the most crippling features of the disease. Fibrosarcoma has been reported to develop in areas of fibrous dysplasia.

X-ray examination reveals an irregular multilocular or scalloped lesion, usually in the shaft of a long bone (Fig. 90). The overlying cortical bone is frequently thinned and expanded around the lesion. The abnormal fibrous tissue within the lesion gives a certain opacity to its reflection on the x-ray film that may be likened to ground glass.

There is no specific treatment for fibrous dysplasia. Biopsy is performed when the diagnosis is in doubt. In a more localized lesion, it might be feasible to perform resection or wide excision of the area. In other instances it might be preferable to scrape out the abnormal tissue surgically and fill the resulting bone defect with fresh bone chips from the ilium.

These surgical techniques are not feasible in the presence of polyostotic fibrous dysplasia, however. Treatment in this instance is directed toward correcting deformities brought about by pathologic fracture, such as bowing of long bones or nonunion of the fracture. Corrective osteotomy and bone grafting may be indicated.

PAGET'S DISEASE (OSTEITIS DEFORMANS)

Paget's disease is a chronic skeletal disease of unknown cause characterized by progressive structural deformities most frequently seen in the pelvis, femur, tibia, lower spine, and skull. It is commonest in males between the ages of 50 and 70. It is estimated to affect 3.5 per cent of the population over 45 years of age, with most patients asymptomatic and the disease discovered only as an incidental finding on a routine x-ray examination. In other patients, however, the

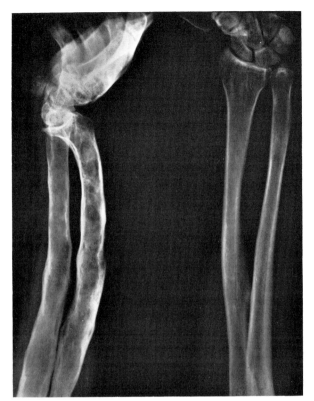

Figure 90. Fibrous dysplasia involving bones of right forearm. Left forearm normal.

disease may appear in an active phase associated with bone pain and skeletal deformity.

Pathologic Findings. The structural changes in Paget's disease are brought about by a disorderly and disorganized combination of accelerated osteolysis and excessive abnormal bone regeneration. The involved areas of bone are extremely vascular and may even exhibit arteriovenous shunts. Grossly these changes cause irregular thickening of the affected bones, which present rough irregular cortical surfaces. Histologically the irregular wavy cement lines that separate areas of bone formed at different periods give rise to the jigsaw mosaic bone pattern that is typical of this disease. The high level of new bone formation is reflected in a rise in serum alkaline phosphatase, often to levels higher than those seen in any other disease. The serum calcium and phosphorus are usually within normal limits.

Clinical Picture. Paget's disease may cause skeletal pain, usually referred to the lower back area or the legs. Involvement of the weight bearing long bones leads to thickening and deformity. The tibia usually bows anteriorly, while the femur tends to bow anteriorly and laterally. Despite the progressive deformity, however, the bones usually remain strong enough for weight bearing, even in the advanced stages of the disease. Involvement of the spine with Paget's disease may be associated with deformity and compression of the vertebral bodies and a kyphosis or scoliosis deformity. Progressive thickening of the external cortex of the skull may lead to enlargement of the head. Prognosis for length of life is good.

X-Ray Picture. On x-ray examination, bones affected by Paget's disease appear thickened and frequently curved. The bone substance appears sclerotic and contains coarse, thick trabeculae that frequently give the involved bone a dense, honeycombed or cystic appearance (Fig. 91). Paget's disease generally begins at one end of a long bone and may spread toward the other end.

Differential Diagnosis. The osteoblastic skeletal metastases from a primary prostatic carcinoma may closely resemble the sclerotic bone lesions of Paget's disease. The finding of an abnormally high serum acid phosphatase value rules out Paget's disease and makes al-

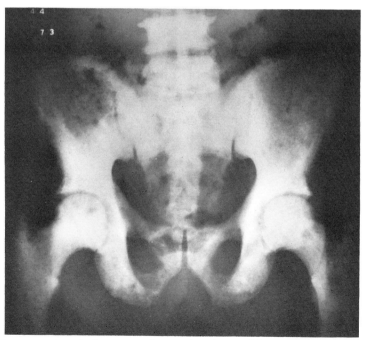

Figure 91. Paget's disease involving pelvis, hip, and femur. Note coarse trabeculation of bone.

most certain the diagnosis of prostatic carcinoma with metastases. In all bone diseases except those due to prostatic carcinoma, it is only the serum alkaline phosphatase value that is increased.

Treatment. At the present time there is no known cure for Paget's disease, and treatment is only symptomatic and supportive. Salicylates, aluminum acetate, parathormone, and x-ray therapy have been used in the past for the relief of pain. More recently, thyrocalcitonin and mithramycin have been reported to be of some value in treatment.

Complications. Two serious complications of Paget's disease are pathologic fracture and malignant degeneration. Pathologic fracture is the commonest complication and may be the earliest clinical sign of Paget's disease. The convex side of the deformed long bone is the usual site of fracture. As a rule the fractures heal but are notoriously slow in uniting.

Malignant degeneration may develop in 5 to 15 per cent of patients with Paget's disease. Osteosarcoma is the malignancy most commonly encountered. This sarcoma is highly malignant and the usual life expectancy after its development is about one year.

Other complications occasionally noted are nerve or spinal cord compression and heart failure secondary to arteriovenous shunts in the affected bones.

SUDECK'S ATROPHY (REFLEX SYMPATHETIC DYSTROPHY, POST-TRAUMATIC PAINFUL OSTEOPOROSIS)

Sudeck's atrophy is a poorly understood painful condition that occasionally develops in an arm or leg following trauma to an extremity or peripheral nerve. The trauma is often quite minor, and the disturbance of function is always greater than that expected from the injury alone. Sudeck's atrophy is thought to represent an irritation of the sympathetic nerve supply which causes a continuous vasospasm of the terminal arterial channels. Patients with this condition complain of burning pain associated with edema, local tenderness, cyanosis, coldness, sweating, frequently trophic changes, and eventually stiffness of the part.

The disorder is associated with an acute atrophy of bone. X-ray examination reveals a spotty osteoporosis involving the bones distal to the site of injury.

Treatment is directed toward increasing the blood flow to the part and preventing stiff, contracted joints. Active exercises, whirlpool baths, and sympatholytic drugs are helpful. Repeated sympathetic ganglion blocks may be curative eventually, but surgical sympathectomy may be required in an occasional patient to effect a cure.

References

Amstutz, H. C., and Carey, E. J.: Skeletal manifestations and treatment of Gaucher's disease. J. Bone and Joint Surg., *48-A*:670, 1966.

Avioli, L. B., Birge, S. J., and Slatopolsky, E.: The nature of vitamin D resistance of patients with chronic renal disease. Arch. Intern. Med., *124*:451, 1969.

Barry, H. C.: Paget's Disease of Bone. Edinburgh: E. & S. Livingstone Ltd., 1969.

Barzel, U. S. (Ed.): Osteoporosis. New York: Grune and Stratton, 1970.

Bricker, N.: Renal osteodystrophy. JAMA, *211*:97, 1970.

DeLuca, H. F.: Vitamin D: New horizons. Clin. Orth. and Rel. Res., 78:4, 1971.

Fairbank, H. A. T.: Atlas of General Affections of the Skeleton. Baltimore: Williams & Wilkins Co., 1951.

Freeman, S.: A brief resumé of calcium and phosphate metabolism. Am. Academy of Orthopaedic Surgeons Instructional Course Lectures, Vol. XII: 165. Ann Arbor: J. W. Edwards, 1955.

Golding, C.: On the differential diagnosis of Paget's disease. J. Bone and Joint Surg., *42-B*:641, 1960.

Harris, W. H., Dudley, H. R., Jr., and Barry, R. J.: The natural history of fibrous dysplasia. An orthopaedic, pathological and roentgenographic study. J. Bone and Joint Surg., *44-A*:207, 1962.

Harris, W. H., and Heaney, R. P.: Skeletal Renewal and Metabolic Bone Disease. Boston: Little, Brown and Co., 1969.

Henry, A.: Monostotic fibrous dysplasia. J. Bone and Joint Surg., *51-B*:300, 1969.

Lichtenstein, L.: Histiocytosis X (eosinophilic granuloma of bone, Letterer-Siwe disease, and Schüller-Christian Disease). J. Bone and Joint Surg., *46-A*:76, 1964.

McGavran, M. H., and Spady, H. A.: Eosinophilic granuloma of bone. J. Bone and Joint Surg., *42-A*:979, 1960.

McKusick, V. A.: The Clinical Behavior of Hereditary Syndromes. Hereditable Disorders of Connective Tissue. St. Louis: C. V. Mosby Co., 1960.

McKusick, V. A., and Scott, C. I.: A nomenclature for constitutional disorders of bone. J. Bone and Joint Surg., *53-A*:978, 1971.

Nicholas, J. A., Saville, P. D., and Bronner, F.: Osteoporosis, osteomalacia, and the skeletal system. J. Bone and Joint Surg., *45-A*:391, 1963.

Norman, A. W., and Henry, H.: The role of the kidney and vitamin D metabolism in health and disease. Clin. Orth. and Rel. Res., *No.* 98, 1974.

Nordin, B. E. C.: Osteomalacia, osteoporosis, and calcium deficiency. Clin. Orthop., *17*:235, 1960.

Ponseti, I. V.: Bone lesions in eosinophilic granuloma, Hand-Schüller-Christian disease and Letterer-Siwe disease. J. Bone and Joint Surg., *30-A*:811, 1948.

Reiss, E.: Primary hyperparathyroidism; A simplified approach to diagnosis. Med. Clin. North Am., *54*:131, January, 1970.

Rodrigues, R. J., and Lewis, H. L.: Eosinophilic granuloma of bone. Review of literature and case presentation. Clin. Orth. and Rel. Res., 77:183, 1971.

Rubin, P.: Dynamic Classification of Bone Dysplasias. Chicago: Yearbook Medical Publishers, 1964.

Stanbury, S. W.: Bone disease in uremia. Am. J. Med., *44*:714, May, 1968.

Strauss, M. B., and Welt, L. G.: Diseases of the Kidney. Boston: Little, Brown and Co., 1971.

Talmage, R. Z., and Munson, P. L. (Eds.): Calcium, Parathyroid Hormone and the Calcitonins. Amsterdam: Excerpta Medica, 1972.

Chapter Nine

Bone Tumors

INTRODUCTION

As in other organ systems of the body, tumor formation may take place in the tissue of the skeletal system. These tumors may arise within the skeletal system as primary growths or may spread secondarily to the skeleton from some distant primary location. Some of these tumors are relatively common; others are quite rare. Some pose no particular threat to the patient's life or function; others are rapidly debilitating and often fatal. It is imperative that the diagnosis of a bone tumor be made with absolute accuracy and that the treatment be planned with extreme care. Diagnosis is best established by a searching history and physical examination, close scrutiny of all essential x-ray views, careful biochemical investigation of the patient's blood and urine, and surgical biopsy with ultimate histologic tissue identification.

Primary bone tumors may be benign or malignant. Benign bone tumors generally are slow-growing, well-circumscribed, noninvading tumors that cause few symptoms, do not spread or metastasize, and do not cause the death of the patient. A few benign bone tumors, however, apparently possess the capability of becoming malignant. Occasionally a lesion is encountered that resembles a benign tumor by its behavior but is not thought to be a true neoplasm by most tumor pathologists. These lesions are believed to represent a self-limiting reaction to some as yet unidentified stimulus and are classified as *reactive lesions.*

Another group of lesions that resemble benign tumors by their behavior, but are not thought to represent true neoplasm, are the *hamartomas.* In these lesions, cells normally present in a local area grow faster than others, but reach cellular maturity as do the normal cells. This results in the formation of a purposeless cellular mass.

Primary malignant bone tumors, fortunately rare, grow rapidly, spread, expand, and invade irregularly, and are associated with pain

189

and disability. They tend to affect children and young adults most frequently. They spread or metastasize to the lungs and other tissues, bringing about a rapid, fatal outcome. Any hope for survival depends upon early diagnosis, usually best established by biopsy.

Tumors that spread secondarily to the skeleton from some distant primary location are malignant, and are called metastatic tumors. They are generally carcinomas arising originally in tissues such as breast, prostate, kidney, thyroid, and lung. As they grow and invade within their tissue of origin, clumps of tumor cells may be carried off by the blood stream or lymph channels to lodge and grow within bone.

Tumor cells in bone generally do not destroy bone tissue, but their presence can evoke several types of host response helpful in diagnosis and identification on the roentgenogram.

Tumor cells in bone may incite local osteoclastic resorption of bone, with the formation of radiolucent areas on the x-ray films. Some tumor cells may evoke the opposite response and cause an osteoblastic response in the host, with the production of a protective wall of dense normal bone around the lesion. This response is known as *reactive bone formation*. Certain tumors are capable of producing osteoid and bone by their own aberrant growth pattern. This bone production within a tumor is called *tumor bone* or *neoplastic bone.*

Several types of periosteal response may also be seen. A tumor that causes expansion of a segment of bone does this by slowly eroding bone from the inside, while at the same time stimulating the periosteum to deposit bone on the outside.

If the periosteum is elevated by a tumor that has broken through the cortex, it is stimulated to produce reactive bone at its remaining point of attachment to the cortex. This produces a triangular-shaped piece of reactive bone on the x-ray film known as *Codman's triangle.*

Elevation of the periosteum in progressive stages stimulates the formation of layers of reactive periosteal bone, giving the so-called "onion-skin" appearance on the x-ray films.

Knowledge of the origin, behavior, and treatment of bone tumors is quite incomplete, and much of the present information is conflicting and controversial. It is known, however, that various cell types comprising the skeletal system may give origin to tumors that vary considerably in their clinical course. The cells of the musculoskeletal tissues all share a common mesodermal origin, but have differentiated along a variety of lines to become osteoblasts, osteoclasts, chondroblasts, fibroblasts, and myeloblasts. This information is of some help in classifying bone tumors. Since the cells of the skeletal system are derived from mesoderm, primary malignant bone tumors are called *sarcomas*. Since most metastatic tumors to bone originate in tissue of epithelial origin, these tumors are known as *metastatic carcinomas.*

Several classifications of bone tumors are available, and most list between 20 and 30 entities, some of extreme rarity. Only the more common tumors are discussed in this chapter. The classification of these tumors, based on Aegerter, is given in Table 2.

TABLE 2. Partial Classification of Bone Tumors

TYPE	BENIGN	MALIGNANT
I. *Reactive Bone Lesions*		
A. *Osteogenic*		
1. Osteoid osteoma		
2. Unicameral bone cyst	All Type I	
3. Benign osteoblastoma		
B. *Collagenic*	and	
1. Subperiosteal cortical defect		
2. Nonossifying fibroma	Type II	
II. *Hamartomas Affecting Bone*	Tumors	
A. *Osteogenic*		
1. Osteoma	are	
2. Osteochondroma		
B. *Chondrogenic*	benign	
1. Enchondroma		
C. *Collagenic*		
1. Angioma		
2. Aneurysmal bone cyst		
III. *True Neoplasms of Bone (Primary)*		
A. *Osteogenic*		
1. Osteosarcoma		Osteosarcoma
2. Parosteal sarcoma		Parosteal sarcoma
3. Giant cell tumor	Giant cell tumor	
(osteoclastoma)	(has malignant	
	potential)	
B. *Chondrogenic*		
1. Benign chondroblastoma	Benign chondroblastoma	
2. Chondromyxoid fibroma	Chondromyxoid fibroma	
3. Chondrosarcoma		Chondrosarcoma
C. *Collagenic*		
1. Fibrosarcoma	None	Fibrosarcoma
2. Angiosarcoma		Angiosarcoma
D. *Myelogenic*		
1. Plasma cell myeloma		Plasma cell myeloma
2. Ewing's tumor		Ewing's tumor
3. Reticulum cell sarcoma	None	Reticulum cell sarcoma
4. Hodgkin's disease		Hodgkin's disease
IV. *Neoplasms Metastasizing to Bone (Secondary)*		
Tumor usually of epithelial origin spreading to bone from a primary growth site in tissue unrelated to skeletal system	None	Primary carcinoma may arise in breast, prostate, kidney, lung, thyroid, etc.

Treatment of tumors of the skeletal system utilizes surgery, radiation therapy, and the chemotherapeutic drugs, which interfere with the growth cycle of the tumor cell. These modalities may be used singly or in thoughtful combination, depending upon the situation presented by each tumor.

Generally, benign bone lesions are treated by surgical excision, with no need for the use of radiation therapy or the cytotoxic drugs. If a large defect remains in the host bone after excision of a benign tumor, it is considered wise to pack the defect with bone chips taken from the ilium in order to accelerate healing of the defect and restore structural integrity to the host bone. The recurrence rate for most surgically excised benign bone tumors is low.

The treatment of malignant bone tumors remains unsatisfactory from the standpoint of long-term patient survival. Surgery, as utilized in the treatment of primary malignant bone tumors, is generally ablative in type, such as limb amputation or hemipelvectomy. Radiation therapy is employed for its local effect if the tumor cells are radiosensitive. The cytotoxic drugs are used for their systemic effect in responsive tumors.

TYPE I.   REACTIVE BONE LESIONS

Osteoid Osteoma

Osteoid osteoma is a relatively infrequent reactive bone lesion, identified by a rather characteristic x-ray and pathologic appearance and causing nagging pain in the patient.

Typically, x-ray examination discloses a small oval clear space in a bone, surrounded by a large area of sclerotic reactive bone (Fig. 92). The small oval clear space is called a *nidus* and contains the neoplastic tissue. Histologically, the lesion consists of varying proportions of osteoid tissue and fine new bone trabeculae in a vascular fibrous matrix.

Osteoid osteoma is seen mostly in children and young adults. Although the lesions may occur anywhere in any bone, they are found most frequently in the lower extremity. These lesions cause pain in the bone, often of a severe degree. If they are located in an accessible region, there may be local tenderness to palpation, although no mass can usually be felt. The pain caused by osteoid osteoma is characteristically worse at night and, surprisingly, is often relieved by aspirin.

Osteoid osteoma is usually treated by operative removal of a block of bone containing the nidus. Some evidence has been presented that indicates osteoid osteoma may undergo spontaneous healing if not treated. In most patients, however, relief of pain requires excision.

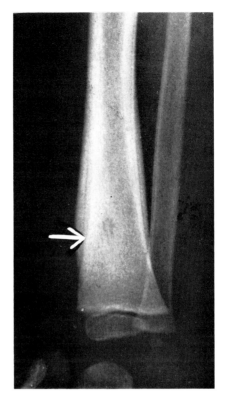

Figure 92. Osteoid osteoma in distal tibia. Note the small oval clear space (nidus) surrounded by an area of sclerotic reactive bone. (Courtesy Dr. Leonard Ellenbogen, Atlantic City, N. J.)

UNICAMERAL BONE CYST

A unicameral bone cyst is a benign cystic lesion of bone found most frequently in the upper end of the humerus and femur. The word unicameral means single chamber. This single chamber cyst is lined with a thin layer of soft tissue and usually contains amber-colored fluid. Bone cysts arise during childhood and adolescence, forming just distal to the growth line but tending to migrate toward the center of the shaft as the bone grows.

X-ray examination discloses a round or oval defect in the bone. This defect is characterized by a circumscribed outline, absence of bone trabeculae within its borders, absence of surrounding reactive bone, a thin overlying cortical shell, and frequently pathologic fracture through the cyst walls (Fig. 93). A typical unicameral bone cyst is a single lesion. Multiple bone cysts may be seen in association with hyperparathyroidism (see p. 179).

A bone cyst may be present in a child's bone for a long time before it is discovered. Frequently, vague symptoms of ache or mild discomfort are overlooked. In about half the patients, the cyst is not

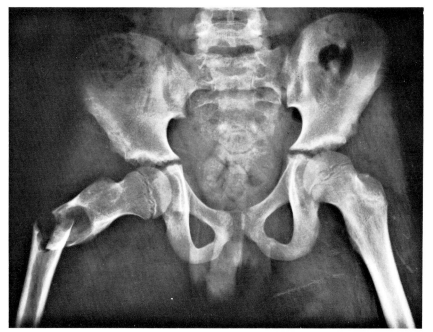

Figure 93.   Unicameral bone cyst of proximal right femur showing pathologic fracture.

discovered until pathologic fracture forces the x-ray examination. Healing of the pathologic fracture frequently occurs and occasionally has been known to bring about spontaneous obliteration of the cyst. Fracture reduction is not in itself dependable treatment, however, because refractures through this area of the bone are common.

Unicameral bone cysts have shown no tendency to undergo malignant change. Their natural pathologic course is toward spontaneous healing.

Treatment of a bone cyst is surgical. For many years, the surgical treatment of choice consisted of opening the cyst cavity at operation and thoroughly scraping the cyst walls down to bleeding bone. The defect was then filled with multiple bone chips taken from the iliac crest. Unfortunately, the recurrence rate following this form of treatment varies from 20 to 40 per cent.

Recently it has been shown that it is possible to elevate the periosteal tube around the segment of diaphysis containing the cyst and surgically remove the entire cyst-bearing segment of diaphysis. Length is maintained by packing the periosteal tube with bone graft and using postoperative traction. It is believed that this and similar treatments will dramatically reduce the recurrence rate for unicameral bone cyst.

Subperiosteal Cortical Defect

Subperiosteal cortical defects are completely asymptomatic, small, eccentrically placed cortical bone craters filled with fibrous tissue. It has been estimated that these lesions can be detected in as many as 20 per cent of all children at some stage during skeletal growth. They are associated with no clinical findings, represent true incidental findings on an x-ray film, and require no treatment. They are sometimes referred to as "bone islands."

Nonossifying Fibroma

Nonossifying fibroma is the name given to an extremely common bone defect found most frequently in the long bones of the lower extremity during the patient's first two decades of life. The lesion consists of a localized area of bone tissue destruction with replacement by collagenous fibrous tissue.

X-ray examination reveals an irregularly circular area of radiolucency, frequently exhibiting a scalloped border of sclerotic bone (Fig. 94). The typical location of a nonossifying fibroma is an eccentric posi-

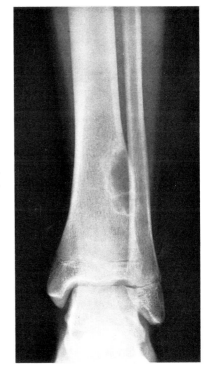

Figure 94. Nonossifying fibroma of distal tibia. Note its characteristic eccentric location.

tion in the distal end of a long bone of the lower extremity. This lesion must be differentiated from bone cyst and fibrous dysplasia.

The majority of these lesions cause no symptoms and are discovered only when an x-ray examination is made for another reason. Occasionally the lesion may cause pain, and rarely it will cause pathologic fracture.

It is believed that the natural course of a nonossifying fibroma is to undergo spontaneous healing. For this reason, definitive treatment of the lesion is rarely necessary.

TYPE II. HAMARTOMAS AFFECTING BONE

OSTEOCHONDROMA

Osteochondroma is a benign hamartoma consisting of a large spur or projection of adult bone topped by a cartilage cap (Figs. 95 and 96). This bone projection usually arises at the joint end of the long bone, and characteristically points away from the joint toward the midpoint of the shaft of the bone. The lesion begins during the growth period and is found most commonly at the knee end of the femur and tibia and at the shoulder end of the humerus. An osteochondroma ceases to grow at about the same time as the nearest growth line closes, and it

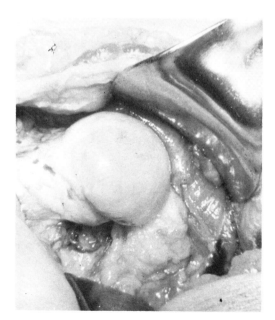

Figure 95. Gross appearance of an osteochondroma of distal femur exposed at surgery.

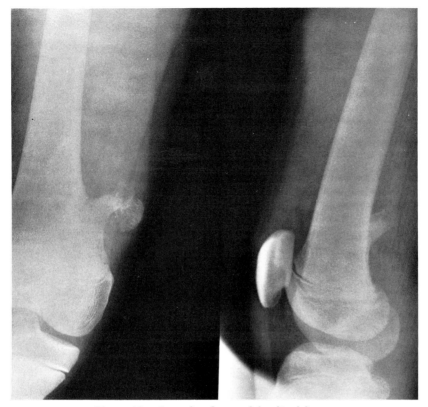

Figure 96. Osteochondroma of the distal femur.

then remains static unless it is disturbed by trauma. The presence of a single osteochondroma is a different, although possibly related, problem from that posed by the condition known as hereditary multiple exostoses (see p. 165).

Osteochondromas arise during childhood. Unless they impinge on sensitive tissues, they are usually asymptomatic. Frequently, the osteochondroma will be discovered quite casually when the patient notices a hard lump near a joint.

On occasion, an osteochondroma has been known to undergo malignant change and become a sarcoma. When this happens, the changes are believed to occur in the cartilage cap. The catalyst for the transformation is believed to be trauma, which could be delivered during physical activity or by inadequate surgical attempts to remove the bone mass.

Treatment consists of complete operative excision of the entire osteochondroma. Incomplete removal may result in recurrence or malignant change.

ENCHONDROMA

Enchondroma is a well-circumscribed, oval-shaped hamartoma containing cartilage cells that are thought to have been left behind by the growing growth line. In time, these cells begin to grow and multiply within the confines of the bone, ultimately creating a cavity for themselves. Enchondroma is the most common bone tumor found in the hand, and is not infrequently discovered in other locations, such as ribs, femur, tibia, humerus, and pelvis. The presence of a single enchondroma is a different, although possibly related, problem from that posed by the condition known as enchondromatosis or Ollier's disease (see p. 182).

Enchondroma is thought to develop during the growth period, but it may lie undetected for years. Although some patients may notice mild ache or pain, the majority have no symptoms relative to the enchondroma. Most of these tumors are discovered after pathologic fracture has occurred, often following very slight injury.

Enchondroma has been known to undergo malignant change and become a secondary chondrosarcoma.

X-ray examination reveals a well-circumscribed round or oval

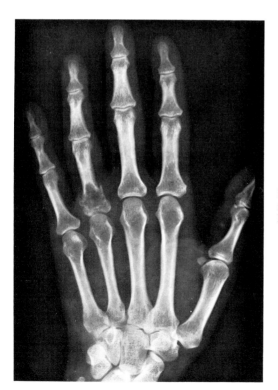

Figure 97. Enchondroma lying in proximal end of proximal phalanx of fourth finger. Note pathologic fracture.

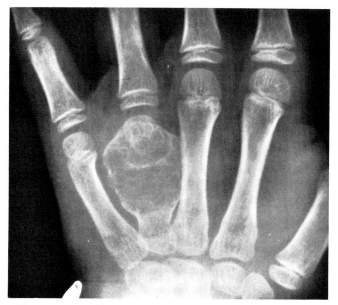

Figure 98. Aneurysmal bone cyst of fourth metacarpal. Note bubble-like appearance.

lytic area in the end of the bone (Fig. 97). It may be difficult or impossible to differentiate on the x-ray film among enchondroma, unicameral bone cyst, and some giant cell tumors.

Treatment of choice consists of opening the cavity and thoroughly scraping out the cartilaginous contents. The defect is then filled with multiple bone chips taken from the iliac crest.

ANEURYSMAL BONE CYST

Aneurysmal bone cyst is a lesion thought to arise from vascular tissue in bone. As it grows, it causes a rather characteristic bubble or ballooning of the overlying cortex. The growth tends to destroy and expand the bone and stretches the overlying periosteum. The periosteal layer, so stimulated, lays down reactive bone, which forms a shell around the tumor and contributes to the bubble-like appearance seen on the x-ray film (Fig. 98).

Aneurysmal bone cysts develop most frequently in adolescents and young adults. They can arise in any bone and are frequently seen in the vertebrae. Pain is the presenting complaint, and a mass may be palpable if the tumor arises in a superficial bone. Extensive bleeding may occur if the overlying cortical bone shell is broken. Pathologic fracture through the aneurysmal bone cyst is not uncommon.

If feasbile, the treatment of choice is surgical curettage and packing of the defect with bone graft material. If the lesion is in a site not easily accessible to surgery, as for example a vertebral body, radiation will control the lesion by sclerosing the blood vessels.

TYPE III. TRUE NEOPLASMS OF BONE (PRIMARY)

OSTEOSARCOMA (OSTEOGENIC SARCOMA)

Osteosarcoma is a primary malignant bone tumor that arises from osteoblasts and primitive cells that have the capacity to form bone. Except for the marrow tumors, osteosarcoma is the commonest and most fatal of the primary malignant bone tumors. It arises most frequently in males under 30 years of age. Only about 20 per cent of patients survive after treatment for as long as five years, with the average patient living for only about 18 months before succumbing to pulmonary metastases.

The tumor usually begins near the growth line of the long bone, although it may arise in flat bones, such as ilium or ribs. It is often found in the metaphyseal region of a long bone, particularly about the knee and shoulder. Because this tumor destroys, erodes, and expands the bone, constant pain is a significant feature. As the tumor grows beyond the confines of the bone, it produces an obvious swelling or enlargement of the part. Pathologic fracture may occur.

X-ray examination discloses an irregular and ill-defined area, usually at the epiphyseal end of a long bone, showing evidence of both bone destruction and bone formation. The tumor destroys bone in irregular fashion and erodes through the overlying cortex to grow out into the soft tissue (Fig. 99). The tumor cells may produce a type of tumor bone that gives a density and a mottling through the tumor area on the x-ray film. Reactive and neoplastic bone may be deposited along the blood vessels running through the tumor, giving the so-called "sun burst" effect frequently seen on the x-ray film. In addition, as the tumor grows it raises the periosteum, which is stimulated to lay down reactive bone. This reactive bone may be reflected on the x-ray film as Codman's triangle, "onion-skin" appearance, or both.

Osteosarcoma has been known to develop secondarily as a complication of other problems affecting bone tissue. It has been seen to develop in Paget's disease, in bone that has been subjected to irradiation, and rarely in an osteochondroma.

Because of the highly malignant nature of this tumor, it is imperative to establish the diagnosis as rapidly as possible. This is best done by surgical biopsy. Once the diagnosis is firmly established, the part containing the tumor is amputated.

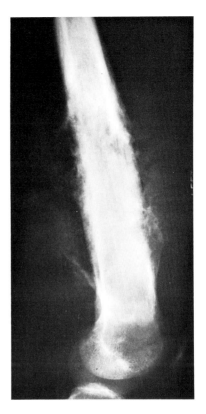

Figure 99. Osteosarcoma of distal femur, showing bone destruction with erosion of tumor into soft parts and the formation of periosteal reactive bone.

Osteosarcoma is not particularly radiosensitive, and beneficial effects from the use of radiation therapy in its treatment are thus doubtful. Radiation may occasionally be used to control local symptoms, however.

Several of the cytotoxic drugs are now being used as adjuvant therapy to surgery. As yet, no good long-term data attesting to their effectiveness have been presented.

Even in the presence of metastases, amputation of a part containing an osteosarcoma may be indicated to relieve pain arising from the enlarging tumor or pathologic fracture.

GIANT CELL TUMOR (OSTEOCLASTOMA)

Giant cell tumor is an aggressive, locally destructive growth of young adults characteristically developing in the region of the former epiphysis of long bones after the growth plate has closed. There is considerable uncertainty about the origin and behavior of this tumor, but little doubt that it is dangerous and shows definite malignant potential.

Giant cell tumor begins as a locally destructive process, partially or entirely within the epiphyseal end of long bones, particularly lower femur, upper tibia, and lower radius. As the lesion grows, it destroys bone and expands the overlying cortex, even to the point of erosion. The tumor may extend to the joint cartilage, but usually not beyond.

X-ray examination discloses an osteolytic expanding lesion appearing at the epiphyseal end of a long bone (Fig. 100). Bone trabeculae divide the tumor into multiple irregular chambers. These chambers are reflected on the x-ray film as a "soap bubble" effect.

Giant cell tumor is found most frequently in patients between the ages of 20 and 40. Growth of the tumor may be slow or rapid, depending on the aggressiveness of each particular tumor. As more extensive bone destruction occurs, pathologic fracture may take place.

Grossly, the tumor consists of soft hemorrhagic material that has been likened to currant jelly. The most conspicuous microscopic fea-

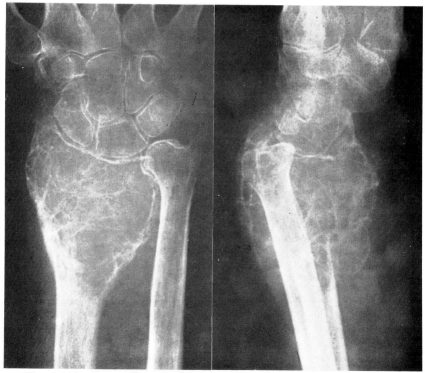

Figure 100.   Giant cell tumor of distal radius. Note "soap bubble" effect. (By permission of Temple University Hospital and Jack Edeiken, M.D.)

ture is the presence of many multinucleated giant cells. It is this feature that gives the lesion its name.

Treatment for this tumor depends upon the bone involved. Irradiation has sometimes been used, particularly if the tumor is in a location that is considered surgically inaccessible. If the tumor is accessible surgically, the traditional treatment has been to curette out thoroughly all the neoplastic tissue and fill the resulting bone defect with iliac bone graft. Unfortunately, recurrence after this type of treatment is relatively common and may be associated with an increase in aggressive behavior and malignant potential. The newest surgical technique for eradicating osteoclastoma involves massive resection of the portion of bone containing the tumor, with fresh cadaver bone being used to replace the removed segment. Occasionally, amputation may be necessary because of the aggressive nature of the tumor or because of malignant change.

BENIGN CHONDROBLASTOMA

Benign chondroblastoma is a relatively rare tumor that arises from cartilage and presents a very characteristic picture on the x-ray film and histologic section. The tumor arises from young chondroblasts in the growth plate before epiphyseal closure occurs; thus the patient with this tumor is invariably young. The epiphysis most frequently affected is the upper end of the humerus, at the shoulder joint. The tumor grows into the bony epiphysis but may extend downward into the metaphysis. Its presence may cause pain, and often an enlargement of the shoulder is noted.

X-ray examination reveals a well-defined area of bone destruction lying within the epiphysis of an adolescent patient. Calcification within the cartilage tissue gives a mottled or speckled appearance to the tumor. In most patients, the lesion is surrounded by a zone of condensed or sclerotic bone.

Treatment of choice consists of opening the cavity and thoroughly scraping out the cartilaginous contents. The defect is then filled with multiple bone chips taken from the iliac crest. Benign chondroblastoma is associated with a very minimal recurrence rate and shows no tendency to undergo malignant degeneration.

CHONDROSARCOMA

Chondrosarcoma is a primary malignant bone tumor that arises from normal cartilage cells to become a large, bulky cartilaginous growth. Except for plasma cell myeloma, chondrosarcoma is the most common primary malignant bone tumor to involve the bones of the trunk, shoulder, and hip. In total frequency, however, chondrosarcoma occurs only about half as often as osteosarcoma. Chondrosarcoma tends to develop mostly in adults over 30 years of age.

As a rule, chondrosarcoma grows slowly and metastasizes later. For this reason, survival rates following treatment of this tumor are generally better than in many of the other malignant bone tumors. Chondrosarcoma apparently may arise as a primary malignant growth from adult cartilage, or it may arise as a secondary malignant change in osteochondroma, enchondroma, or Paget's disease.

Chondrosarcoma may involve the epiphyseal ends of long bones, such as femur, tibia, or humerus, but is much commoner in the pelvic and shoulder girdle areas. Because of the destructive nature of the growth, pain is usually the main symptom. Since the tumor tends to form a large mass, visible and palpable enlargement of the part may be noted. Although the tumor destroys bone, pathologic fracture is unusual because the periosteum frequently lays down new bone which protects against fracture.

X-ray examination reveals the presence of a multichambered area of bone destruction containing scattered areas of calcification (Fig. 101). Periosteal new bone formation may be seen around the tumor, and the outline of a bulky mass may be noted beyond the confines of the bone.

Treatment of choice in the majority of patients is amputation of the part containing the tumor. Radiation is not used because chondrosarcoma is a radioresistant tumor. The cytotoxic drugs are apparently also ineffective in the treatment of chondrosarcoma.

FIBROSARCOMA

Fibrosarcoma is a relatively infrequent, slow-growing primary malignant bone tumor arising from fibrous connective tissue elements of bone. Fibrosarcoma occurs about one-third as often as osteosarcoma and exhibits a tendency to recur locally rather than spread to the lungs. With adequate treatment, the prognosis for survival is better with this tumor than with osteosarcoma or chondrosarcoma.

Fibrosarcoma may develop at any age and usually involves long bones, such as femur and tibia. It may arise from the periosteum as a palpable tumor mass, but most frequently it develops as a bone destroying tumor from the fibrous tissue within bone itself. The principal symptom is pain. Pathologic fracture is infrequent.

X-ray examination reveals an irregular, poorly defined area of bone destruction showing no evidence of bone formation either within the tumor proper or in the surrounding bone tissue.

Treatment of choice is usually amputation of the affected part

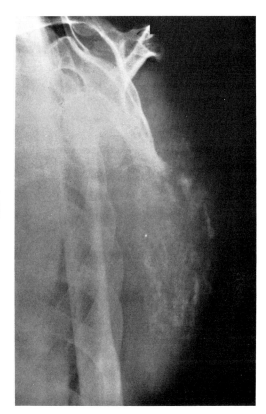

Figure 101. Chondrosarcoma of scapula, showing bone destruction and scattered areas of calcification.

above the level involved. Several of the cytotoxic drugs are now being used as adjuvant therapy to surgery. As yet, however, no good long-term data attesting to their effectiveness have been published. Radiation therapy is not used because fibrosarcoma is a radioresistant tumor.

Ewing's Tumor

Ewing's tumor is a highly malignant primary sarcoma of bone thought to arise from cells of the marrow reticulum. Characteristically, it affects children and adolescents and usually involves the flat bones, such as ilium, ribs, and vertebrae, and the shafts of long bones. Ewing's tumor is the third most frequent primary malignant bone tumor, following multiple myeloma and osteosarcoma in statistical frequency.

Ewing's tumor begins in the medullary region of the bone and destroys bone from within. It may gradually erode to the cortex to grow out into the surrounding soft tissues. Spread of the tumor within the marrow cavity frequently causes a great deal of bone necrosis, which may result in pathologic fracture.

Extensive bone necrosis produced by Ewing's tumor may cause pain, swelling of the part, and local heat, in addition to leukocytosis and an elevated sedimentation rate. These features, suggestive of infection, in association with radiologic evidence of bone destruction may lead to a mistaken diagnosis of osteomyelitis.

X-ray examination reveals an irregular area of bone destruction, usually in the shaft of a long bone and involving both the marrow cavity and overlying cortex (Fig. 102). As the tumor bursts through the confines of the bone, it raises the periosteum and so stimulates it to lay down strips of reactive bone. This is reflected on the x-ray film as lamellation of the cortical bone or "onion-skin" appearance.

The microscopic picture of Ewing's tumor is fairly characteristic, consisting of sheets and circles of intact and degenerated small round cells.

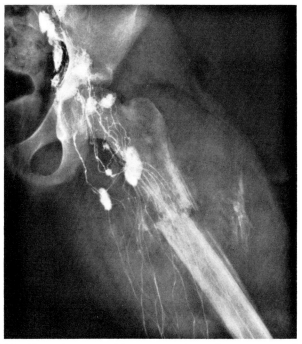

Figure 102. Ewing's tumor of femur. Note bone destruction involving marrow cavity and cortex, pathologic fracture, and "onion-skin appearance" along lateral cortex. Radiopaque material represents a lymphangiogram performed to detect regional lymph node metastasis. (Courtesy Dr. John Hope, The Children's Hospital, Philadelphia, Pa.)

Treatment for Ewing's tumor involves a combination of irradiation and long-term cytotoxic drug therapy. Irradiation is used for its local effect and drug therapy for its systemic effect. Other than for biopsy, surgery plays a very limited role in the treatment of Ewing's tumor.

The mortality rate with Ewing's tumor is extremely great, because the tumor is highly malignant and exhibits a propensity to spread to other bones as well as to the viscera and lungs. The average patient has a life expectancy of less than two years after onset of the tumor.

RETICULUM CELL SARCOMA

Reticulum cell sarcoma, a relatively uncommon tumor, is a lymphoma arising in bone. Reticulum cell sarcoma is the slowest growing and least malignant of the marrow tumors. Histologically its cellular picture is often quite difficult to distinguish from that of Ewing's tumor. Reticulum cell sarcoma, however, affects an older age group than Ewing's tumor, is less malignant, and may be associated with a 50 per cent 10-year survival rate.

The tumor is found in both long and flat bones. It may produce widespread bone destruction with expansion into the surrounding soft tissues. It frequently causes pain, and may be associated with a palpable lump and pathologic fracture. Unlike in Ewing's tumor, however, bone necrosis is not a feature of reticulum cell sarcoma, and consequently a systemic response suggesting infection is absent.

X-ray examination reveals an irregular destructive process, usually in the shaft of long bones, involving medullary cavity and cortex. The presence of the tumor may cause an expansion of the affected shaft. Reactive bone formation within the tumor area gives the lesion a characteristic granular or mottled appearance on the x-ray film.

Treatment for reticulum cell sarcoma consists of a combination of irradiation and long-term cytotoxic drug therapy. Irradiation is used for its local effect and drug therapy for its systemic effect. Surgery is limited to biopsy and possibly to treatment of pathologic fractures of long bones.

PLASMA CELL MYELOMA

Plasma cell myeloma arises from plasma cells in the bone marrow and is the most common of the primary malignant bone tumors. Since the site of origin is bone marrow, tumors may appear in multiple bones simultaneously. For this reason, the disease is also called *multiple myeloma*.

Myeloma is seen mostly in the 40 to 60 age group and affects males more frequently than females. Unlike those of other tumors, the earliest lesions of myeloma are frequently found in flat bones, such as skull, pelvis, and vertebral bodies. The bone lesions cause erosion of the marrow cavity and overlying cortex, giving rise to pain and resulting quite frequently in pathologic fracture. Involvement of the lumbar vertebrae may cause compression fracture of the vertebrae and back pain.

Laboratory examination is great help in establishing the diagnosis of multiple myeloma. The tumor produces large amounts of abnormal protein belonging to the globulin fraction. This abnormal protein, called Bence Jones protein, is excreted through the urine, and its presence may be detected in approximately 50 per cent of patients with multiple myeloma by examining a collected 24 hour urine sample. The production of abnormal protein results in an elevation of the value of total serum protein and a reversal of the normal albumin-globulin ratio. The electrophoretic pattern for total serum protein gives a characteristic tracing in patients with myeloma. Examination of marrow tissue taken by biopsy from the sternum or iliac crest may demonstrate myeloma cells.

X-ray examination characteristically reveals multiple discrete "punched-out" areas frequently affecting multiple bones, such as skull, vertebrae, pelvis, and shafts of long bones (Fig. 103). The lesions cause destruction of bone and appear as rounded, sharply demarcated "holes" in the bone. As a rule, no associated bony sclerosis or reactive bone formation around the lesions is seen on the x-ray film.

Treatment for multiple myeloma consists of a combination of irradiation and long-term cytotoxic drug therapy. Radiation is used for its local effect and drug therapy for its systemic effect. Surgery plays no definitive role in the treatment of multiple myeloma except for biopsy purposes or in the treatment of pathologic fractures.

The prognosis is poor, with the average patient surviving only one to three years after onset of the disease.

TYPE IV. NEOPLASMS METASTASIZING TO BONE (SECONDARY)

Primary carcinomas arising particularly in breast, prostate, kidney, thyroid, and lung may secondarily invade the bone tissue by direct extension or by way of blood stream or lymphatic transportation. Metastatic malignant tumor deposits in bone are more common than any of the primary malignant bone tumors. The tumor that most frequently metastasizes to bone is adenocarcinoma of the breast.

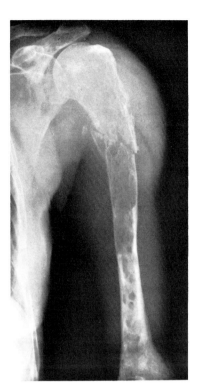

Figure 103. Multiple myeloma involving humerus. Note pathologic fracture.

Some metastatic cancer deposits in bone, such as breast cancer, may cause purely destructive lesions, while others, such as prostatic carcinoma, may cause lesions characterized by reactive bone formation (Fig. 104). The bones most often affected are skull, spine, pelvis, and femora. It is believed that metastatic cancer deposits may be present in bone tissue for some time before causing enough destruction to be detectable on the x-ray film.

Usually the first symptom to be noted is bone pain. This is particularly suggestive if the patient has had a prior diagnosis of a primary malignancy of a tissue such as breast or prostate. Pathologic fractures are rather common with metastatic carcinoma, because these lesions are frequently associated with marked bone destruction.

In some patients, aspiration biopsy of the metastatic lesion can be carried out to establish the diagnosis and identify the primary site, while in other patients, open surgical biopsy may be required. Metastatic deposits in bone usually reproduce some of the cellular patterns characteristic of the tissue of origin.

Treatment depends to a great extent on the type and origin of the primary carcinoma that has metastasized to bone. Irradiation, hor-

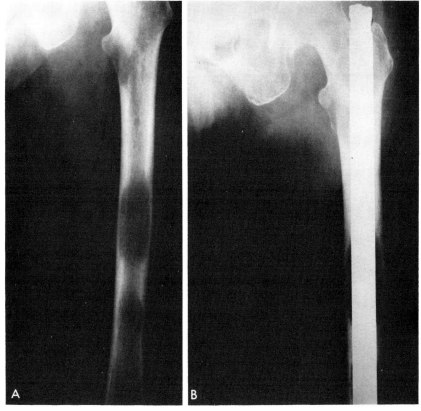

Figure 104. A, lytic lesions in femoral shaft due to metastatic adenocarcinoma of breast. *B*, same patient after "prophylactic" nailing using "stacked" intramedullary rods.

mones, cytotoxic drugs, and surgery all play some role in the treatment program.

Surgery is most effective in the treatment of pathologic fractures, particularly of the major long bones. Whenever possible, "prophylactic" internal fixation of major long bones should be considered if the presence of a large lesion presages an impending pathologic fracture. This spares the patient the excruciating pain of a long bone fracture.

The development of methyl methacrylate or "bone cement" has added another dimension to the palliative treatment of metastatic tumors of long bones with or without pathologic fracture. Large segments of diseased bone can be replaced by "bone cement" used in conjunction with sturdy internal fixation. Although not curative or even definitive, such surgical methods help to improve the quality of survival for patients with metastatic carcinoma.

References

Aegerter, E. E., and Kirkpatrick, J. S., Jr.: Orthopaedic Disease, 3rd Edition. Philadelphia: W. B. Saunders Co., 1968.

Barnes, R., and Catto, M.: Chondrosarcoma of bone. J. Bone and Joint Surg., *48-B*:729, 1966.

Bhanasli, S. K., and Desai, P. B.: Ewing's sarcoma. Observations on 107 cases. J. Bone and Joint Surg., *45-A*:541, 1963.

Coventry, M. B., and Dahlin, D. C.: Osteogenic sarcoma: A study of 600 cases. J. Bone and Joint Surg., *49-A*:101, 1967.

Dahlin, D. D., and Ivins, J. D.: Fibrosarcoma of bone: A study of 114 cases. Cancer, *23*:35, 1969.

Donaldson, W. F., Jr.: Aneursymal bone cyst. J. Bone and Joint Surg., *44-A*:1450, 1963.

Friedman, B., and Hanoaka, H.: Round-cell sarcomas of bone. J. Bone and Joint Surg., *53-A*:1118, 1971.

Goldenberg, R. R., Campbell, C. J., and Bonfiglio, M.: Giant cell tumor of bones: An analysis of 218 cases. J. Bone and Joint Surg., *52-A*:619, 1970.

Griffiths, D.: Orthopaedic aspects of myelomatosis. J. Bone and Joint Surg., *48-B*:703, 1966.

Johnson, R., and Humphries, S. R.: Past failures and future possibilities in Ewing's sarcoma. Cancer, *23*:161, 1969.

Lichtenstein, L.: Bone Tumors, 3rd Edition. St. Louis: C. V. Mosby Co., 1965.

Marcove, R. C., and Lewis, M. M.: Prolonged survival in osteogenic sarcoma with multiple pulmonary metastases. A case report and review of the literature. J. Bone and Joint Surg., *55-A*:1516, 1973.

McLean, F. C.: The use of isotopes in orthopaedics. Part I: The atomic nucleus and isotopes. Am. Academy of Orthopaedic Surgeons Instructional Course Lectures, J. Bone and Joint Surg., *45-A*:1067, 1963.

Moore, M.: Tumor-specific antigens: Their possible significance in the etiology and treatment of malignant disease. J. Bone and Joint Surg., *53-B*:13, 1971.

Neer, C. S., et al.: Treatment of unicameral bone cysts, a follow-up study of 175 cases. J. Bone and Joint Surg., *48-A*:731, 1966.

Watt, J.: The use of cytotoxic drugs in the surgery of malignant disease. J. Bone and Joint Surg., *50-B*:511, 1968.

Chapter Ten

Disorders of the Shoulder

INTRODUCTION

The term shoulder is used clinically to encompass the entire shoulder region. The more descriptive term, shoulder girdle, is used to identify the glenohumeral joint and its lesser auxiliary joints and components. The shoulder girdle comprises the upper humerus, scapula, clavicle, and sternum, articulating through the glenohumeral, acromioclavicular, and sternoclavicular joints (Fig. 105). Although the glenohumeral joint, or shoulder joint proper, is the major and most important element of the shoulder girdle, all component parts play a role in successful arm trunk movements. Injury or disease affecting any part of the shoulder girdle may result in disturbances of shoulder motion or pain.

As an element of the shoulder girdle, the clavicle acts as an outrigger to hold the arm and the scapula outward and backward. Full elevation of the arm, in the direction of either forward flexion or abduction, takes place chiefly through the glenohumeral joint but must be accompanied by rotation of the scapula on the thorax to be completed. Rotation of the scapula is dependent upon movement through the acromioclavicular joint and rotation of the clavicle through the sternoclavicular joint. Thus it can be seen that an apparently simple maneuver, such as raising one's arm, depends upon a complicated interdependence of several joints working in rhythm and involves all the component parts of the shoulder girdle.

GENERAL CONSIDERATIONS

The shoulder joint proper, or glenohumeral joint, is the pivotal joint of the upper extremity. Consider how difficult everyday motions,

212

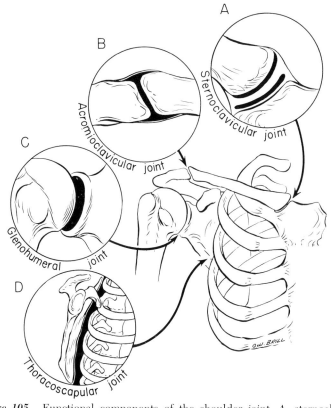

Figure 105. Functional components of the shoulder joint. *A*, sternoclavicular joint. *B*, acromioclavicular joint. *C*, glenohumeral joint. *D*, thoracoscapular joint. (From DePalma, A. F.: Surgery of the Shoulder, 2nd ed. Philadelphia: J. B. Lippincott Co., 1973.)

such as reaching up to a shelf or scratching one's back, would be without an extremely movable shoulder joint. A price has to be paid for this mobility, however, and it is obtained at the expense of stability. A glance at the anatomy of the joint shows that it is indeed constructed for mobility rather than stability.

The shoulder joint, like the hip, is a ball and socket joint. In contrast to the hip joint, however, the humeral head presents a small area of bony contact to the glenoid which, in turn, constitutes a very shallow socket. Both bony parts are enclosed in a loose capsule. The overhanging coracoacromial arch prevents upward displacement of the humerus at the shoulder joint, but the joint depends mainly upon muscles for its stability. Four short muscles, the teres minor, the infraspinatus, the supraspinatus, and the subscapularis, arise closely around the humeral head and support it. Their tendons blend with one another and with the joint capsule to form a conjoined tendon that inserts in and about the greater tuberosity of the humerus. This conjoined tendon is spoken of as the *musculotendinous* or *rotator cuff* of the shoulder, and its chief function is to stabilize the humeral head in the glenoid cavity. The long muscles that pass across the joint, such as the biceps, coracobrachialis, deltoid, latissimus dorsi, triceps, pectoralis major, and teres major, are the prime movers of the joint.

A joint that presents loose bony contact and depends upon muscles for stability will indeed be flexible but also weak. For this reason, the majority of orthopaedic problems encountered about the shoulder joint involve the soft tissue components of the joint rather than the bony part. Degenerative arthritis of the shoulder joint, for example, is most unusual. It should also be noted that the shoulder is the only joint in the body in which recurrent dislocation is common.

Contrast the function and behavior of the shoulder joint with that of the hip joint, which is the counterpart pivotal joint of the lower extremity (see p. 337). In the hip joint, mobility is sacrificed to stability.

INTERVIEWING AND EXAMINING THE PATIENT

The majority of patients presenting with a shoulder problem do so because of pain, ache, or some type of discomfort. Less commonly the presenting complaint is stiffness, weakness, or deformity. Pain in the shoulder area may arise from a problem primary in the joint, or it may be referred to the part from a problem originating elsewhere in the body. Referred pain can usually be traced to cervical spine disorders, cardiac disorders, gallbladder disease, or diseases involving the mediastinum or diaphragm. Referred pain, however, is less likely to be accompanied by local tenderness and limitation of motion. A good searching history and complete physical examination should enable the examiner to distinguish between primary and referred causes of shoulder pain.

THE INTERVIEW

The patient should be asked to describe his complaint and to point to the area involved. Many times an important clue can be obtained immediately. If the complaint is pain, its type should be determined. Pain in some shoulder disorders is brought on only by movement, while in others the pain is present constantly. The type and location of any radiating pain should be ascertained.

A clear statement should be obtained about the duration of symptoms, beginning with the type of onset and the subsequent progress. It is important to determine if the patient has previously had similar episodes, and if so, how they were treated. The patient should be questioned concerning a history of trauma or possible occupational diseases.

Primary shoulder disorders present symptoms that are definitely related to shoulder and arm motions. This point should be clearly delineated by the history. Many shoulder problems are characteristically aggravated by certain activities, such as combing the hair, putting on a coat, reaching into the back pocket, or finding a comfortable position for the arm in bed at night. It is also important to question the patient about activities that relieve the complaint.

THE EXAMINATION

It is necessary that the patient be sufficiently undressed for the examination. Males may be stripped to the waist. Females should be gowned in such a manner that both arms and shoulders and the upper chest area are exposed. The local examination of a patient with shoulder complaint begins at the sternal notch and covers the entire shoulder girdle, utilizing the unaffected side as the control.

Inspection. The examiner should look for any evidence of deformity, atrophy, redness, swelling, or any abnormality that might distinguish one shoulder from the other.

Palpation. The area is palpated for evidence of swelling, deformity, muscle spasm, or local painful areas, with special reference to the sternoclavicular joint, clavicle, acromioclavicular joint, shoulder joint, rotator cuff, and bicipital groove.

Range of Motion. The range of joint motion is assessed both actively and passively. Both shoulder joints are put through a full active range of flexion, extension, abduction, adduction, and internal and external rotation, and any differences are noted. Observation is made of the shoulder rhythm in relation to glenohumeral motion and scapular rotation (Fig. 106). The same motions are checked passively to uncover any joint tightness.

Special Maneuvers. Special maneuvers are required for specific diagnoses, such as evaluating the strength of the rotator cuff in case of suspected cuff tear, or seeing if forced supination of the forearm gives pain in the bicipital groove.

Neurologic Examination. The examiner should evaluate muscle power and look for evidence of clonus or spasticity and for evidence of sensory changes. The biceps, triceps, and brachioradialis reflexes should be compared.

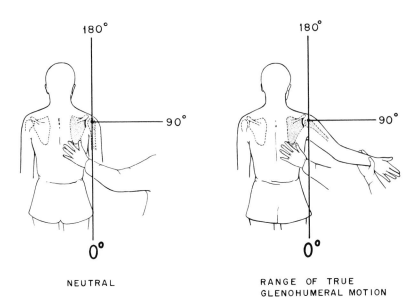

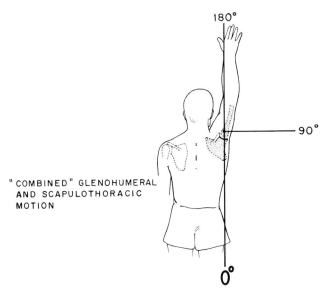

Figure 106. Elevation of the arm at the shoulder joint involves both the glenohumeral and scapulothoracic components. (Courtesy of American Academy of Orthopaedic Surgeons.)

X-ray Examination.   The most useful routine views are antero-posterior projections taken with the shoulder in internal and external rotation.

DISORDERS OF THE STERNOCLAVICULAR JOINT

DISLOCATION

A force applied to the arm, shoulder, or chest may cause a traumatic dislocation of the medial end of the clavicle at the sternoclavicular joint. The displaced clavicle rides upward, causing a visible and palpable prominence of the joint. The prominence is apparent when the injured joint is compared with its counterpart joint on the opposite side. X-ray examination confirms the diagnosis.

Injuries to the sternoclavicular joint may be treated by open reduction, with the reduction maintained by metallic pin fixation. The pin is removed after healing is completed.

OLD DISLOCATION

Occasionally a patient presents with an unreduced sternoclavicular dislocation of long standing. No treatment is attempted if the dislocation is asymptomatic. If it is causing pain or distress because of its instability, reconstruction of the joint, aided by temporary internal fixation, may be carried out. Some orthopaedic surgeons prefer to excise the dislocated end of the clavicle as an alternative procedure to relieve pain.

DEGENERATIVE ARTHRITIS

Degenerative arthritis may affect the sternoclavicular joint and give rise to a painful thickness and swelling of the joint. A patient may seek attention because of a "lump" in the neck area.

In the acute stage the joint may be warm, thickened, and tender. Later all symptoms and signs may subside, but the thickness and enlargement usually remain. This condition may be related to Tietze's syndrome, which is characterized by pain, swelling, and tenderness of the second and third costochondral junctions (see p. 291).

Pain may be relieved by warm applications and by the use of orally administered anti-inflammatory agents. Sometimes it is necessary to inject hydrocortisone into the sternoclavicular joint. Surgical treatment is unnecessary.

DISORDERS OF THE ACROMIOCLAVICULAR JOINT

The acromioclavicular joint is frequently involved by athletic and industrial injuries that tear the supporting ligaments and cause varying degrees of disruption of the joint. After this type of injury, the weight of the dependent arm pulls the acromion down, and the lateral end of the clavicle may displace out of the joint and become prominent beneath the skin.

Degenerative arthritis may also affect the acromioclavicular joint to cause shoulder girdle pain.

SUBLUXATION

If an injury tears the joint capsule and overlying musculature, but spares the conoid and trapezoid ligaments linking the coracoid process to the clavicle, the degree of joint disruption is minimal and the injury is described as a subluxation of the joint. To demonstrate incomplete displacement of the acromioclavicular joint on x-ray, the film must be taken with the patient in the standing position and holding a weight in his hand. This tends to pull the acromion downward and allows some upward migration of the lateral end of the clavicle.

Most subluxations can be treated by a combination of a pressure strapping centered over the joint and sling support for the arm. This holds the joint together until healing occurs. Occasionally the strapping will have to encircle the joint and elbow completely in order to elevate the acromion enough to bring about a reduction.

DISLOCATION

Complete dislocation of the acromioclavicular joint occurs when the injury ruptures the joint capsule and overlying musculature along with the conoid and trapezoid ligaments. This is the "shoulder separation" so often sustained by athletes. With the arm dependent, displacement of the clavicle is obvious both clinically and by x-ray examination (Fig. 107).

Treatment for this injury varies with the experience and judgment of the physician. Nonoperative treatment utilizes an encircling bandage of tape or plaster designed to reduce the dislocation and hold the parts together until healing occurs. Operative treatment may consist of open reduction of the dislocation with repair of the ruptured conoid and trapezoid ligaments. An alternative method is open reduction maintained by threaded metal pins introduced through the acromion into the clavicle. A satisfactory operative treatment in older patients or those in sedentary occupations is excision of the distal third of the clavicle.

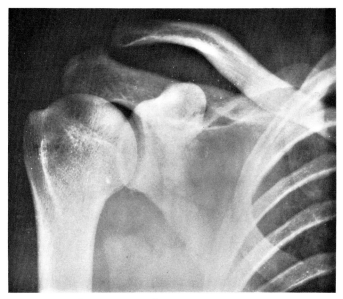

Figure 107. Complete traumatic dislocation of acromioclavicular joint (shoulder separation). (Courtesy Dr. Phillip Marone, Methodist Hospital, Philadelphia, Pa.)

ACQUIRED DEGENERATIVE ARTHRITIS

Acquired degenerative arthritis of the acromioclavicular joint may be a cause of shoulder area pain seen, for the most part, in the older patient. The condition is more frequent in males, particularly those who have subjected the joint to repeated trauma from either athletic or occupational demands. Movement through the acromioclavicular joint is limited to its role in the shoulder girdle mechanism, but the joint can be subjected to compression and shearing forces. For this reason, adduction of the arm across the chest and abduction above the horizontal are the motions that cause shoulder pain. For the same reason, these patients frequently experience pain in the affected shoulder when they sleep on that side.

In most patients the joint margins will be felt to be enlarged and roughened, and visible enlargement of the joint is frequently observed. Direct pressure on the joint may elicit pain. Often surprisingly little actual damage to the joint is noted on x-ray examination, even in patients presenting marked clinical findings. This is because the majority of the changes involve the soft tissue and cartilage components of the joint, which are not visible on the x-ray film. Thus there is usually no direct proportional relationship between the severity of the clinical findings and the degree of degenerative change noted on the x-ray film. The pain due to acquired degenerative arthritis of the acromioclavicular joint can be relieved in the majority of patients by hydrocortisone injected into and around the involved joint. Local hydrocortisone may be combined with appropriate oral doses of an anti-inflammatory agent and with local heat applied to the joint. If the symptoms cannot be controlled by these measures, the distal end of the clavicle may be removed by operation. This widens the joint and relieves the pain.

FRACTURE OF THE CLAVICLE

The clavicle may be broken by a fall on the arm or shoulder. Occasionally the clavicle of a newborn infant is fractured during a difficult delivery. The bone usually breaks through its mid-portion, but rarely protrudes through the skin or damages the subclavian artery. The shoulder girdle nevertheless loses its outrigger strut, and the shoulder tends to droop downward and forward, adding to the displacement of the fracture fragments.

TREATMENT IN CHILDREN

Fracture of the clavicle is a fairly common injury in children. Perfect reduction of the fracture is not necessary because of the capacity of growing bone to reshape and remodel its contours. Satisfactory reduction can be achieved in most children by applying a figure-of-eight bandage made of elastic bandages or plaster; this tends to hold the shoulders upward and backward. Open reduction is not necessary in children.

TREATMENT IN ADULTS

In adults it is important to obtain and maintain good apposition of the fracture fragments. It may be possible to reduce the fragments satisfactorily by moving the shoulders upward and backward. The reduced position, once obtained, may be maintained by a plaster of paris figure-of-eight bandage.

If satisfactory reduction or efficient immobilization cannot be obtained in adults, open reduction may be carried out with the position maintained by an intramedullary threaded pin (Fig. 108).

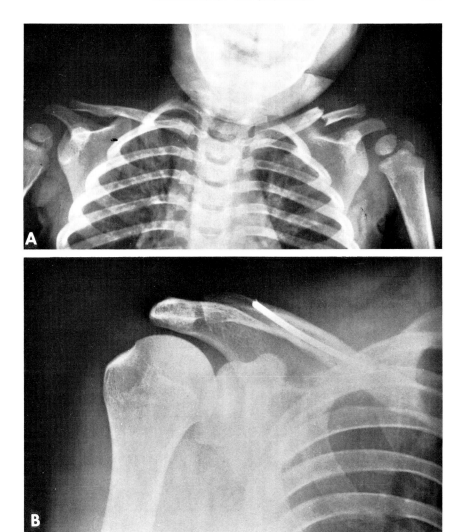

Figure 108. A, Fracture of left clavicle in child. B, Fracture of clavicle in adult, transfixed with intramedullary pin.

FRACTURE OF THE SCAPULA

Fracture of a portion of the scapula is an unusual injury and is caused most frequently by a direct blow. It is usually seen in association with other injuries in patients sustaining severe trauma.

Most fractures of the scapula heal readily when treated with simple support to the arm and local measures to the scapular area to relieve pain and swelling.

DISORDERS OF THE SHOULDER JOINT (GLENOHUMERAL)

Trauma

SPRAIN

An injury caused by twisting the upper extremity or shoulder region can result in a stretching of the capsule and muscles about the shoulder joint that may produce a temporary painful disability. This may be associated with bleeding into the joint (hemarthrosis) that will give the shoulder region a swollen appearance. X-ray examination will be negative, except for possible capsular swelling. Simple sling support, combined with cold compresses, is helpful in relieving pain. Motion should be encouraged as soon as comfort permits. Moist heat to the area is beneficial as motion begins to return.

FRACTURE

In an elderly person, a fall on the hand or arm frequently causes a fracture of the humerus through the surgical neck region. Immediate pain and disability are noted by the patient. Although the x-ray film may disclose varying degrees of impaction, comminution, or displacement of the fragments, the position is usually acceptable in the majority of these older patients, and no actual reduction is necessary (Fig. 109). The arm and shoulder are immobilized in a Velpeau bandage for three weeks, after which activity may be resumed. Satisfactory use of the shoulder may be obtained even if the fragments heal in a moderately deformed position.

If the displacement of the fragments is too severe to expect return of a functional range of shoulder motion, open reduction can be carried out to replace the fragments in a more anatomic position. If comminution is so severe that open reduction is impractical, the fragments can be excised and replaced with a humeral head prosthesis. Total shoulder prostheses are now being developed for use in those few patients in whom severe trauma or disease has resulted in loss of the rotator cuff. The units of a total shoulder prosthesis are fixed to the humeral shaft and scapula with methyl methacrylate bone cement.

Occasionally fractures through the greater tuberosity of the humerus require open reduction. In this instance, the attached musculotendinous cuff has retracted and pulled the tuberosity fragment up toward or under the acromion. The only treatment of value is to reattach the fragment in its proper location by suture or screw fixation (Fig. 110).

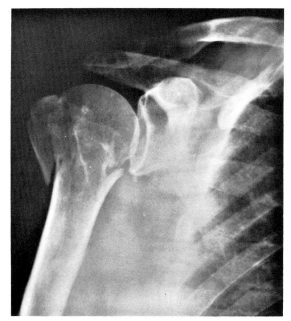

Figure 109. Comminuted fracture through surgical neck region of humerus.

DISLOCATION

A force applied to an upper extremity may result in an abnormal degree of abduction and external rotation to the humerus and force the humeral head to tear out of the joint and lodge beneath the coracoid process of the scapula (Fig. 111). This injury is called an anterior shoulder dislocation and may occur in any age group. Rarely, the shoulder may dislocate posteriorly. In order for the joint to dislocate anteriorly, the subscapularis muscle must stretch or tear along with the anterior joint capsule.

The patient with this injury seeks attention because of shoulder pain and severe disability. Inspection reveals a typical flattening of the normally rounded shoulder contour. Palpation reveals displacement of the humeral head from its normal position beneath the acromion to the subcoracoid region. Both before and after reduction, the examiner must always check the integrity of the axillary, radial, median, and ulnar nerves, and the arterial circulation.

As soon as the diagnosis is confirmed by x-ray examination, the dislocation is reduced by manipulation and the arm and shoulder are immobilized in a Velpeau bandage for three or four weeks.

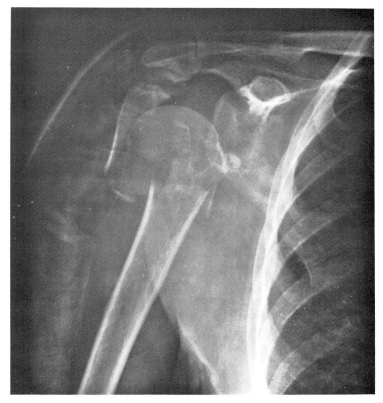

Figure 110.   Fracture through the surgical neck of the humerus with marked upward displacement of the greater tuberosity fragment. (Compare with Fig. 109).

Associated fracture of the humeral head or greater tuberosity sometimes accompanies dislocation of the shoulder joint in middle-aged or elderly patients. In most of these patients, however, successful reduction of the dislocation also reduces the accompanying fracture.

Less frequently, a complete fracture through the upper shaft of the humerus may be seen in association with dislocation of the humeral head. This is a serious injury, and open reduction with internal fixation is required to secure the fragments in position.

RECURRENT DISLOCATION

Dislocation of the shoulder joint in a younger patient carries with it a high recurrence rate, estimated at as great as 40 per cent. This predilection for redislocation is unique to the shoulder joint. Recurrence is not common in middle-aged or elderly patients because of the normal tendency of the subscapularis muscle to tighten with age, thereby effectively limiting the motion of external rotation. Authorities are not agreed upon the cause of recurrent dislocation. Undoubtedly some type of capsular or tendinous stretching occurs with the initial dislocation that does not completely heal, but there is no universal agreement about its exact nature. The tendency for redislocation is definitely related to the inherent anatomic instability of the shoulder joint. Although recurrent dislocation may occur posteriorly, the great majority of patients with this disorder sustain recurrent anterior dislocations.

Anterior dislocation may occur on abduction and external rotation of the arm. Some patients experience multiple shoulder dislocations following unguarded movements of the arm, and many patients become adept at reducing their own dislocations. Recurrence can be-

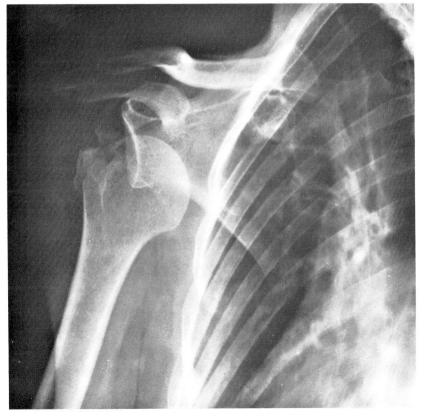

Figure 111. Anterior dislocation of the right shoulder with fracture through greater tuberosity.

come so frequent as to preclude vigorous physical activity in an otherwise healthy person.

No amount of immobilization will cure the tendency for the shoulder joint to dislocate repeatedly. Operative repair, such as transplanting the subscapularis tendon to a different location on the humerus to form an anterior soft tissue buttress for the humeral head, is necessary for permanent correction of this condition.

RUPTURE OF THE BICEPS TENDON

The tendon of the long head of the biceps brachii muscle lies in the bicipital groove of the humerus, where it may undergo degenerative changes with resulting loss of tensile strength. Shoulder pain may be noticed by the patient as the degenerative tendon and tendon sheath changes occur. Some evidence has been presented that implicates the use of hydrocortisone injections into the tendon sheath of the biceps tendon in degenerative changes of the tendon tissue (see bicipital tenosynovitis, p. 231).

By lifting or lowering a heavy object, a patient may apply a sudden force to this weakened tendon that may cause it to fray apart in the bicipital groove with resulting pain and weakness in the arm. The small proximal piece of tendon remains in position in the bicipital groove, but the distal fragment with the attached muscle belly retracts toward the elbow. The torn biceps muscle belly shortens, giving a ball-like appearance to the arm muscle. The lower shoulder and upper arm area is tender to palpation, and a muscular gap can be felt. The tissues appear swollen and indurated, and the overlying skin becomes ecchymotic. Weakness in flexion of the elbow and supination of the forearm are noted by the patient.

Operative repair may be carried out. The distal tendon fragment with the attached muscle belly is located and fastened to the bicipital groove of the humerus with sutures or a metallic staple.

Less commonly, the rupture may occur at the elbow where the biceps tendon inserts distally on the bicipital tuberosity of the radius. In this instance, the muscle belly retracts toward the shoulder and must be reattached to the bicipital tuberosity by operation.

TEARS OF THE ROTATOR CUFF

The musculotendinous or rotator cuff of the shoulder, which acts to stabilize the humeral head in the glenoid cavity so that the motion of shoulder abduction can be initiated, normally undergoes some degenerative changes with advancing age. Asymptomatic "worn-out" spots may appear in the cuff. If a sudden adduction force is applied to such a cuff while the arm is being held in abduction, particularly in a patient over 40 years of age, traumatic tears of the cuff tissue can occur that may make it impossible for the patient to initiate the movement of shoulder abduction.

The patient may be aware of immediate pain in the shoulder. Local tenderness may be noted over the cuff, and the patient may be unable to initiate or maintain active abduction of the arm at the shoulder joint. If the examiner passively places the arm in abduction at the shoulder, the patient may be unable to sustain this position and the arm will drop to the side. Full passive mobility of the shoulder joint, however, is never lost.

Routine x-ray examination of the shoulder is negative unless there is an associated fracture. The diagnosis may be confirmed by injecting air or dye into the shoulder joint and observing its escape into the subdeltoid bursa on an x-ray film. This study is called an *arthrogram*.

The initial treatment of a tear of the rotator cuff is conservative, because many patients sustain only incomplete ruptures and may gradually recover strength and motion spontaneously. The arm is supported in a sling, and hot applications may be applied to the shoulder. Surgical exploration of the rotator cuff area is reserved for those patients who do not recover on a conservative program after a four- to six-week trial. These patients have usually sustained massive tears or complete ruptures of the rotator cuff that will necessitate operative repair.

Derangements of the Subacromial Mechanism

The painful shoulder is a complaint that is fairly common to all age groups in both sexes, and in order to treat these patients satisfactorily, diagnosis of the exact cause must be determined in each case. The use of "bursitis" as an all-inclusive term denoting the diagnosis and basis for therapy in the painful shoulder syndrome is irrational. Excluding the traumatic causes already discussed, shoulder pain may radiate from a lesion of the cervical spine or may represent irritation from some other organ, such as gallbladder or heart. Most frequently, however, it originates in the shoulder joint proper as some derangement of what is known as the subacromial mechanism.

The subacromial mechanism of the shoulder joint is bounded above by the acromion and the coracoacromial ligament and below by the humeral head. Its component structures include the subacromial or subdeltoid bursa, the musculotendinous or rotator cuff, the articular capsule of the shoulder joint, and the tendon–tendon-sheath gliding

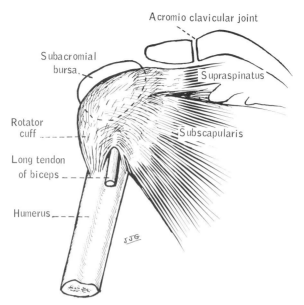

Figure 112.   Subacromial mechanism of shoulder.

mechanism of the tendon of the long head of the biceps brachii muscle (Fig. 112).

The majority of patients with shoulder pain will be found to have some lesion involving a component of this mechanism. The use of the blanket term "bursitis" to explain all the derangements of the subacromial mechanism constitutes the most important single factor mitigating against successful management of the painful or stiff shoulder. All lesions of the subacromial mechanism may secondarily involve the subdeltoid bursa, but only rarely is a true primary subdeltoid bursitis encountered. The most frequently seen derangements of the subacromial mechanism causing shoulder pain are calcific deposits in the musculotendinous cuff, bicipital tenosynovitis, lesions of the acromioclavicular joint, and frozen shoulder deformity or adhesive capsulitis of the shoulder joint.

CALCIUM DEPOSITS

Amorphous calcium deposits may occur in many soft tissue sites throughout the body, giving rise to pain and dysfunction. By far the most common site for the deposition of amorphous calcium is the musculotendinous or rotator cuff of the shoulder. The calcification usually occurs in the supraspinatus portion of the cuff. This is the condition most commonly referred to erroneously as "bursitis."

Calcification is seen most frequently during the third, fourth, and fifth decades of life and is slightly more common in the male. There is a high incidence in "white collar" workers and housewives. It is believed that repeated small injuries sustained by the cuff cause degenerative and necrotic areas to appear in the tendon tissue. In the presence of necrosis, the local tissue reaction becomes alkaline, thus inducing precipitation of calcium into the area. The physical characteristics of the calcium deposit will greatly influence the type of pain felt by the patient. If the calcium is in a liquid or soft state, an acute process will ensue characterized by severe throbbing shoulder pain and marked disability. If the deposit is dry, gritty, and hard, a chronic picture is produced characterized by less intense shoulder ache and a "catching" pain on certain motions associated with raising the arm above the horizontal plane.

Acute Stage. The acute stage is characterized by severe, disabling shoulder pain that has been known to reduce an adult to tears. It is often described as a constant throbbing or beating type of pain. Although markedly aggravated by motion of the shoulder, the pain is constantly present, even when the shoulder is immobile. This point is useful in distinguishing the acute stage from the chronic stage or from a bicipital tenosynovitis. In the latter two conditions, shoulder pain is not present constantly but rather is brought on by movement of the arm and shoulder.

The onset of shoulder pain may be sudden and surprising or may be preceded by a few days of shoulder ache. The pain originates in the shoulder cuff region, but it may radiate up into the neck or down into the forearm and hand. Exquisite tenderness may be produced by palpation over the area of the calcium deposit. The patient usually holds the arm splinted to the side.

Anteroposterior x-ray films of the shoulder joint, taken with the arm in both external and internal rotation, reveal the amorphous calcium deposit in the rotator cuff (Fig. 113).

Chronic Stage. The chronic stage is characterized by ache or pain in the shoulder brought on by movement of the arm. The patient may be aware of a constant ache or an uncomfortable sensation in the shoulder, but it is never as severe or disabling as an acute process. Usually the patient can get along quite well if certain motions of the shoulder, such as raising the arm above the horizontal plane in throwing a ball, are avoided. This type of motion produces the so-called "painful arc syndrome," in which pain is caused by impingement of the hard calcified material beneath the coracoacromial ligament as the arm is raised in abduction. The patient with a chronic calcium deposit usually has had discomfort for many months and has learned to avoid painful movements. Most patients notice pain when they attempt to

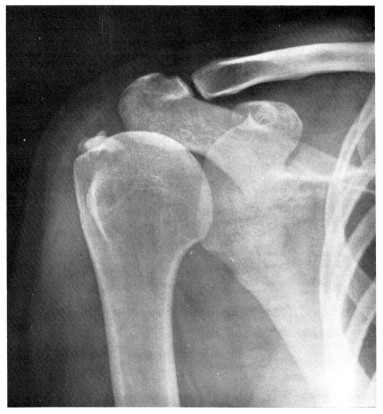

Figure 113. Calcium deposit lying in the rotator cuff just above the greater tuberosity of the right humerus.

lie on the affected shoulder at night or complain of difficulty in finding a comfortable position for the arm in bed. X-ray examination of the shoulder joint will reveal the presence of the calcium deposit.

Mixed Stage. Occasionally a patient with a dry, hard calcium deposit in the rotator cuff (chronic stage) will sustain fresh trauma to the affected shoulder and, in the space of a few hours, develop severe disabling shoulder pain. In this instance, the fresh trauma has caused the hard, dry calcified material to pass into the liquid or soft state. The clinical picture produced is identical to that described for the acute stage. Gardening, lifting heavy objects, shoveling, and carrying heavy suitcases are activities that frequently bring about this change in the physical characteristics of the calcium deposit.

Treatment. "Needling" of the calcium deposit is frequently very effective treatment. Once the site of the calcification has been localized by clinical and x-ray examination, the deposit is entered with an 18-gauge needle under local anesthesia. Multiple needle puncture of the calcium deposit is carried out by moving the point of the needle rapidly into and out of the deposit. This maneuver serves to break up the localized calcium deposit and lessen its tension, and it also tends to change the local tissue pH to the acid side by bringing fresh blood to the area. This is helpful because calcium tends to go into solution in an acid medium. Calcium can sometimes be aspirated into the syringe, although this is not necessary in order to effect a cure. Before the needle is withdrawn, 50 mg. of hydrocortisone may be injected into the deposit area for its "anti-inflammatory" effect. Some physicians combine "needling" with the oral administration of anti-inflammatory drugs. If this treatment is successful, the patient will notice a rapid disappearance of the constant, beating pain and a gradual return of normal shoulder motion and function.

Surgical excision of the calcium is advised when the deposit is too large to be needled effectively, when there are repeated recurrences, or when the x-ray film shows the calcium deposit to be burrowing into the bone.

X-ray therapy has been used with benefit in many patients. Such therapy is not without its dangers, however, and at best it only serves to convert an acute stage into a chronic stage by "drying out" the deposit.

Under no circumstances should heat in any of its forms be applied to a shoulder during the acute stage of a calcium deposit. This usually results in increased shoulder pain. Ice packs to the shoulder are more soothing. After the acute stage has been treated, heat is helpful in restoring motion to the joint.

BICIPITAL TENOSYNOVITIS

Mechanical tenosynovitis involving the tendon–tendon-sheath gliding mechanism of the long tendon of the biceps in the bicipital groove of the humerus is a common cause of shoulder pain. The long tendon of the biceps muscle arises from the supraglenoid fossa of the glenoid cavity, extends through the space between the superior part of the capsule of the shoulder joint and the humeral head, and passes into the fibrous tunnel formed by its theca, covering the bicipital groove. The tendon is ensheathed in a synovial membrane that extends as an outpocketing from the joint into the bicipital groove and makes up the tendon sheath part of the gliding mechanism..Actually, the tendon does very little gliding within the groove. It is the humerus that glides on the tendon and irritates the inflamed tendon sheath.

This gliding mechanism is readily disturbed by excessive activity of the arm, particularly when the arm is made to work at a disadvantage, or by direct trauma to the area of the bicipital groove. Once the process is precipitated, all activities that require much motion of the humerus on the tendon will produce pain. Abduction and external rotation, as well as internal rotation and extension, are the movements of the arm most likely to irritate the biceps tendon and cause pain. Such movements are required, for example, in combing the hair, putting on a shirt or coat, fastening a brassiere, or reaching for a telephone.

Clinical Picture. The onset of pain in this condition may be slow and gradual, or it may be more acute, following sudden vigorous activity of the arm such as in shoveling snow. Trauma to the arm may produce a strain or "snap" of the tendon in the bicipital groove, causing an irritation of the tendon sheath. The pain originates in the anterior and medial aspect of the shoulder but may radiate along the course of the biceps muscle to the elbow or even to the forearm and fingers. Occasionally, pain may radiate to the posterior aspect of the shoulder joint and to the neck.

Bicipital tenosynovitis is more common in the female, and its greatest incidence is in 45 to 65 year old patients. The pain is always brought on by the motions previously described and is relieved by resting the arm.

Invariably, these patients describe great difficulty in finding a comfortable position for the affected arm in bed. Point tenderness may be found over the biceps tendon in the bicipital groove or along the anterior aspect of the humerus. A combination of abduction, external rotation, and extension of the arm at the shoulder may cause pain in the region of the bicipital groove. Forced flexion of the elbow against resistance and forced supination of the forearm against resistance, with the elbow flexed, frequently cause pain in the area of the bicipital groove. If bicipital tenosynovitis is present for several weeks, it may cause a frozen shoulder deformity. Since bicipital tenosynovitis involves the soft tissues of the shoulder joint, x-ray examination is negative.

Treatment. A period of rest to the arm and shoulder is helpful. This may be supplied by a sling. Too much immobilization must be avoided, however, to prevent the complication of a frozen shoulder or adhesive capsulitis. Moist heat applied to the area of the bicipital groove is quite soothing to the patient. Hydrocortisone, in doses of 50 to 75 mg. injected directly into the tendon sheath within the bicipital groove, is effective in relieving the tendon sheath irritation if it is not given too frequently. In some patients, injected hydrocortisone may cause degenerative lesions of the biceps tendon and may be associated with eventual rupture of the biceps tendon. Injected hydrocortisone may be combined with orally administered anti-inflammatory drugs. Diathermy and ultrasound treatment to the painful area have been used, but they do not seem to be as effective as the anti-inflammatory agents.

Rarely, operative intervention may be required for relief of pain if all other treatment methods have failed. At operation, the biceps tendon is permanently anchored to the bicipital groove of the humerus by suture or by means of a metal staple. Anchoring the tendon firmly to the underlying bone obliterates the tendon–tendon-sheath gliding mechanism and the stimulus for pain.

Disorders of the Acromioclavicular Joint

Disorders of the acromioclavicular joint may be classified under trauma or under derangements of the subacromial mechanism. They may occur frequently and, if not readily recognized and treated, may result in considerable shoulder pain and discomfort. These disorders have already been discussed on page 218.

Frozen Shoulder Deformity, Adhesive Capsulitis of the Shoulder

The term "frozen shoulder" is not the title of a specific disease process but, like the term "jaundice," indicates the objective manifestations of some causative factor. The primary causative factor for the development of a frozen shoulder is pain associated with elevating the arm in a person who tends to self-protect the extremity. The pain may arise in the shoulder joint itself and may follow dislocation, fracture or other upper extremity trauma, bicipital tenosynovitis, calcium deposits in the rotator cuff, or painful lesions of the acromioclavicular joints. The pain may arise primarily away from the shoulder but radiate to this region with enough intensity to result in a frozen shoulder. Such pain transference may be seen after myocardial infarction, radical mastectomy, and thoracoplasty. Regardless of cause, the pain is of sufficient unpleasantness to discourage shoulder and arm movements. Continued immobility of the shoulder joint allows the capsule to adhere to the proximal humerus, resulting in a stiffened or frozen shoulder deformity.

Most authorities agree that the pain which limits or prevents elevation of the arm must occur in a patient of a peculiar personality type for a true frozen shoulder to develop. These are thought to be persons who react poorly under stress. They have been described as having "periarthritic personalities." It is noticed that in this type of individual the shoulder, self-protected from painful elevation, gradually and insidiously becomes stiff and more painful.

Clinical Picture. The patient with a frozen shoulder presents with a tight stiff shoulder joint that developed following some primary cause of shoulder pain (Fig. 114). The original cause of pain, as noted, may be one of several possibilities and may already have been corrected. Passively, the glenohumeral joint is tight and contracted in all planes of motion. Actively, the patient may superficially appear to have a greater range of motion than passively, but this appearance is the result of compensatory scapulothoracic motion. The overlying shoulder muscles may appear atrophic. Many times these tense patients present with associated muscle spasm that produces pain running from the occiput to the wrist. Frequently associated vasomotor effects in the hand and fingers are seen. The combination of neck, chest wall, and arm pain sometimes mimics cervical radiculitis (see p. 285).

Treatment. The treatment of a frozen shoulder involves locating and treating the primary cause of pain, if it is still present, and paying sympathetic attention to the psychological difficulties of the patient.

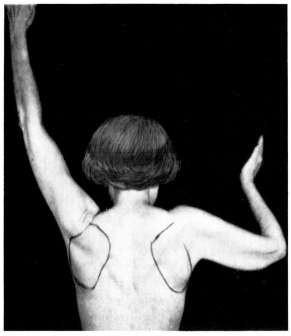

Figure 114. Patient with frozen shoulder deformity on right: glenohumeral rhythm is grossly disturbed on the right side. The scapula on the right side rotates outward with elevation of the right humerus, indicating loss of glenohumeral joint motion. (From DePalma, A. F.: Surgery of the Shoulder, 2nd ed. Philadelphia: J. B. Lippincott Co., 1973.)

Friendly interest and encouragement often accomplish a great deal. Exercises within painless arcs of motion must be encouraged.

Inflating the shoulder joint with a relatively large volume of normal saline solution mixed with local anesthetic and a corticosteroid frequently peels the adherent capsule from the humeral head. Combined with gentle manipulation of the shoulder, this treatment, called *infiltration brisement*, is often quite beneficial. Manipulation of the tight shoulder joint under anesthesia is not favored, because it may cause fracture or rupture of an important tendon. In an occasional patient, the tightness may be sufficiently severe to require surgical release of the tight structures about the shoulder joint.

References

Abbott, L. C., and Lucas, D. B.: The function of the clavicle. Its surgical significance. Ann. Surg., *140*:583, 1954.

Bailey, R. W.: Acute and recurrent dislocation of the shoulder. J. Bone and Joint Surg., 49-A:767, 1967.

DePalma, A. F.: Surgery of the Shoulder, 2nd Edition. Philadelphia: J. B. Lippincott Co., 1973.

Graham, W., and Rosen, P.: The shoulder-hand syndrome. Bull. Rheum. Dis., 2:277, 1962.

Inman, V. T., Saunders, J. S., deC., M., and Abbott, L. D.: Observations on the function of the shoulder joint. J. Bone and Joint Surg., 26:1, 1944.

Chapter Eleven

The Upper Extremity

In Chapter 10, the reader's attention was drawn to the great mobility of the shoulder joint. This mobility characterizes the entire upper extremity. Man's upper limbs are free and possess great range of movement. His ability to survive and flourish depends, to a considerable extent, on this capability. Unfortunately, man is also prey to many diseases or disorders that may seriously impair this mobility through pain, deformity, or muscle weakness. This impairment may arise primarily in a segment of the upper extremity, or it may radiate secondarily to the part from a primary focus in the neck or shoulder.

When a complaint is referable to the upper extremity, the examiner must be prepared to differentiate between the primary and secondary causes. It is well to remember that the examination of the upper extremity begins at the sternal notch and works out gradually to the finger tips. For this reason the patient should be suitably draped so that the neck, shoulders, and both upper extremities are exposed for examination and comparison.

For descriptive purposes, disorders of the upper extremity are presented under the headings of upper arm, elbow, forearm, wrist, and hand.

THE UPPER ARM

GENERAL CONSIDERATIONS

Frequently, pain in the arm will be a radiating type with its origin in the neck or shoulder. Pain arising in the neck is discussed on page

279, that arising in the shoulder on page 217. Two conditions affecting the shoulder, bicipital tenosynovitis and rupture of the biceps tendon, overlap anatomically into the arm area and may cause arm symptoms predominantly.

Bone tumors may involve the humerus. The more common benign bone tumors seen in this area include unicameral bone cyst, osteochondroma, and giant cell tumor. Primary malignant bone tumors, such as osteosarcoma, fibrosarcoma, and Ewing's tumor, occasionally arise in the humerus. Metastatic carcinoma from a primary site, such as the breast, kidney, prostate, or lung, not infrequently involves the humerus. The presence of a tumor in the bone may be a cause of pathologic fracture (see p. 25).

Although more rare, benign and malignant soft tissue tumors may also be found in the upper arm area.

FRACTURE OF THE HUMERUS

Injury to the humerus may result in a transverse or spiral fracture through the mid-shaft of the bone (Fig. 115). Whenever possible, closed reduction is the treatment of choice, using a sugar-tong splint

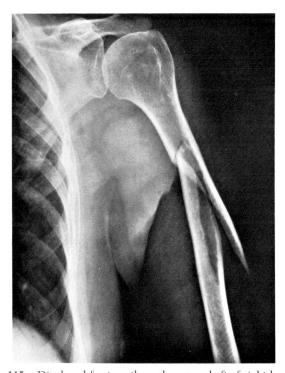

Figure 115.   Displaced fracture through upper shaft of right humerus.

with a Velpeau bandage, a hanging cast, or a shoulder spica as the immobilizing agent. If open reduction is deemed necessary, either intramedullary pin fixation or compression plate fixation is usually employed.

The two major complications of fracture of the humerus are nonunion of the bone and radial nerve palsy. Nonunion occurs in 5 to 12 per cent of patients and requires bone graft operation for its cure.

Injury to the radial nerve adjacent to the musculospiral groove may accompany humeral shaft fractures. This may result in the patient's losing the power actively to dorsiflex the wrist and elevate the thumb. The wrist hangs limply in a flexed position, and the condition is called "wrist drop." This complication occurs in about 12 per cent of patients. However, nerve function returns in the majority of these patients within a three- to nine-month period—unless there is further trauma from the treatment itself—because it is likely that the radial nerve is only bruised and not ruptured in association with the humeral shaft fracture. The wrist should be splinted in the dorsiflexed position (position of function) while awaiting nerve regeneration.

RADIAL NERVE PALSY

Radial nerve palsy, as previously noted, may complicate a humeral shaft fracture. A penetrating wound of the arm may damage or sever the radial nerve, resulting in a temporary or permanent wrist drop. Temporary radial nerve palsy may also result from direct pressure against the nerve trunk. This is occasionally caused by improper use of crutches or by a person's falling asleep with his arm draped over the back of a chair or bench. Complete return of nerve function can be expected in instances of temporary radial nerve palsy. Complete severance of the radial nerve requires surgical repair—or if this is impossible, wrist fusion and tendon transfers—to restore dorsiflexion ability to the paralyzed wrist.

THE ELBOW

From an anatomical standpoint, the elbow is the most complicated joint of the upper extremity. This consideration accounts for many of the complications that follow involvement of the elbow by trauma or disease. The distal end of the humerus and the proximal ends of the radius and ulna are specially constructed to fit together to form the elbow articulation (Fig. 116). Normal appearance and normal range of motion of the elbow require that this structural relationship be maintained.

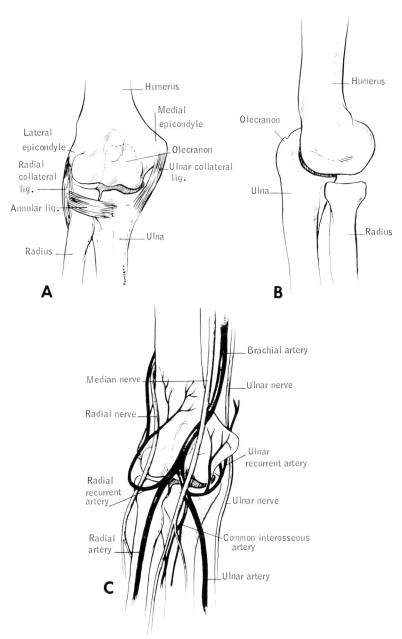

Figure 116. Skeletal anatomy of elbow. *A*, ligaments. *B*, bones, lateral view. *C*, nerves and arteries.

Basically, the elbow is a hinge joint and allows only flexion and extension through an arc of 150 degrees (see Fig. 4). Mechanically, this motion occurs through the humero-ulnar component of the joint, with the radius playing only a passive role. The radius is more directly concerned with the motions of pronation and supination of the forearm. Like the knee joint, the elbow depends upon strong collateral ligaments for lateral stability. The muscles are massed in front and behind in order to flex and extend the joint.

When the elbows are flexed to a right angle and held firmly at the sides, the forearms can be rotated into almost 90 degrees of pronation and supination. A normal range of pronation and supination requires smooth rotation of the radial head on the capitellum of the humerus, in addition to mobility through the superior radio-ulnar joint and the inferior radio-ulnar joint at the wrist. A bone block at any of these levels will obliterate the motion of pronation and supination.

When the forearm is viewed from the front with the elbow joint completely extended, it is seen that the forearm projects outward from the arm at an angle of 10 to 15 degrees. This is known as the *carrying angle* and depends for its existence on a proper relationship between the various bones making up the elbow joint. The carrying angle can best be appreciated when the subject is standing erect, both arms stiffly at his side with palms facing forward. It can then be seen that the forearms project away from the sides of the body. This allows one to carry an object without bumping it against the legs. If the carrying angle is abnormally increased by trauma or disease, the deformity is called *cubitus valgus.* Decrease in the carrying angle is known as *cubitus varus* (see Fig. 49).

The relationship of the ulnar nerve, median nerve, and brachial artery to the elbow must be continually borne in mind in considering problems involving this joint. The ulnar nerve lies in a vulnerable position as it passes beneath the medial epicondyle. At the level of the elbow joint, the brachial artery and median nerve overlie the anterior aspect of the humerus and the brachialis muscle.

GENERAL CONDITIONS

The elbow joint may fall victim to the same general problems that beset all joints.

Arthritis. Rheumatoid arthritis may destroy the joint, causing deformity and stiffness. Degenerative arthritis is not a common problem at the elbow, since this disorder tends to involve weight bearing joints primarily. Bleeding into the elbow joint is a frequent occurrence in hemophilia and may result in permanent joint damage.

Infection. Pyogenic infection and tuberculosis may involve the elbow joint and must be quickly recognized and vigorously treated if permanent joint damage is to be avoided.

Tumors.   Benign and malignant bone and soft tissue tumors may appear in the elbow joint area, although none has a particular affinity for the site.

Traumatic Myositis Ossificans.   On occasion, hemorrhage into a muscle may produce irregular masses of bone, complete with cortex and medullary cavity. This condition, known as traumatic myositis ossificans (Fig. 117), is most commonly seen over the anterior surface of the femur following hemorrhage into the quadriceps muscle, and over the flexor surface of the elbow following hemorrhage into the brachialis anticus muscle. In almost all instances the hemorrhage is produced by injury, and the resulting bone mass lies alongside the bone or may be attached in part to the underlying bone.

The process is thought to represent metaplasia of fibroblasts and is characterized by heterotopic calcification and ossification. As time passes, the bone becomes more mature and dense. It can complicate fractures and dislocations at the elbow and can become a major functional problem by acting as a block to flexion.

Traumatic myositis ossificans must be differentiated from osteosarcoma and myositis ossificans progressiva, a rare congenital disease characterized by the formation of sheets of bone in muscles, ligaments, and fascia. Careful study of the physical fractures

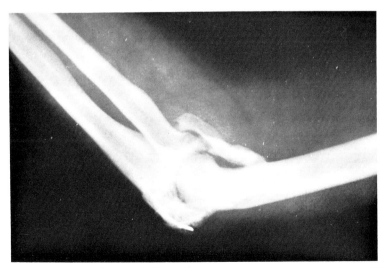

Figure 117.   Lateral x-ray of elbow, showing an area of mature myositis ossificans overlying the flexor aspect of the joint.

characteristics of the bone mass, its x-ray appearance, and the histologic sections should permit this essential distinction.

Treatment depends on the stage of activity of the process. During the active phase, rest and immobilization are essential. Misguided attempts at forceful exercise or early surgical removal will be rewarded with further bone formation. If there is functional impairment, surgical excision of the mass should be carried out, but only after the ectopic bone has become dense and mature, a state reached six months to one year after its first appearance.

Trauma

Subluxation of the Radial Head. This condition, known as "nursemaid's elbow," is seen exclusively in infants and young children. Forceful pulling on a child's hand or forearm may cause the cartilaginous radial head to slip partially out of encircling orbicular ligament. As a result, the child refuses to use the arm because of pain and holds it in a semiflexed and slightly pronated position. X-ray examination is of no help because the radial head, at this age, is cartilage and will not show on the film.

Reduction is quite easy, requires no anesthesia, and is achieved by first rapidly turning the forearm into full supination and then following with sudden flexion of the elbow. As the maneuver is carried out, the radial head can be felt to "click" back into place. The reduction is usually stable, and no immobilization is required. The child can be encouraged to use the arm normally.

Dislocation of the Elbow Joint. A fall on the outstretched hand in a child or adult not infrequently causes a traumatic dislocation of the elbow joint. The joint gives way under the force and, most commonly, the lower end of the humerus is driven over the coronoid process of the ulna and out through the torn anterior capsule. The ulna and radius are forced backward, and the ulna finally lodges behind the lower end of the displaced humerus. This is described as a posterior dislocation of the elbow. Anterior dislocation of the elbow joint is quite rare.

The injury results in a painful deformity of the elbow soon accompanied by marked swelling. Normally, the point of the olecranon lies ahead of a line connecting the medial and lateral humeral epincondyles. In the presence of a posterior dislocation of the elbow, the point of the olecranon typically lies behind this line. X-ray examination will confirm the diagnosis of dislocation (Fig. 118). The possibility of associated nerve or circulatory damage must always be considered.

Closed manipulative reduction under adequate anesthesia should be carried out as soon as possible. The elbow is immobilized in a pos-

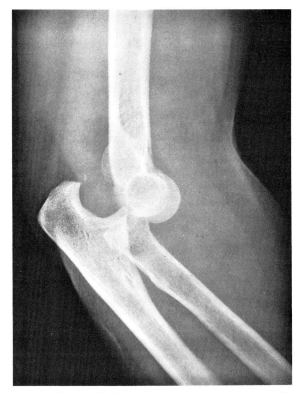

Figure 118. Lateral view of elbow, showing traumatic posterior dislocation of the joint.

terior plaster splint in a safe degree of flexion for three weeks. The elbow joint has poor tolerance for injury and immobilization, and it may be months before full motion returns.

Unlike the shoulder joint, however, the elbow joint rarely suffers recurrent dislocation. Occasionally dislocation is accompanied by circulatory or nerve damage. Traumatic myositis ossificans may be seen as a complication.

Supracondylar Fracture of the Humerus. The supracondylar area of the humerus is the lower flared end of the bone just above the elbow joint. Fractures through this area occur commonly in children and uncommonly in adults. They are occasionally accompanied by frightening complications and distressing physical deformity. The immediate deformity may superficially resemble that caused by a posterior dislocation of the elbow, except that the relationship between the olecranon and the epicondyles is not disturbed. X-ray examination serves to differentiate the two.

On the lateral x-ray view, it can be recognized that normally the lower end of the humerus, containing the condyles, tilts forward at an angle of approximately 30 degrees with the shaft. A fracture through the supracondylar area results in a broken bone of two fragments (Fig. 119). The small distal fragment consists of the lower flared condylar portion of the humerus, to which are attached the elbow joint and forearm. The larger proximal fragment is the remainder of the humeral shaft. Most often following fracture, the small distal fragment is displaced backward, but rarely it may be displaced forward, depending on the direction of the fracturing force. This displacement results in a loss of the normal forward angulation of the lower end of the humerus. In addition to being displaced backward, the small distal fragment usually rotates on the larger proximal fragment. If the backward displacement of the distal fragment is not corrected and the forward angulation restored, permanent alteration in the range of flexion and extension at the elbow joint will occur. If the rotatory displacement is not corrected, it will result in permanent abnormality of the carrying angle, with the appearance of a cubitus valgus or cubitus varus deformity.

Every child with a suspected elbow fracture should have an x-ray

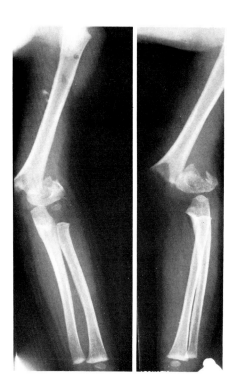

Figure 119.   AP and lateral views of supracondylar fracture of the humerus. (Compare with Fig. 120.)

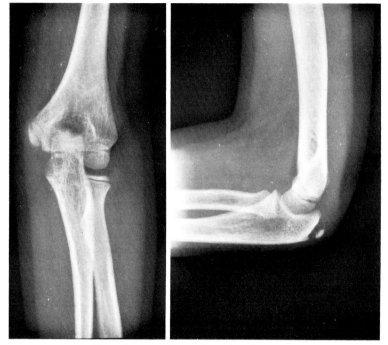

Figure 120.   AP and lateral views of normal child's elbow. Note open growth lines.

examination of both elbows for comparison. The normally present cartilage growth lines (epiphyseal cartilage) at the lower end of the humerus sometimes make the detection of a fracture line difficult. If the child has an x-ray of the uninjured elbow for comparison, detection can be facilitated (Fig. 120). Such comparison is usually not necessary in an adult, however, because growth lines are no longer present to cause confusion.

Immediate check should be made to determine the existence of any circulatory embarrassment or nerve damage. Treatment of the fracture should be undertaken as soon as the x-ray films are reviewed and the diagnosis is established. This is one injury that brooks no delay. Swelling about the elbow enlarges rapidly and increases the danger of bony and vascular complications.

Reduction of a displaced supracondylar fracture involves restoring the normal forward angulation of the distal end of the humerus, in addition to correcting the rotational spin of the distal fragment. If these objectives are not accomplished, permanent limitation of motion or deformity will result. The choice of a method of reduction depends on the severity of the individual fracture and the training and experience of the operator. Many of these fractures can be successfully reduced by closed manipulative methods; others require skin or skeletal traction. Post-reduction fixation of the fragments by percutaneous pinning is favored by some orthopaedic surgeons. Open reduction is not usually considered necessary. Immobilization in plaster for a total of six weeks is normally sufficient to insure adequate bone healing. The prognosis for return of normal function is excellent in a well-reduced fracture that heals without complication.

Complications may arise following a supracondylar fracture of the humerus because of: (1) inadequate or incomplete reduction of the fracture, (2) damage to nerves passing over the fracture site, or (3) circulatory impairment heralded by weak or absent radial pulse.

Inadequate reduction will result in permanent limitation of motion or an obvious physical deformity, such as cubitus valgus or cubitus varus (Fig. 49).

Stretching or contusion injuries to the median and ulnar nerves and deep muscular branch of the radial nerve have been reported. The nerve damage in almost all cases is temporary and disappears in time without any specific treatment. It is important, however, to recognize evidence of nerve damage, if present, before fracture treatment is started.

The most dreaded complication of a supracondylar fracture of the humerus is circulatory embarrassment, which is expressed as an extremely weak or absent radial pulse. If present before reduction, such embarrassment is usually due to antecubital edema, impingement of a bone fragment against the brachial artery, or rarely, a torn or lacerated brachial artery. If the embarrassment appears after reduction, it is probably due to vascular obstruction secondary to tight bandages or to a position of acute or extreme flexion. An absent radial pulse in the presence of a supracondylar fracture of the humerus demands maximum effort to determine its cause and bring about correction. If it is ignored or not corrected within a four- to eight-hour period, a severe deforming and crippling condition of the hand and forearm known as *Volkmann's ischemic contracture* may result.

Volkmann's Ischemic Contracture. This tragic condition is due, basically, to ischemia that results in massive infarction of muscle tissue. It is seen most commonly after supracondylar fractures of the humerus, but it may also follow other fractures about the elbow joint and forearm bones. It may involve the lower extremity following fractures of the femur and tibia, and it has been described subsequent to the use of Bryant's traction in small children.

It is thought that acute venous obstruction, coupled with arterial spasm, is the cause of the ischemia. If allowed to continue unchecked, the ischemia leads to massive muscle infarction with a gradual replacement of muscle by fibrous tissue and a binding down of tendons and nerves with scar. In the upper extremity, the final result is a hard atrophic forearm with a stiff clawhand deformity. If the nerves are involved, the hand may be anesthetic and paralyzed.

If recognized early, this catastrophe is avoidable. The first rule is to think of the possiblity when dealing with any condition of the extremities that might be complicated by impaired peripheral circulation. Avoid tight casts and bandages or severely flexed positions that could cause acute venous obstruction. Check the peripheral circulation frequently with special reference to the arterial pulses and the color, temperature, and swelling of the fingers or toes. Be alert to the complaint of pain in the forearm or leg, particularly if pain is associated with inability to extend the digits. This could indicate the beginnings of muscle ischemia.

If ischemia is suspected, all constricting bandages should be released immediately and the extremity elevated. If the ischemia shows no signs of correcting itself after one to two hours of close observation, emergency surgery is performed to open the fascial planes for decompression.

Fractures of the Olecranon. Fracture of the olecranon is more common in adults than in children and is caused by a direct fall on the elbow or by forced contraction of the triceps muscle following a fall on the hand with the elbow flexed. Many times associated laceration of the lateral aponeurosis of the triceps tendon allows marked separation of the fragments. Since this fracture involves the humero-ulnar component of the joint, an inadequate reduction may result in a limitation of extension at the elbow.

Although many olecranon fractures can be reduced satisfactorily by immobilizing the extremity in a cast with the elbow in complete extension, it may take two or three months for the fracture to heal and several more months for the patient to regain elbow joint motion. This has led to a general tendency toward operative treatment because it offers the advantage of earlier motion. In general, two surgical methods are in use:

1. Open reduction of the fracture may be performed with the fragments held in position by means of internal metallic fixation devices, such as wire, nails, or screws.

2. If the proximal fragment is not too large, it may be excised and discarded, and the triceps may be resutured to the ulnar shaft.

Fracture of the Radial Head. Fracture of the radial head is common in adults and is caused, usually, by a fall on the outstretched hand. Because this fracture tends to cause joint stiffness if immobilized, the key to its successful treatment is early motion. The choice of treatment depends on the degree of displacement of the fragments, but all methods have in common the use of early joint motion.

If displacement of the fragments is minimal or absent, the fracture is ignored and early motion is stressed. Pain can be controlled by aspirating blood from the distended radiohumeral joint and keeping the elbow at rest in a posterior plaster splint for 48 hours. After this period, immobilization is eliminated and motion started.

If the fracture is comminuted or if the displacement is such that interference with pronation and supination can be anticipated, operative excision of the radial head is carried out, preferably within 24 hours of injury. No immobilization is used and early motion is encouraged.

Although not as frequently, similar injuries may be seen in children. In this instance, trauma causes a fracture of the radial neck or a separation of the upper radial epiphysis. In either case, reduction must be carried out if there is displacement of the fragments. If closed reduction is unsuccessful, open reduction is used. The radial head should not be removed in the child because a growth deformity might develop. Subsequent overgrowth of the ulna at the wrist might produce a clubhand deformity.

SPECIFIC CONDITIONS

Osteochondritis Dissecans. Osteochondritis dissecans is a joint condition in which a fragment of articular cartilage, with or without subchondral bone, becomes partially or completely separated from the parent bone. It occurs most commonly in the knee joint, but it may also be seen in the elbow, ankle, and hip joints. The area of involvement in the elbow joint is usually the capitellum of the humerus. The condition is described in more detail in the discussion of the knee joint (see p. 376).

The presence of osteochondritis dissecans in an elbow joint may cause pain, joint swelling, and restriction of motion. If the separated piece becomes a loose body, it may wedge between the bones of the joint and cause locking or a block to extension. The lesion is visible on clear x-ray films.

If the diagnosis is made before the fragment completely separates, healing by "creeping substitution" may take place if the joint is put at rest. If this does not occur or if the fragment becomes a loose body, surgical excision is indicated.

Loose Bodies. Joints, on occasion, may be found to contain loose fragments of bone or calcified tissue which, by their presence and mobility, cause pain, joint irritation, and "locking." These fragments are known as loose bodies or "joint mice" and arise as a result of trauma or disease.

Loose bodies are most commonly found in the knee joint, but the elbow, shoulder, hip and ankle joints may also contain them. As we have seen, osteochondritis dissecans may be a cause of loose bodies. Other causes may be fracture of the articular surface, fracture of an osteoarthritic spur, fracture of articular hyaline cartilage, and osteochondromatosis (see p. 376). Treatment is operative removal in order to relieve the symptoms caused by the presence of these fragments and to save the joint from further damage.

Tennis Elbow. The term "tennis elbow" refers to a common condition that is characterized by pain in the region of the lateral epicondyle of the humerus with radiation down the extensor surface of the forearm. This predicament is brought on by activity that combines excessive pronation and supination of the forearm with an extended wrist, particularly in a person not accustomed to it. Thus tennis, badminton, sculling, or using a screwdriver may be inciting causes.

Although the mechanism producing "tennis elbow" is understood, the actual cause of the pain has never been clearly established. Several causes probably exist; among them are radiohumeral bursitis, tendinitis of the common extensor origin, and traumatic epicondylitis or periostitis at the lateral epicondyle. The patient exhibits an area of palpable tenderness over the lateral epicondyle of the humerus or the radiohumeral joint. Pain can be characteristically aggravated by forced dorsiflexion of the wrist against resistance, which puts tension on the common extensor origin and reproduces pain.

X-ray examination of the elbow is usually negative, but calcium deposits have been noted on rare occasions.

Most patients respond to moist heat and local injections of the corticosteroids at the site of maximum tenderness. Occasionally it is necessary to rest the extensor tendons in a plaster splint with the wrist fixed in dorsiflexion. In a few patients, operative release of the common extensor origin from the lateral epicondyle of the humerus may be required.

Medial Epicondylitis. On rare occasions, the region of the medial epicondyle of the humerus may become painful as a result of activity that puts excessive strain on the common flexor origin. Local palpable tenderness will exist in the region of the medial epicondyle. Pain is aggravated by forced palmar flexion of the wrist against resistance. This motion places tension on the common flexor origin and reproduces pain.

The same modalities used in treating lateral epicondylitis or

tennis elbow can be used in a patient suffering from medial epicondylitis.

Olecranon Bursitis.   Trauma to the point of the elbow often
results in marked swelling of the olecranon bursa, giving rise to a
large knob in this area. Following trauma, the fluid contained in the
bursal sac is frequently bloody, and the bursal walls become permanently thickened. Tender swelling of the olecranon bursa is also seen
with gout and rheumatoid arthritis.

Treatment consists of aspiration of the fluid and local instillation
of hydrocortisone, followed by application of a pressure dressing. If
the problem cannot be controlled locally, operative excision of the
thickened bursa may be carried out.

Traumatic Ulnar Neuritis.   Because of its vulnerable position in
the ulnar groove behind the medial epicondyle of the humerus, the
ulnar nerve may be impinged upon by deformities of the elbow, giving rise to a traumatic ulnar neuritis.

It is known that the ulnar nerve is unusually mobile in some people and will, as a consequence, dislocate across the tip of the medial
epicondyle on flexion and return to its normal location on extension of
the elbow. A certain percentage of these patients ultimately develop a
traumatic ulnar neuritis from friction alone. Other causes of traumatic
ulnar neuritis include osteoarthritic spur formation growing into the
ulnar groove, scarring following laceration or contusion of the soft tissues near the medial epicondyle, and any congenital deformity of the
elbow that increases the carrying angle.

The most common cause of traumatic ulnar neuritis, however, is
residual deformity of the elbow from a previous fracture, specifically,
a cubitus valgus deformity following a supracondylar fracture of the
humerus or displaced fractures of the medial epicondyle of the humerus. In these instances, it may be years before the ulnar neuritis develops. In one reported case, neuritis developed 50 years after the
elbow fracture. For this reason, the condition is known as tardy ulnar
neuritis.

The patient with ulnar neuritis may complain of numbness,
tingling, and pain over the ulnar distribution, particularly the fourth
and fifth fingers. He frequently notes a feeling of clumsiness in the affected hand. This can progress from the stage of interossei weakness
with muscle wasting to complete interossei paralysis.

Traumatic ulnar neuritis is treated by displacement of the ulnar
nerve from the area of irritation, preferably before motor changes
occur and while sensory complaints are still reversible. This is accomplished by surgically transposing the nerve anteriorly to the front
of the medial epicondyle and burying it beneath the mass of soft flexor
muscle tissue.

THE FOREARM

The forearm is the lever for the hand and as such is an important segment of the upper extremity. Trauma or disease affecting the forearm may therefore seriously impair the function and efficiency of the entire part. The motions of flexion and extension of the forearm are, for the most part, controlled by the elbow joint. The motions most often limited by forearm problems are pronation and supination. This range of motion is usually limited in the direction of pronation.

GENERAL CONSIDERATIONS

The motion of pronation and supination requires a rolling of the radius and the ulna on each other along their longitudinal axes. Equal amounts of motion take place at the superior and inferior radio-ulnar joints, which requires that the radial head not impinge on the capitellum of the humerus. Fracture or dislocation of the radial head or trauma involving the superior or inferior radio-ulnar joints may seriously impair this forearm motion.

TRAUMA

Fracture of the Forearm Bones. Because of the intimate relationship between the radius and the ulna, a force strong enough to break either forearm bone commonly breaks both bones simultaneously. Fracture of a single forearm bone usually results from a direct blow applied to the bone. Fractures of both bones of the forearm are often the consequence of a fall on the outstretched arm and are more common in children than in adults. Their management, however, poses a more difficult problem in the adult.

In children, closed reduction with immobilization in a long-arm plaster cast is usually sufficient for a good result with correction of the forearm bowing deformity. Frequently in children the bones will be broken on the convex side of the deformity, but the cortex will appear intact on the concave side. Such fractures are spoken of as "greenstick" fractures. To obtain complete reduction and stabilization of a "greenstick" fracture, it is necessary to complete the fracture of both cortical surfaces manually during reduction. If this is not done, the bowing deformity of the forearm bones may recur within the cast.

In adults, nonunion is relatively common following treatment of fractures of both bones of the forearm. Strong muscle pull results in marked positional deformity of the fragments, and interposition of muscle tissue between the fragments frequently makes adequate closed reduction impossible. As a result, more than half of all forearm fractures in adults require open reduction. At the time of surgery, some form of internal fixation, such as compression plate fixation, is used. Frequently, the use of internal fixation is combined with the addition of bone graft material around the fracture site. For better function results, the decision to employ open reduction should be made within a few days of injury.

An occasional complication of fracture of both bones of the forearm is *synostosis* or cross union between the two bones. This bony growth connecting the two forearm bones may occur at either radio-ulnar joint or anywhere along the shafts, usually opposite the site of fracture. It arises along injured periosteum or interosseous membranes or within a hematoma. Its presence may effectively limit the motion of pronation and supination by preventing one bone from rolling on the other. Surgical release at the point of obstruction may successfully restore a functional range of pronation and supination.

Mechanical Tenosynovitis.   Acute post-traumatic tenosynovitis of the flexor tendon sheaths in the forearm may be seen following strenuous and unaccustomed use of the hand and wrist. As a result of the overactivity, serous fluid accumulates in the flexor sheaths, and the distension results in severe temporary discomfort and disability of the part.

Clinically, the flexor compartment of the forearm may appear swollen and may be tender. Motions of the wrist and hand may be markedly limited by pain. There is usually no vascular or nerve complication.

The condition usually responds rapidly to local heat and rest. The rest may have to be afforded by plaster immobilization.

THE WRIST

The wrist is the movable bridge that connects the hand to the forearm. It comprises the distal end of the radius and ulna plus eight carpal bones arranged in a proximal and distal row. The stability of the wrist joint is maintained by strong ligaments that lash the bones together.

The lower end of the radius is broad and thick and articulates with the proximal row of the carpal bones (Fig. 121). This is the radiocarpal joint, which is responsible for the major portion of the motions of dorsiflexion or extension, palmar flexion, radial deviation, and ulnar deviation of the wrist joint. As previously described, pronation and supination at the wrist joint is dependent upon a movable forearm. The distal ulna does not articulate with any of the carpal bones and can be surgically removed, if necessary, without causing any particular disturbance to wrist joint mechanics.

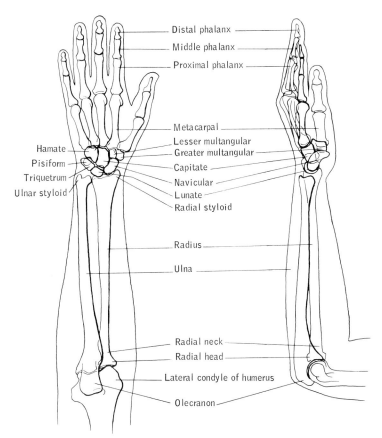

Figure 121. Bones of the forearm and hand. (Redrawn from Marble, H. C.: The Hand.)

It is important to note that normally the tip of the radial styloid lies ahead of the tip of the ulnar styloid at the wrist. Fractures in this region are frequently accompanied by an alteration in the relationship of these landmarks.

The carpal bones on the volar aspect of the wrist are bridged by the volar carpal ligament. The deep passage beneath this wide transverse band is called the *carpal canal* or *carpal tunnel*. The structures that pass through this canal are the median nerve and all the flexor tendons of the fingers (Fig. 122). The radial artery, ulnar artery, and ulnar nerve lie outside the carpal tunnel.

On the dorsal or extensor surface of the wrist, the dorsal carpal ligament contributes to the formation of the osteofibrous tunnels, which house the extensor tendons as they pass over the dorsal surface of the radius.

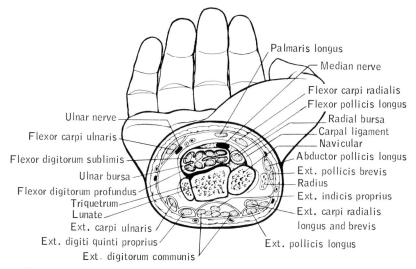

Figure 122. Cross-sectional anatomy of the hand through the proximal row of carpal bones. (Redrawn from Marble, H. C.: The Hand.)

GENERAL CONSIDERATIONS

Because malposition of the wrist can seriously impair the use of the hand, every effort must be made to keep this joint in the position of function during the treatment period of an injury or disease. The position of function for the wrist is 30 degrees of dorsiflexion or extension and 10 degrees of ulnar deviation.

Arthritis. Rheumatoid arthritis may involve the wrist, leading to progressive loss of motion and ankylosis. Disability is greatly lessened if the wrist stiffens in the position of function. Osteoarthritis, unless induced by trauma, is not a frequent problem here, since the wrist is not a weight bearing joint.

Infection. Pyogenic infection may affect the wrist proper or the tendon sheaths lying in relation to it. Acute suppurative tenosynovitis may involve the wrist area by extension from the hand. Pyogenic arthritis and acute suppurative tenosynovitis are serious problems that require immediate treatment, including surgical drainage when necessary.

Tuberculous tenosynovitis is occasionally seen as a diffuse granulomatous thickening of the tendon sheaths around the wrist, particularly on the extensor surface. Excision of the tuberculous tissue, combined with adequate chemotherapy, frequently arrests the process and preserves joint mobility.

Tumors. Benign and malignant bone and soft tissue tumors may appear in the wrist joint area, but none are particular to the location.

Ganglion. Ganglion is a term used to describe a smooth cystic swelling that may appear in relation to any of the extremity joints but is seen most frequently about the wrist. Ganglia are thought to arise from degeneration in the connective tissue close to joints and tendon sheaths. They subsequently become unilocular or multilocular encysted swellings containing thick, colorless viscid fluid. Although they may cause symptoms of pain and weakness secondary to the pressure of the local swelling, they have never been known to become malignant.

About the wrist, ganglia most commonly arise from the joint capsule and present on the dorsal surface as visible and palpable cystic tumors. They may also appear on the volar wrist surface. The patient may be aware of a gradual onset, or the swelling may arise suddenly. Trauma seems to be a factor in about half the cases.

Ganglia can be treated by aspiration or by excision. Aspiration of the fluid contents through a large bore needle, with the instillation of hydrocortisone and the use of a pressure dressing, is successful in decompressing the cystic swelling in a high precentage of patients. However, it may be necessary to repeat the treatment several times before a clinical cure is obtained.

If surgical excision is elected, it is well to remember that a ganglion is like an iceberg with the greatest amount of its mass submerged. Surgery is thus carried out in a field made bloodless by the use of a tourniquet. The surgeon must be prepared to expose the joint capsule in order to excise the entire ganglion and its capsular base.

TRAUMA

Because of its exposed position and its role as a defensive shield for the rest of the body, the wrist is frequently subjected to trauma, including lacerating injuries, dislocation, and fractures.

Laceration. The wrist is the narrowest segment of the upper extremity. The tendons that flex and extend the fingers and the nerves that motivate these tendons, plus the arterial and venous circulation, must pass through this narrow neck on the way to the hand. Lacerating injuries at this level, therefore, possess the capability of severing tendons, arteries, and nerves, and of inflicting grievous damage to the hand.

The hand is well supplied with blood by arterial arches formed by the radial and ulnar arteries. A lacerated or severed artery can be ligated without danger of compromising the circulation.

Severed tendons and nerves must be repaired in order to restore function to the hand. This is often a task of the greatest magnitude and is certainly no job for the surgical novice. Successful restoration of hand function following such an injury requires detailed knowledge of the anatomy of the area and sound surgical judgment.

Dislocation of the Wrist.   A fall on the palm may displace the hand dorsally and cause a dislocation of the wrist joint. The actual dislocation may occur at the radiocarpal joint or through the bones of the carpus. Careful x-ray examination, with films of the normal wrist for comparison, should reveal the type of dislocation present.

Usually dislocations of the wrist joint can be readily reduced by closed manipulation followed by immobilization for three or four weeks. If closed reduction is unsuccessful, open reduction of the dislocation is carried out.

Dislocation of the Lunate Bone.   A fall on the palm of the hand that forces the wrist into sudden extension may dislocate the lunate bone out of its position in the proximal row without causing any other damage to the wrist. The lunate dislocates forward, tearing the capsule, and comes to rest in the carpal tunnel. In this position, the bone presses against the flexor tendons, causing the hand to be held with the wrist and fingers in semiflexion. Motion of the wrist and fingers is painful.

The dislocated bone also presses against the median nerve, causing a median neuritis characterized by pain, paresthesias, atrophy, and weakness or paralysis of the muscles of opposition.

This injury occasionally goes unnoticed on the x-ray film and must be considered in evaluating trauma to the wrist.

If diagnosis is made early, closed reduction may be successful. If it is not, operation will be necessary to reduce the dislocated lunate bone and repair the capsular tear.

Some authorities favor excising the lunate bone if it has been dislocated for a period longer than three weeks, because of the likelihood of the development of avascular necrosis of the bone.

Colles' Fracture.   The most common bone injury produced by a fall on the outstretched hand is Colles' fracture, defined as a fracture through the distal end of the radius with or without a fracture of the ulnar styloid. An associated fracture of the elbow or shoulder may accompany a Colles' fracture. As a rule, there are not accompanying nerve or circulatory complications with Colles' fracture.

Clinically, the wrist appears puffy and deformed. The distal radial fragment is displaced and tilted dorsally, giving rise to the characteristic hump or "silver fork" deformity seen when the wrist is viewed from the side. Backward displacement of the distal radial fragment causes shortening of the radius and an alteration in the normal position of the radial styloid in relation to the ulnar styloid. The normal volar concavity of the radius is lost, and the area feels distended to the touch.

X-ray examination will confirm the diagnosis and will also show if impaction or comminution of the fragments is present (Fig. 123).

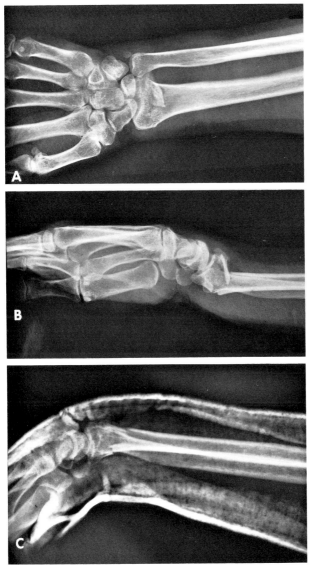

Figure 123. A and B, AP and lateral views of wrist, illustrating the typical deformity of a Colles' fracture. C, lateral view of same wrist after closed manipulative reduction and plaster fixation.

Many Colles' fractures can be adequately reduced by closed manipulative reduction, provided effective muscular relaxation can be supplied by anesthesia. The goal of the reduction is to restore radial length and to replace the distal radial fragment in its normal anatomic position. Immobilization should include the elbow to prevent pronation and supination, and can be achieved by the use of a sugar-tong splint or long-arm plaster cast. Every effort should be made during the healing period to maintain motion and flexibility in the fingers and knuckles.

In some patients, the Colles' fracture may be quite comminuted and unstable. It may be impossible to maintain satisfactory reduction with plaster cast fixation. In this instance, a treatment technique such as pins and plaster fixation can be utilized. This technique is described in Chapter 2.

Fracture of the Navicular.   Fracture of the navicular is the injury most frequently sustained by the carpal bones and is found mainly in young adult males. Pain and disability are not great, and many of these injuries are erroneously diagnosed and treated as "wrist sprains." For this reason, nonunion of the fracture occurs in a high percentage of patients. In one series, 76 per cent of the patients presented x-ray evidence of an established nonunion of the navicular at the time of initial examination by an orthopaedic surgeon.

The fracture may be missed on routine anteroposterior and lateral x-ray views, but can be seen on the oblique view of the wrist (Fig. 124).

If the diagnosis of a fracture of the navicular is made early, plaster immobilization for three to six months is usually followed by healing. If the patient is seen after nonunion has become established, some type of surgical treatment, such as bone grafting, is required.

SPECIFIC CONDITIONS

Madelung's Deformity.   Madelung's deformity is a relatively rare malformation of the wrist that gives the joint the cosmetic appearance of having sustained a forward dislocation. It is thought to arise from an epiphyseal growth defect at the lower end of the radius that causes the radius to shorten and grow in a volar and ulnar direction. Comparative overgrowth of the ulna results in marked dorsal prominence of the lower end of this bone and instability of the distal radio-ulnar joint. The patient may present because the deformity causes a feeling of weakness and insecurity in the wrist.

The deformity can be greatly lessened by excising the distal end of the ulna and straightening the radius by surgical osteotomy.

Osteochondrosis of the Carpal Bones.   As previously described,

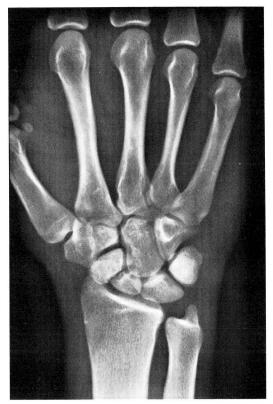

Figure 124. AP view of the wrist, illustrating an established nonunion of the navicular bone.

the osteochondroses are characterized by avascular necrosis of bone, with involvement limited to pressure epiphyses and the tarsal and carpal bones (see p. 84). Avascular necrosis of the lunate bone is known as *Kienböck's disease;* involvement of the navicular bone is known as *Preiser's disease.*

The process probably starts during the growth period, but symptoms at this age may be minimal or absent. Symptoms usually arise secondary to mechanical disturbance or induced degenerative arthritic changes in the wrist joint. For this reason, the majority of patients presenting with this problem are adults. The chief complaint is aching pain or discomfort in the wrist with use. There may or may not be restriction of joint motion. A history of trauma is frequently obtained.

Occasionally, the bone may become revascularized following prolonged immobilization. In certain selected patients, it may be beneficial to excise the flattened dense bone and fill the resulting defect with a silastic prosthesis. If there is much secondary degenerative arthritis in the wrist joint, arthrodesis or fusion of the wrist may be required for pain relief.

Carpal Tunnel Syndrome. As mentioned previously, the carpal bones on the volar aspect of the wrist are bridged by the transverse carpal ligament, forming the carpal tunnel for the passage of the finger flexor tendons and the median nerve. Normally, the carpal tunnel becomes tight and narrow when the fingers and wrist are held in forced flexion. If any soft tissue or extrusion of bone is insinuated into this tight canal, symptoms of median nerve compression may be experienced. Abnormal pressure on the median nerve in the tunnel gives rise to the clinical condition known as the carpal tunnel syndrome.

Causes of the abnormal pressure include dislocation of the lunate bone, malunited Colles' fracture, certain fractures of the navicular bone, arthritic deformities and spurs, hypertrophy of the volar ligament, soft tissue masses such as lipomas and ganglia, and thickening of the flexor tendon sheaths secondary to rheumatoid arthritis or chronic tenosynovitis. In occasional patients, no definite cause can be determined.

Symptoms are produced by motions that tend to constrict the carpal canal, such as forced flexion and extension of the wrist. The patient may complain of pain with median nerve radiation, associated with numbness and paresthesia of median nerve distribution. Manual compression of the carpal tunnel may accentuate the symptoms. Thenar atrophy and weakness of opposition of the thumb may develop.

Symptoms may subside following a period of immobilization of the wrist and avoidance of work that requires flexion of the joint. If this is not successful, the transverse carpal ligament may be divided surgically in order to decompress the median nerve.

THE HAND

The hand is man's universal tool, functioning at the end of a long jointed lever known as the upper extremity. Anatomic study of the hand reveals it to be a mechanism of extreme delicacy, refinement, and specialization. For this reason, trauma or disease affecting the hand is capable of causing severe functional impairment.

Considering the clearly evident importance of the hand, it is surprising to note that hand problems received little special attention for many years. During this period, treatment was often haphazard and results were uncertain. The past three decades, however, have seen the emergence of a new surgical specialist, the hand surgeon.

Trauma or disease affecting the hand may implicate skin, bones, joints, tendons, and nerves. The problems may overlap the fields of orthopaedic surgery, plastic surgery, and neurosurgery. The hand surgeon brings knowledge of all three specialties to bear on the problem for the maximum benefit of the patient.

GENERAL CONDITIONS

Pyogenic Infection.   Pyogenic infections in the hand are serious problems because of their potential for causing severe tendon damage. Infection may destroy tendon sheath gliding mechanisms or cause actual tendon slough with resulting finger stiffness.

PARONYCHIA.   Paronychia is a pyogenic infection of the tissues just lateral to the fingernail. Pus accumulates and forms a small abscess. The infection may spread around the base of the nail to the other side, or it may burrow beneath the nail to involve the nail bed.

Treatment entails hot soaks, antibiotics, and adequate surgical drainage, including removal of part or all of the nail if necessary.

FELON.   Felon is a pyogenic abscess in the distal pulp space of a finger characterized by exquisite pain. The connective tissue of the distal phalanx forms a closed sac that includes part of the bone of the distal phalanx. An abscess in this area is, therefore, a closed space infection, and pus may accumulate under considerable pressure. The pressure may cause an avascular necrosis of the bone, or infection may invade the bone tissue, resulting in osteomyelitis of the distal phalanx.

Treatment involves early recognition and adequate surgical drainage of the abscess.

TENDON SHEATH INFECTIONS.   Puncture wounds of the fingers may introduce pyogenic organisms, particularly staphylococcus, into the flexor tendon sheaths. Infection here is called *acute suppurative tenosynovitis* and may result in permanent loss of finger function through tendon necrosis and slough.

Tendon sheath infection causes a rapid uniform swelling of the finger, which is held stiffly in a semiflexed position. There is marked tenderness to palpation over the length of the tendon sheath, and attempts to extend the finger passively cause severe pain.

If unchecked, tendon sheath infection may spread into the palm and forearm. Infection in the index, middle, and ring fingers spread to the mid-palmar space. Infection in the thumb and index finger may rupture into the thenar space. The forearm may be invaded by infection spreading through the tendon sheaths of the thumb and little fingers.

Tendon sheath infections are serious problems and true surgical emergencies. Incision and drainage should be carried out immediately in a bloodless field. Adequate antibiotic coverage is essential. Inadequate or delayed treatment may result in tendon slough and a stiff finger.

Tuberculous Tenosynovitis. The extensor or flexor tendon sheaths of the hand may become involved with tuberculosis. In contradistinction to pyogenic infection, tuberculous tenosynovitis is usually characterized by a slow onset with gradual progressive swelling of the involved tendon sheaths over a long period of time. Often it causes little or no disturbance of hand function.

Tuberculous tenosynovitis is treated similarly to other skeletal tuberculous infections, utilizing immobilization, chemotherapy, and surgical excision of the diseased tissue in selected cases.

Tumors. Benign tumors of soft tissue and bone are relatively common in the hand. Fortunately, malignant tumors are rare.

GIANT CELL TUMOR (XANTHOMA). The most common benign soft tissue tumor seen in the hand is the giant cell tumor or xanthoma, which orginates from tendon sheaths and other fibrous structures. It arises most frequently on the flexor or extensor surface of a finger and appears beneath the skin as a firm, nodular painless swelling. It may produce a pressure erosion of the underlying bone. On cross section, it presents a characteristic yellow-brown color when examined grossly. Treatment is complete surgical excision (Fig. 125).

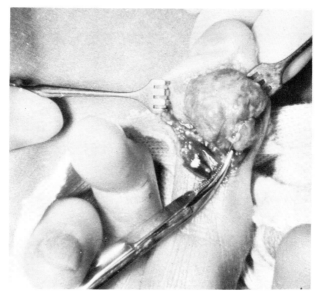

Figure 125. A soft tissue giant cell tumor, arising from flexor tendon sheath, exposed at operation.

GLOMUS TUMOR. This is a benign tumor involving the neuro-myoarterial glomus, which is a heat regulatory mechanism located in the skin. The tumor frequently, but not always, appears beneath a fingernail as a purplish dot. It causes exquisite pain on pressure and is extremely sensitive to temperature changes. Treatment is surgical excision.

GANGLION. The wrist joint area is the most common site for ganglia, with the fingers ranking second (see p. 255). Ganglia are often discovered accidentally as painless, firm cystic masses arising from flexor tendon sheaths. Occasionally the patient will notice pressure pain when an object is grasped firmly in the hand. Treatment is complete surgical excision.

Other benign soft tissue tumors and masses that may be seen about the hand include lipomas, hemangiomas, solitary fibromas, and foreign body granulomas.

ENCHONDROMA. Enchondroma is a benign tumor of carti-laginous origin that is the commonest bone tumor seen in the hand (see p. 198). This x-ray appearance in a phalanx is of a circular area of radiolucency with a bulging and thinned cortical border (Fig. 97). Often this tumor is asymptomatic until minimal trauma causes a pathologic fracture through the weakened shell of bone. Once it is diagnosed, treatment consists of complete currettage of the bone cavity, which is then filled in with chip bone grafts.

Primary malignant bone tumors are quite rare in the hand. Very infrequently an osteosarcoma, chondrosarcoma, or Ewing's tumor may be seen. Metastatic carcinoma may occasionally involve the bones of the hand.

TRAUMA

Because the hand plays a role in almost every human endeavor, it is not surprising that it is often injured. It has been stated that more than 75 per cent of all injuries resulting in permanent partial disability occur in the hand and fingers. Joint dislocations and fractures are not uncommon. Lacerating and crushing injuries to the hand may sever tendons and nerves. The treatment of hand trauma frequently poses perplexing problems that require specialized knowledge for their solution.

Dislocations. Dislocation of finger joints can occur at the in-terphalangeal or metacarpophalangeal level. As a rule, these disloca-tions reduce quite readily with manipulation. The affected finger is immobilized for one week (Fig. 27).

Occasionally, the end of a dislocating bone will "button-hole" through the capsule of the joint. When this occurs, the torn capsule may fold around the bone end, making closed manipulative reduction impossible. This situation is seen most commonly with dislocations of the metacarpophalangeal joint of the thumb and requires an open reduction with repair of the capsule for its treatment.

Fractures. Fractures of the phalanges and metacarpals may be spiral or transverse. Often there is no displacement of the fracture fragments and simple immobilization will suffice to insure healing. Finger fractures are immobilized for a 10 to 14 day period in gentle flexion; the positions of extension and acute flexion are unphysiologic, and prolonged immobilization will lead to joint stiffness. Nondisplaced metacarpal fractures are immobilized for a three to four week period with the hand and wrist in the position of function.

Displacement of the fracture fragments leads to shortening and rotation of the involved finger. If the displacement cannot be reduced and held by closed methods, a more vigorous form of treatment must be sought. Some treating physicians elect skeletal traction, while others favor open reduction with intramedullary pin fixation. Regardless of the type of treatment used, the deformity caused by the fracture must be overcome, and every effort must be directed toward early motion to minimize residual joint stiffness.

Occasionally, a patient presents with a severely traumatized hand with extensive skin damage, lacerated tendons and nerves, and multiple fractures. In this instance, the fractures are best treated by intramedullary pin fixation. This provides a stable skeletal framework for the rest of the reconstructive procedures.

BOXER'S FRACTURE. The term boxer's fracture applies to a frequently seen fracture through the neck of the fifth metacarpal, most often obtained by striking an object with a clenched fist. The head of the fifth metacarpal is displaced into the palm, and the patient presents with a flattening or loss of the knuckle prominence (Fig. 126).

It may be possible to reduce the depressed metacarpal head into normal alignment by pushing upward on the flexed proximal phalanx of the fifth finger and pushing downward on the metacarpal shaft simultaneously. If it proves impossible to reduce the fracture, open reduction and intramedullary pin fixation may be carried out. If it proves possible to reduce the fracture but impossible to maintain position, percutaneous pinning of the fracture fragment may be carried out.

BENNETT'S FRACTURE. Bennett's fracture is a fracture through the base of the thumb metacarpal with a proximal displacement of the first metacarpal shaft away from the greater multangular bone. It is caused by a force applied to the end of the thumb and, if not accurately reduced, can result in permanent disability to the thumb.

If the displacement is minimal, reduction may be obtained by immobilizing the hand and wrist with the thumb in wide abduction;

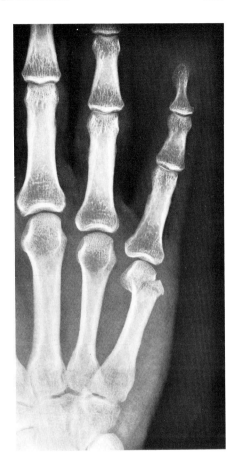

Figure 126. Displaced fracture through the neck of the fifth metacarpal bone (boxer's fracture).

but in most cases the fragments are displaced and unstable, and the fracture will require skeletal traction or open reduction with pin fixation for its correction.

Tendon Lacerations. Industrial and household accidents can result in lacerating injuries to the hand and fingers that sever flexor tendons (Fig. 127). Although these are potentially crippling injuries requiring specialized skill and knowledge for their repair, a few general principles concerning their management should be known to all physicians.

Each finger contains two flexor tendons: the flexor sublimis inserts on the middle phalanx, and the flexor profundus inserts on the distal phalanx. The thumb has only one long flexor tendon inserting on the distal phalanx. These flexor tendons are contained in dense fibrous tunnels or sheaths in the area from the distal flexion crease of the palm to the distal finger joints. This is the area known to the

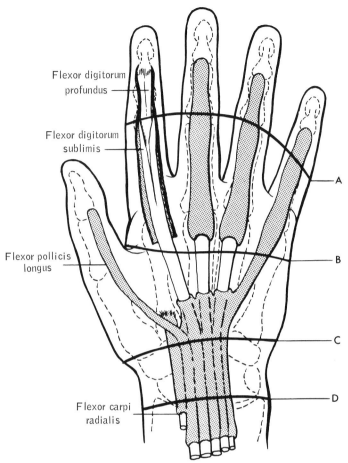

Figure 127. Flexor tendons and tendon sheaths on palmar surface of hand. Zones indicate common areas of tendon laceration: Zone A, flexor tendons may be repaired primarily distal to line A. Zone A-B, no man's land. No primary tendon repairs here. Delayed management requires a tendon graft. Zone B-C, repair one tendon only. If both are cut, repair flexor digitorum profundus. Zone C-D, may repair more than one tendon. Open carpal ligament. Zone D, more than one tendon may be repaired proximal to line D in forearm. Repair of median nerve takes precedence. Flexor pollicis longus may be repaired throughout its length, but leave tendon sheath open at repair site.

hand surgeon as "no man's land," because primary repair of lacerated flexor tendons gives uniformly poor functional results owing to scar adherence between the tendon and the sheath. In this region, it is considered better initial treatment to cleanse and close the wound, leaving the tendon unrepaired. Later, after complete wound healing, tendon grafting is performed. In this way, the tendon does not become adherent to the fibrous sheath by scar formation. If a tendon does become adherent to the fibrous sheath by scar formation, resulting in a finger that has no motion, treatment includes complete excision of the tendon and replacement with a silastic tendon prosthesis around which a new sheath can form. Months later, the tendon prosthesis can be removed and a new tendon graft inserted in the new tendon sheath.

A laceration may sever both the flexor sublimis and flexor profundus tendons at the same level in the hand. If both tendons are repaired at the same level, they will become adherent to each other with resulting finger stiffness. The proper treatment is repair of the profundus with excision of the sublimis tendon. This is feasible because the profundus runs to the distal phalanx and has sufficient strength to flex the entire finger, even in the absence of the sublimis.

In some areas of the hand and fingers, primary tendon repair is the treatment of choice. However, timing is important. In cleanly incised wounds or in wounds with only minimal tissue damage or contamination, tendons may be repaired safely up to six or eight hours following injury. If the wound is contaminated or contused, or if the surgeon is in doubt about proper treatment, the best course of action is to cleanse and close the wound without tendon repair. Later, after complete wound healing, tendon grafting can be performed.

Occasionally, a patient will present with a severely mangled hand, including loss of skin covering, multiple fractures, and severed tendons and nerves. The initial treatment of severe trauma to the hand involves meticulous surgical debridement, intramedullary pin fixation of fractures, and skin closure, using skin grafts if necessary. The major nerves and the digital nerves should be sutured primarily if possible. If this is not feasible, they can be repaired at a second stage. In the severely mangled hand, severed flexor tendons are never repaired at the time of initial treatment. They are allowed to go unrepaired until complete wound healing has occurred; then they are treated by tendon graft replacement.

SPECIFIC CONDITIONS

Mallet Finger (Baseball Finger, Dropped Finger). Mallet finger is the term applied to the deformity that results when a direct blow on the tip of an extended finger forces the distal phalanx into sudden flexion and avulses the extensor tendon from its insertion. The extensor tendon may pull away cleanly, or it may tear away along with a chip of bone from the distal phalanx.

The end of the finger exhibits a characteristic "droop," and the patient loses the ability to extend the finger tip actively. Initially, the distal interphalangeal joint is swollen and painful. Later, the deformity may be annoying only because of the propensity of the dropped finger to get in the way or catch in clothing or pockets.

If the deformity is treated soon after onset, the distal phalanx may be splinted in the position of hyperextension, with the proximal interphalangeal joint flexed, for a period of six weeks. A return to adequate function is usually obtained. In patients with a deformity of long duration, surgical repair is often unsatisfactory. However, fusion of the distal interphalangeal joint in the position of function gives good results in the occasional patient who is seen late and whose symptoms are sufficient to warrant surgery.

Trigger Finger.   A trigger finger or snapping finger is one that locks in a flexed position and can be extended only with some difficulty associated with a "snap" or "pop." This curious behavior involving fingers and thumb is due to a narrowing or constriction of the flexor sheath at the level of the metacarpal neck. There is accompanying nodular enlargement of the tendon that is probably secondary to the constriction. This "trigger mechanism," which is almost always located at the level of the metacarpal head, blocks free passage of the tendon, and if the tendon passes the point of obstruction, a click or snap is produced.

Occasionally the condition is relatively painless, but most often it is accompanied by an aching pain as a mechanical tenosynovitis develops. Pressure on the trigger mechanism is painful.

In children, involvement of the thumb is seen, but rarely involvement of the fingers. Because trigger thumb has been seen in newborns, it is suspected that the condition may be congenital in many instances. In the adult, the condition may involve fingers or thumbs, with the thumb being involved more frequently.

In many instances hydrocortisone, injected into the sheath at the level of the trigger mechanism, may reduce local edema sufficiently to allow free tendon gliding to resume. If this does not occur, surgical excision of the constricted portion of the sheath will effect a cure.

De Quervain's Disease.   This is a term applied to a commonly seen, painful, mechanical tenosynovitis that affects the abductor pollicis longus and extensor pollicis brevis in their common sheath passing over the radial styloid to the thumb. The cause may be either trauma or repeated mechanical irritation. If the condition becomes chronic, the sheath may thicken and become stenotic.

De Quervain's disease is more common in women. The patient may complain of pain in the region of the radial styloid and thumb with use of the hand. Motions such as wringing out wet clothes and removing lids from jars may aggravate the pain. The patient may frequently drop lifted objects because of the pain. There may be tenderness to pressure over the affected tendon sheath and the radial styloid. The radial styloid may frequently appear sharply prominent because of the thickness of the overlying tissue, which results from the inflammatory lesion. A confirmatory maneuver to elicit pain in this condition is forcibly to snap the wrist into ulnar deviation with the thumb folded into the palm (*Finklestein test*).

If the condition is of only a few weeks' duration, it may rapidly respond to local heat and plaster splint immobilization of the thumb and wrist or to local instillation of hydrocortisone into the tendon sheath. Chronic cases, or those not responding to local hydrocortisone, may need surgical release of the tendon sheath at the wrist.

Dupuytren's Contracture. This term is applied to a chronic hyperplasia of the palmar fascia that leads to progressive fibrosis and contracture of the hand. As the contracture matures, the pretendinous bands of the palmar aponeurosis to the fingers shorten and pull the fingers into positions of fixed flexion. The fingers most frequently affected are the ring finger and little finger (Fig. 128). The fibroblastic proliferation of the palmar fascia involves the skin and draws it down into tight puckers and nodules. Firm nodules may be palpated in the palm or the base of the fingers.

Dupuytren's contracture is most common in men past middle age

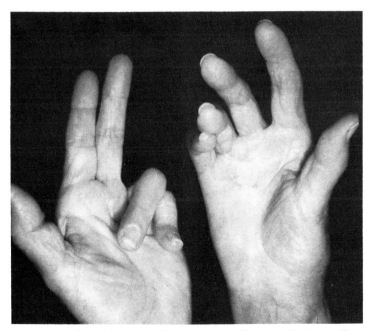

Figure 128. Bilateral Dupuytren's contracture. (Courtesy Dr. James Hunter and Dr. Lawrence Schneider, Thomas Jefferson University Hospital, Philadelphia, Pa.)

and is usually bilateral. The exact cause is unknown, but a hereditary pattern has been noted. Trauma is not thought to play a significant role, since the condition occurs frequently in those who do not do heavy manual labor. A higher incidence in those with gout and diabetes has been observed. The condition, as a rule, is relatively painless, but it may be associated with disabling functional impairment.

There is no known effective conservative therapy except stretching exercises to the fingers. The treatment of choice is usually operative resection of all the involved palmar fascia. Some surgeons favor a limited or conservative resection, while others favor a radical resection of the palmar fascia with skin grafting if necessary.

Rupture of Extensor Pollicis Longus Tendon. A tendon may rupture as a result of excessive tension or secondary to degenerative or attritional changes in the tendon tissue. Examples already discussed are rupture of the biceps tendon and the mallet finger deformity. Another area that is sometimes affected is the thumb, with rupture of the extensor pollicis longus tendon.

Rupture of this tendon may follow a Colles' fracture and is secondary to attritional or degenerative changes in the tendon substance induced when the tendon rubs against irregular bony surface. It sometimes occurs in certain occupations, such as those of drummer, polisher, and carpenter. It results in loss of extension of the distal thumb joint and partial loss of extension in the proximal joint, with consequent impairment of grasp.

Direct suture of the tendon through the ruptured area is not feasible because of loss of length. Treatment consists of a free tendon graft or a tendon transference operation.

References

Boyes, J. H.: Bunnell's Surgery of the Hand, 5th Edition. Philadelphia: J. B. Lippincott Co., 1970.

Bradley, K. C., and Sunderland, S.: The range of movement at the wrist joint. Ant. Rec., *116*:139, 1953.

Eyler, D. L., and Markee, J. E.: Anatomy and function of the intrinsic musculature of the fingers. J. Bone and Joint Surg., *36-A*:1, 1954.

Garden, R. S.: Tennis elbow. J. Bone and Joint Surg., *43-B*:100, 1961.

Gartland, J. J.: Management of supracondylar fractures of the humerus in children. Surg. Gynecol. Obstet., *110*:145, 1959.

Kaplan, E. B.: Functional and Surgical Anatomy of the Hand, 2nd Edition. Philadelphia: J. B. Lippincott Co., 1965.

Landsmeer, J. M. F.: The coordination of finger-joint motions. J. Bone and Joint Surg., *45-A*:1654, 1963.

Leao, L.: de Quervain's disease. J. Bone and Joint Surg., *40-A*:1063, 1958.

Luck, J. V.: Dupuytren's contracture. J. Bone and Joint Surg., *41-A*:635, 1959.

Markee, J. E.: Anatomy of the hand. Am. Academy of Orthopaedic Surgeons Instructional Course Lectures, Vol. XIV: 149. Ann Arbor: J. W. Edwards, 1957.

Pennsylvania Orthopaedic Society: Evaluation of treatment for non-union of the carpal navicular. A report made by the Scientific Research Committee, Pennsylvania Orthopaedic Society. J. Bone and Joint Surg., *44-A*:169, 1962.

Stark, H. H., Boyes, J. H., and Wilson, J. N.: Mallet finger. J. Bone and Joint Surg., *44-A*:1061, 1962.

Steel, F. L. D., and Tomlinson, J. D. W.: The "carrying angle" in man. J. Anat. (Lond.), *92*:315, 1958.

Tanzer, R. C.: The carpal tunnel syndrome - A clinical and anatomical study. J. Bone and Joint Surg., *41-A*:626, 1959.

Chapter Twelve

Disorders of the Jaw, the Neck, and the Thorax

THE JAW

The orthopaedist is rarely confronted with problems involving the jaw. He may be consulted regarding fractures, tumors, or infections of the mandible, but in most instances these conditions are treated by oral surgeons. He is more likely to be consulted by patients complaining of pain, snapping, locking, or stiffness involving the temporomandibular joints.

TEMPOROMANDIBULAR JOINT

A patient may be seen with the complaint of pain accompanied by a snapping or "popping" sound in the region of one or both temporomandibular joints. Medical attention is sought when it becomes difficult for the patient to eat because of pain and the accompanying loud noise. Examination may disclose local tenderness over one or both temporomandibular joints, and a palpable click or snap may be felt in the area when the mouth is opened and closed. On a few occasions a patient may present with locking of the jaw.

It is believed that the most common cause of pain in the temporomandibular joint is chronic joint subluxation resulting from dental malocclusion. This is not difficult to understand when it is realized that, unlike other paired joints in the body, both temporomandibular joints must move simultaneously and in harmony, being at the com-

272

plete mercy of the teeth. Two situations may develop, either in association with the dental malocclusion or independently of it, to cause the pain, snapping, and occasional locking. (1) The articular disc of the temporomandibular joint may develop a mechanical derangement, similar to a semilunar cartilage in the knee, to cause pain, snapping, or locking of the joint. (2) Recurrent dislocation of the temporomandibular joint may develop, with the condyles of the mandible slipping forward when the mouth is opened. Repeated joint subluxation over a long period of time gradually leads to joint degeneration.

X-rays of the temporomandibular joints, taken with the mouth in the opened and closed positions, are necessary for proper investigation of the complaint.

Replacement of missing teeth and correction of malocclusion may be curative if treatment is started before joint degeneration begins. Acute pain in the joint may be effectively treated by local heat and rest to the jaw, and occasionally by the use of intra-articular corticosteroids. Chronic symptoms, particularly if associated with locking, may require surgery. If an internal derangement of the articular disc is found, the disc is removed. Chronic subluxation or dislocation can be treated by condylectomy or a bone block operation.

A sensation of stiffness in the temporomandibular joint may accompany subluxation. True stiffness with actual loss of joint motion may be seen with rheumatoid arthritis, as a late result of trauma, or occasionally as a result of osteomyelitis of the temporal bone secondary to middle ear infection. As a consequence of these disease states, bony ankylosis of one or both of the temporomandibular joints may occur. This results in a serious deformity with profound nutritional implications.

Some motion may be restored to the jaw by resecting the condyles or by performing a surgical arthroplasty of the temporomandibular joint.

THE NECK

The neck, or cervical spine, is an extremely flexible segment of the vertebral column, bridging the space between the head and the relatively rigid thorax. Anatomically, the neck consists of seven cervical vertebrae with their intervertebral discs and articulations, anterior and posterior ligaments, and the anterior and posterior cervical musculature. These structures are compactly associated with the spinal cord, the nerve roots, and the two vertebral arteries with their associated sympathetic nerves.

The cervical vertebrae are shaped primarily to give extreme flexibility to this segment of the spine. The upper two cervical vertebrae are structurally different from the rest of the vertebrae to allow free mobility to the head. The cervical spine is not only a flexible support between two rigid elements, the head and the thoracic spine, but when normal acts as a protective bony encasement for the spinal cord, nerve roots, and vertebral arteries with their associated sympathetic nerves.

GENERAL CONSIDERATIONS

Most complaints about the neck develop as a result of congenital deformities or acquired problems such as degenerative joint conditions and trauma, including the controversial "whiplash" injury. Infection and tumor may involve the cervical spine, but this is less common.

Problems arising in the neck produce mainly pain and restriction of neck motion. Radiation of pain from the cervical area may involve the head, the anterior chest, the interscapular area, the shoulders, and the upper extremities. Pain of neck origin is frequently aggravated by the use of a pillow while lying in the recumbent position. For this reason, patients often describe great difficulty in achieving comfort in bed. It is also a common observation that patients suffering from neck problems declare the morning hours to be the time of their worst pain and stiffness. Unguarded movements of the head during sleep and the propped-up position of the head in relation to the shoulders produced by the pillow are believed to irritate the neck.

EXAMINATION OF THE NECK

The position of the head and neck in relation to the shoulder girdle and trunk should be observed and any deviation from normal posture noted. As a result of pain or deformity, the head may be held rigidly in a neutral posture or may be carried in a tilted or rotated position. The presence or absence of spasm or tenderness in the anterior or posterior cervical musculature should be ascertained.

The range of motion allowed by the neck is next determined (Fig. 129). Motions of the cervical spine are flexion, extension, rotation to the right and left, and lateral tilt or bend to the right and left. It is important to note whether the neck motions are unrestricted and whether movements of the head on the neck aggravate or reproduce pain.

Any areas of local tenderness along the anterior or posterior column of the neck are noted. It is not uncommon to find areas of local tenderness to palpation in the region of the scalene muscles anteriorly

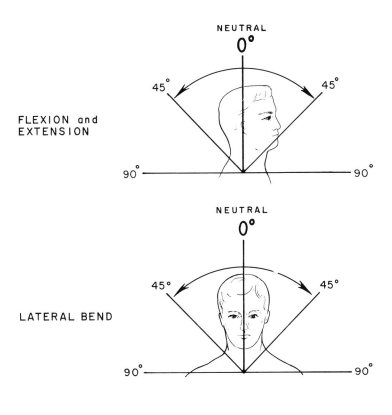

FLEXION and
EXTENSION

LATERAL BEND

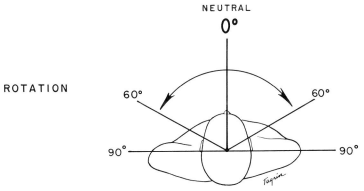

ROTATION

Figure 129. Motions of the cervical spine. (Courtesy American Academy of Orthopaedic Surgeons.)

or the trapezius muscles posteriorly, or along the spinous process and interspinous area of the cervical spine.

The pattern of any radiating pain must be carefully analyzed and the motion causing it accurately noted. Arm pain does not necessarily originate in the arm itself but rather may radiate to the arm from the neck or shoulder region. It is important for the examiner to make this distinction carefully. In addition, neck pain may radiate to the head, anterior thorax, interscapular area, and shoulder. Almost always any radiating pain originating in the cervical spine area will be reproduced or aggravated by motions of the head or by a compressive force on the head.

If the symptoms suggest spinal cord or nerve root involvement, neurologic examination of both upper extremities is routinely carried out. This should include evaluation of the biceps, triceps, and brachioradialis reflexes, as well as the detection of any abnormalities in the motor and sensory pattern.

Examination of the cervical spine is not considered complete without an x-ray study of the area. Anteroposterior, oblique, and lateral views with the neck in neutral position are the most useful. Special views are obtained when indicated.

Congenital Deformities

TORTICOLLIS (CONGENITAL WRY NECK)

Torticollis is a congenital abnormality of the sternocleidomastoid muscle that results in a typical positional deformity of the head. In almost all patients there is an obstetrical history of some type of abnormal delivery, such as breech presentation. The most widely held theory of etiology postulates intrauterine malposition of the fetus, causing a pressure ischemia of the sternocleidomastoid muscle. This frequently results in fibrosis and ultimate contracture of the muscle. Not infrequently a firm lump representing a hyperplastic fibrous mass can be palpated in the substance of the sternocleidomastoid muscle.

Clinical Picture.   The infant lies with his head in a characteristic position. The head is tilted to the side of the deformity and the chin points toward the opposite shoulder (Fig. 130). The mother usually notices some restriction of the infant's neck motion. A firm lump may be palpated in the substance of the sternocleidomastoid muscle, but the lump usually regresses in size and ultimately disappears in a few months. Regression may be complete, with ultimate resolution of the deformity. In many instances, however, regression is apparently incomplete, and a fibrous contracture ensues, resulting finally in secondary contracture of most of the soft tissues of the neck.

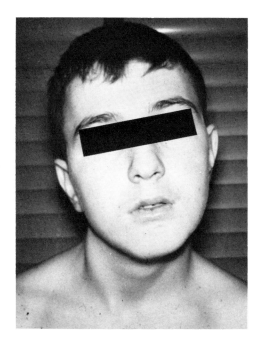

Figure 130. Residual torticollis, right, in older boy.

After several months of deformity, in the more severe cases, a flattening and asymmetry of the face may develop on the side of the contracture. This facial asymmetry usually corrects itself if treatment is completed by about the third year of life. If untreated, the deformity of the head tends to increase with age because of the inability of the fibrotic sternocleidomastoid muscle to grow at relatively the same rate as the cervical spine. If allowed to persist, torticollis will eventually be accompanied by a compensatory curvature of the cervical and upper thoracic spine, elevation of one shoulder, and ocular imbalance.

A significant number of infants with congenital torticollis have an associated congenital dislocation or congenital subluxation of the hip.

X-ray examination usually reveals a normal-appearing cervical spine. Occasionally, a torticollis deformity is seen in association with a congenital skeletal abnormality of the cervical or upper thoracic vertebrae, such as hemivertebrae or Klippel-Feil syndrome.

Acquired torticollis may appear later in life as the result of trauma or infection in the throat, neck, or cervical spine. It may also be caused by disease of the central nervous system or by psychogenic factors.

Treatment. When the deformity is relatively mild and noted shortly after birth, it can frequently be corrected by gently stretching the head and neck into the overcorrected position. This is done several times daily by the mother.

Surgical treatment is advised for all patients in whom contracture has not been corrected by the age of two years, or earlier if the deformity is severe. Usually surgical division of the sternal and clavicular insertions plus all tight facial structures is sufficient to obtain correction. In late or very tight cases, the insertion of the muscle into the mastoid process may also have to be cut. A collar, brace, or traction device is used in the immediate postoperative period, followed by the continuation of stretching exercises. Recurrence of the deformity may occur because of reattachment of the tight fibrotic muscle ends, necessitating further surgical correction.

CERVICAL RIB

A cervical rib is a congenital overdevelopment of the transverse process of the seventh cervical vertebra and may vary in size from simple enlargement of the process to a complete supernumerary rib. The process attaches to the first rib either by a fibrous band or by bone. The deformity is frequently bilateral.

This abnormality may be significant because the subclavian artery and lowest trunk of the brachial plexus arch over the rib. If local pressure occurs, neurologic and vascular symptoms may develop in the arm. However, a cervical rib may be completely asymptomatic.

Clinical Picture. The patient may complain of pain and paresthesia in the forearm and hand, particularly on the ulnar side. An area of sensory loss or anesthesia may be detected in the forearm or hand. Weakness of the hand may be associated with wasting of the thenar, interosseous, or hypothenar muscles. Vascular manifestations may range from dusky cyanosis of the forearm and hand to gangrene of the fingertips associated with a diminution of the radial pulse. The patient characteristically notices aggravation or relief of symptoms in relation to the the position of the arm.

Treatment. No treatment is indicated in the asymptomatic patient. Symptoms can frequently be relieved by the use of a Thomas collar and by various physical therapy devices, such as cervical traction. If symptoms persist, surgical excision of the rib is indicated.

KLIPPEL-FEIL SYNDROME

Klippel-Feil syndrome is a rare congenital malformation of the cervical spine that combines elements of many skeletal deformities. All or part of the cervical vertebrae are fused together. Frequently many of the laminar arches are open and spina bifida is present. In addition, other developmental deformities of the cervical vertebrae, such as hemivertebra, may be present, and there may be an associated cervical rib.

The clinical result is extreme shortness of the neck, with the head appearing to rise from between the shoulders. Cervical spine motion is markedly restricted.

There is no effective treatment.

Acquired Conditions

SCALENUS ANTICUS SYNDROME

Spasm or hypertrophy of the anterior and middle scalene muscles is occasionally seen, producing pain in the neck along with neurologic and vascular symptoms in the arms.

The tendon of the anterior and middle scalene muscles inserts onto the first rib, enveloping the brachial plexus and subclavian artery. Spasm or hypertrophy of the scalenus muscles may produce compression of the brachial plexus and subclavian artery, giving rise to symptoms similar to those produced by a cervical rib.

This condition is seen most often in tense young females, but it may also be seen following trauma to the neck or in connection with certain occupations. Poor posture with sagging of the shoulder girdle is thought by some to be important in its production.

The patient with scalenus anticus syndrome may complain of neck pain with radiation into the shoulder and arm. There may be tenderness to palpation over the course of the muscle. Numbness, tingling, and muscle weakness, if present, correspond roughly to the ulnar nerve distribution. The radial pulse may be diminished in volume when the arm is dependent.

The use of a cervical collar frequently relieves symptoms. In an occasional patient surgical release of the scalene muscle is required.

DEGENERATIVE DISEASE OF THE CERVICAL SPINE

Degenerative disease of the cervical spine is an extremely common clinical problem. Three more or less separate clinical states can be recognized under the general heading of degenerative disease of the cervical spine. These three clinical states are *cervical disc degeneration, degenerative arthritis of the cervical spine,* and *herniated cervical disc.* Although the basic etiologic cause for these conditions has not yet been defined, it is quite likely that it is similar for all three. The eventual pathologic changes seen in these conditions are quite similar, differing only in degree.

Cervical disc degeneration and degenerative arthritis of the cervical spine basically cause symptoms of pain and stiffness in the neck.

In addition, degenerative arthritis of the cervical spine and herniated cervical disc may cause compression of the adjacent spinal nerve roots. If this complication occurs, the patient may complain of pain radiating to the shoulder, arm, or hand and may exhibit signs and symptoms of nerve root compression.

Cervical Disc Degeneration. Degeneration of a cervical intervertebral disc represents premature aging of this particular tissue. The pathophysiology of disc degeneration has been adequately described, (see p. 325), but the reason why one patient has it and not another is still unclear.

Rapid depolymerization of the acid mucopolysaccharide and dehydration of the nucleus pulposus of the disc convert this normally gel-like substance into a thinned fibrous scar tissue that can no longer function as an adequate shock absorber. This change most frequently involves the C5-C6 intervertebral disc. Characteristically, disc degeneration results in narrowing of the involved interspace that can best be appreciated on the lateral x-ray view of the cervical spine.

CLINICAL PICTURE. The patient with symptoms related to cervical disc degeneration is generally younger than the patient with symptoms caused by degenerative arthritis of the cervical spine. Females appear to be affected more frequently than males.

The patient will present with acute onset of neck pain, usually localized to one side of the neck, with extension of the pain into the interscapular area. Symptoms may come on spontaneously or may be induced by some traumatic episode. The neck pain is reproduced or aggravated by motions of the head. Typically, the neck pain is worse in the morning upon arising from bed. The neck pain is commonly associated with occipital headache. Frequently there is a diffuse radiation of pain into the area of the trapezius muscle and into the general area of the shoulder.

On examination, neck motion is usually restricted because of pain. Palpation along the paracervical muscle masses and over the trapezius muscle generally elicits tenderness. Tenderness over the spinous processes and the interspinous ligaments of both the cervical and the upper thoracic spine is a common finding. The neurologic examination is negative.

X-ray examination typically reveals a normal-appearing cervical spine, except for narrowing of the involved interspace (Fig. 131).

TREATMENT. The neck is put to rest and pressure is removed from the involved interspace by the use of a soft collar. It is especially important for these patients to wear the collar during sleeping periods. Moist heat to the neck in the form of hot applications or hot showers is most beneficial.

The anti-inflammatory drugs, particularly Butazolidin (phenylbu-

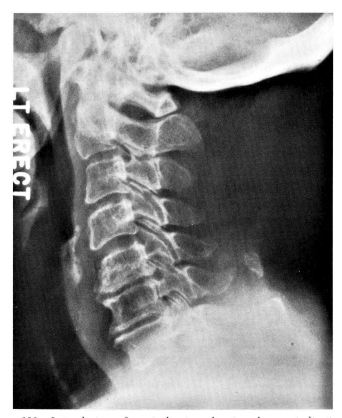

Figure 131. Lateral view of cervical spine, showing changes indicative of disc degeneration at C5-C6 and C6-C7 levels.

tazone) and Tandearil (oxyphenbutazone), seem to have almost a specific quieting effect on the symptoms. Cervical traction is not indicated in these patients, since they do not have cervical radiculitis.

The vast majority of patients with symptoms caused by cervical disc degeneration obtain relief with conservative measures. Interbody fusion of the affected interspace can be carried out through the anterior cervical approach in those few patients who do not satisfactorily respond to a conservative program.

Degenerative Arthritis of Cervical Spine. Degenerative arthritis of the cervical spine is a diffuse degenerative process that appears simultaneously to involve the intervertebral discs, vertebral bodies, ligamentous structures, and apophyseal joints. With multiple disc degeneration and narrowing of multiple disc spaces, hypertrophic bone changes appear in the form of osteophytes or spurs. These osteophytes form circumferentially about the marginal attachments of the anulus fibrosus to the vertebral bodies, but they are usually more prominent anteriorly than posteriorly. As the narrowing process continues, the apophyseal joints sublux, resulting in additional degeneration of these synovial joints with osteophyte formation at their margins.

CLINICAL PICTURE.   The typical patient with symptoms related to degenerative arthritis of the cervical spine is past middle life and complains of stiffness and neck pain. The stiffness is characteristically worse following periods of immobility of the head and is relieved, to a certain extent, by motion. The pain, on the other hand, is characteristically aggravated by movement of the head and by certain sleeping positions. The pain may localize in the neck but may radiate to the head, the anterior chest, the thoracic spine region, or the shoulders.

Motions of the cervical spine are restricted by both pain and stiffness. There is usually diffuse tenderness to palpation over the posterior neck structures and the trapezius muscles.

Radiation of pain to the arm or hand may signal the complication of nerve root compression by bony encroachment on the adjacent spinal nerve roots.

X-ray examination reveals involvement of multiple cervical interspaces (Fig. 132). The involved intervertebral disc spaces are narrowed, and spur formation may be present along the anterior and posterior aspects of the vertebral bodies. The subjacent bone shows hypertrophic changes, with involvement including the apophyseal joints. The C4-C5, C5-C6, and C6-C7 interspaces are the most frequently involved. Narrowing of the intervertebral foramina, reactive bone changes about the apophyseal joints, and bone spurs projecting posteriorly into the nerve root foramina may be present to account for the signs and symptoms of cervical nerve root compression if this is disclosed by examination of the patient.

It is interesting that many patients demonstrate these typical x-ray changes indicative of degenerative arthritis of the cervical spine yet are completely asymptomatic. The fact that almost all persons in the seventh and eighth decades of life show x-ray signs of degenerative change in the cervical spine indicates the correlation between such degeneration and the aging process.

Not infrequently patients may be seen for the first time with complaints of pain and stiffness in the neck dating from a recent injury.

X-ray examination reveals the changes typical of degenerative arthritis, which are thought to take years to develop. Is there any connection in this instance between x-ray evidence of previously existing degenerative arthritis and recent trauma to the neck that can bring about a clinical state characterized by stiffness and pain?

As mentioned previously, a patient may show x-ray evidence of

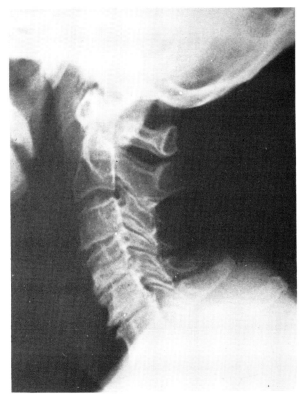

Figure 132.   Lateral x-ray of cervical spine, showing changes indicative of degenerative arthritis.

degenerative arthritis in the cervical spine segment, yet be completely asymptomatic as far as normal activities are concerned. Flexibility of the involved spinal segment, however, is decreased by the joint narrowing and spur formation. The addition of trauma, particularly of the "whiplash" variety, to this less resilient cervical segment may upset the functional balance of the neck. The neck may be unable to adjust to the additional insult, and the symptoms of neck pain and stiffness may present. In this instance, then, previously existing asymptomatic degenerative changes in the cervical spine may be sufficiently aggravated by trauma to produce the typical symptoms of stiffness and pain.

TREATMENT.   In the vast majority of instances, the symptoms caused by degenerative arthritis of the cervical spine can be alleviated by a nonoperative treatment program. Support to the head with a Thomas collar, particularly during sleeping periods, is especially beneficial. Moist heat applied to the neck musculature is most helpful.

The orally administered anti-inflammatory agents, particularly Buta-zolidin (phenylbutazone) and Tandearil (oxyphenbutazone), are effective in the relief of pain and stiffness due to degenerative arthritis if no medical contraindication to their use exists. The dosage schedule is similar to that described for degenerative arthritis of the lumbar spine (p. 324). The blood count should be checked periodically if long-term use of these drugs is contemplated. The use of cervical traction is not indicated unless the complication of cervical radiculitis is present.

Surgery is rarely required in the treatment of degenerative arthritis of the cervical spine, unless the problem is complicated by an intractable cervical radiculitis. If spinal fusion is felt to be necessary to control chronic neck pain, the procedure can be carried out through either an anterior or a posterior approach, depending upon the requirements of the individual case.

Herniated Cervical Disc. Herniation of an intervertebral disc may occur in the cervical spine, but this is much less common than lumbar disc herniation. If frank herniation does occur, however, it is usually secondary to rather severe trauma to the cervical spine and is seen most commonly in younger individuals. The reason for the rarity of this lesion in the cervical spine is that the spinal canal and foramina have relatively strong anatomic barriers to posterior and posterolateral herniation. Posteriorly, the posterior longitudinal ligament is much heavier than that found in the lumbar region. Posterolaterally, the uncus, which contributes to the so-called *joints of Luschka*, provides a bony barrier to nuclear herniation. Thus, in contradistinction to disc herniation in the lumbar spine, frank herniation of the nuclear material in the cervical spine through a defect in the anulus fibrosus and through the posterior longitudinal ligament is quite rare.

Occasionally, however, a piece of disc material escapes the protective anatomic barrier and protrudes laterally to compress an adjacent cervical nerve root. Symptoms of neck pain, with radiation into the shoulder, arm, and hand, are produced as a result of cervical nerve root compression. In other instances the herniation may be blocked by anatomic barriers and cannot protrude posterolaterally to press on cervical nerve roots. Instead it may protrude posteriorly in the midline through a bulging or rupture of the posterior longitudinal ligament to produce cord tract pressure symptoms with manifestations in the low back and legs.

When present, disc protrusions are found most commonly at the C5-C6 and C6-C7 interspaces because that is where maximal motion occurs. Routine films of the cervical spine may be negative. Myelography is helpful in confirming the diagnosis and in localizing the level of involvement. Electromyography is useful in confirming the presence or absence of nerve root irritation.

TREATMENT.   Effective conservative treatment is based on de-compressing the nerve root by the use of cervical traction and a head halter, preferably with the patient recumbent in bed. The neck is supported with a collar during periods when the patient is out of the traction. Local moist heat to the neck, muscle relaxant drugs, and appropriate analgesic drugs are beneficial.

Surgical treatment is reserved for those patients who fail to respond to an adequate conservative program and for those showing a neurologic deficit significant in degree or progressive in nature.

CERVICAL NERVE ROOT COMPRESSION SYNDROME (CERVICAL RADICULITIS, CERVICAL ROOT SYNDROME)

Any condition in the neck that causes impingement or entrapment of a cervical nerve root or encroachment on its intervertebral foramen may be accompanied by signs and symptoms of a cervical nerve root compression syndrome (Fig. 133). The most frequent causes of this condition are degenerative arthritis and herniated intervertebral disc. In the cervical spine, degenerative change with posterior spur formation is a more common cause of nerve root irritation than is protrusion of an intervertebral disc. The opposite is true in the lumbar spine. Less frequent causes include cervical subluxations and dislocations, cervical fractures with backward displacement of the fragments, congenital anomalies of the cervical spine, and tumors.

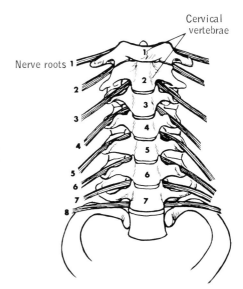

Figure 133. Relationship of cervical nerve roots to cervical vertebrae.

Clinical Picture. The characteristic complaint of the patient with cervical nerve root compression or cervical radiculitis is shoulder and arm pain associated with numbness and tingling in the hand and fingers. The pain is described as severe and sharp and usually follows a radiating pattern from the shoulder to the arm and frequently into the forearm to the fingers. The pain may also radiate to the anterior chest or subscapular area.

Pain is characteristically aggravated by certain motions of the head, particularly turning toward the side of the pain. It is also intensified by coughing, sneezing, straining, or by jarring the neck, as in coming down heavily on the heels or in the application of pressure to the top of the head. In general, the pain is related to movements of the head and the neck; it is not produced by movements of the shoulder and arm.

The objective signs presented by the patient are determined by the level of involvement. The most common areas of involvement are C5-C6 and C6-C7, with entrapment of the sixth and seventh cervical nerve roots.

If the compression involves the sixth cervical nerve root, the sensation of numbness and tingling will predominate over the lateral aspect of the forearm and hand and into the base of the thumb and index finger. Sensory loss may be noted over the dorsal and radial aspects of the thumb and hand. Weakness of the biceps muscle may be found with a diminished or absent biceps reflex.

If the seventh cervical nerve root is involved, the sensation of numbness and tingling will predominate over the dorsal surface of the wrist and hand and into the base of the index and middle fingers. Sensory loss may be noted over the dorsal surface of the hand and index and middle fingers. Weakness of the triceps muscle may be found with diminished or absent triceps reflex.

Diagnosis is established by an attentive history, a thorough physical examination, and a careful study of the x-ray films. Electromyography or myelography may be indicated to aid in localizing the level of involvement.

Treatment. Treatment of cervical nerve root compression syndrome is determined to a certain extent by the cause of the nerve root compression. Surgical treatment is frequently required if the cause is tumor, cervical dislocation, or displaced cervical fractures.

If the cause is arthritic spur impingement or herniated intervertebral disc, the patient is put to bed in head halter cervical traction. A period of several weeks in traction may be required to relieve the nerve compression. Local heat, muscle relaxant drugs, and appropriate analgesics may be added to the program. A Thomas collar is used when the patient is allowed out of bed. Surgical treatment is reserved for those who fail to respond to an adequate conservative program and for those showing neurologic deficit of significant degree.

Traumatic Deformities

Flexibility of the cervical spine is gained at the expense of stability, making the intricate soft tissue structures and the slender vertebral column of the neck extremely prone to injury. The cervical vertebrae are mechanically vulnerable to trauma, not only because of their shape but also because of their function. Automobile accidents, falls from high places, diving accidents, and trauma incurred in body contact sports frequently produce injury to the neck.

Trauma to the neck may result in cervical sprain, subluxation or dislocation of one vertebra upon another, fracture of the bony parts, or fracture-dislocation of a vertebra. Some of these conditions result in damage only to muscles, ligaments, and bones. Others may be associated with the grave complication of spinal cord damage.

In the cervical region, the proximity of the spinal cord and nerve roots to the vertebral elements makes neurologic damage an ever-present possibility with many of these injuries. Severe cord involvement is more common following cervical spine trauma than following trauma to the thoracic or lumbar regions. Any injury to the cervical spine that results in a decreased anteroposterior diameter of the vertebral canal may be accompanied by spinal cord or nerve root damage. Thus, dislocation of one vertebra upon another, fracture-dislocations of vertebrae, and vertebral fractures in which bone fragments are displaced backward into the vertebral canal are serious injuries associated with varying degrees of temporary or permanent paralysis.

A high percentage of patients, following injury to the neck, present with bizarre complaints including dizziness, nausea, headache, transitory deafness, blurred vision, and loss of balance. There is reason to suspect that irritation of the cervical sympathetic nervous system and of the vertebral artery gives rise to a somatoautonomic reflex that accounts for these accompanying symptoms. This is known as the *posterior cervical sympathetic syndrome* or *Barré-Lieou syndrome*.

CERVICAL SPRAIN

The joints of the cervical spine, like other joints in the body, may be subjected to sprain injuries. Force applied to the head or neck may cause a stretching injury to the anterior and posterior cervical ligaments and muscles, with production of the clinical state known as cervical sprain.

The majority of cervical sprains occur as a result of "rear-end" automobile collisions, the impact from which causes hyperextension then hyperflexion of the neck. This is the injury frequently designated "whiplash" — a confusing and misleading term that should not be used by physicians, since it does not accurately describe either the injury itself or the clinical state produced.

The symptoms and signs of acute cervical sprain are those resulting from ligamentous and muscular damage. The initial symptoms may be slight and may go unnoticed in the excitement of the accident. However, after a lag period of hours or days, the patient becomes aware of increasing pain and stiffness in the neck.

The mechanism seems similar to the production of the muscle spasm seen in low back disorders (p. 311). The anterior and posterior cervical ligaments and muscles are stretched at the moment of injury. These sprained tissues are then required to support the weight of the head while the patient remains ambulatory. This added demand upsets the muscular balance and, after a time (lag period), the paracervical muscles go into spasm, with an accompanying increase in pain and stiffness.

The pain may radiate to the shoulders, chest, and upper extremities. It is aggravated by movement or jarring of the head. Injury to the neck muscles may cause pain upon swallowing. Many patients have associated complaints of headache, dizziness, blurred vision, nausea, and loss of balance.

On examination the patient may be seen to splint the neck and voluntarily restrict motion of the head. When asked to turn the head, the patient may turn trunk, shoulders, and head together as a unit. The neck muscles usually feel tense and tight and may be tender to palpation.

The neurologic examination usually fails to reveal any alteration in sensory, motor, or reflex pattern.

X-ray examination is negative for evidence of bone or joint damage. The usual finding is loss of the normal lordotic curve regularly seen on the lateral x-ray view. This extension of the cervical spine is always seen in association with spasm of the long neck muscles.

Effective treatment is dependent upon adequate and prolonged rest to the neck. This can often be obtained by the use of a Thomas collar. If this is not sufficient, collar support should be combined with bed rest. These measures may be supplemented with local heat, analgesics, and muscle relaxant drugs. Cervical traction is not indicated in the presence of acute post-traumatic muscle spasm.

Subluxation of a Vertebra

Subluxation is an incomplete forward or lateral dislocation of one vertebra upon the one below. Trauma to the head and neck may result in a stretching or tearing of the supporting ligaments, allowing one cervical vertebra to drift partially away from another.

Because the dislocation is incomplete, there is usually no spinal cord involvement. However, pressure or traction on cervical nerve roots typically occurs, and the signs and symptoms of a cervical nerve root compression syndrome are often produced.

Subluxation or partial dislocation of one vertebra upon another can be demonstrated on lateral x-ray views of the neck taken in flexion and extension.

Reduction of the subluxation can often be achieved by allowing the patient's head to hang free over the edge of a bed or an examining table. The weight of the head may be sufficient traction to pull the vertebrae back into normal alignment. If this procedure is not successful, mechanical traction or manipulative reduction is carried out. After reduction of the subluxation has been achieved, the neck is immobilized in a brace to allow the soft tissues to heal.

Dislocation of a Vertebra

Anterior dislocation of one vertebral body upon another is a relatively common injury of the cervical spine and is frequently complicated by spinal cord damage with temporary or permanent paralysis below the level of the lesion. This injury results from a fall on the back of the head, which causes rupture of the normally weak posterior ligaments, allowing one vertebra to displace forward upon another.

Routine anteroposterior and lateral x-ray films will disclose the dislocation (Fig. 134).

Skeletal traction applied to the skull is needed to reduce the dislocation. If this is unsuccessful, open surgical reduction is carried out and the part is immobilized in a plaster cast. In some patients the reduction will prove to be unstable, allowing the dislocation to recur. Spinal fusion of the involved segment must then be carried out in order to regain stability of the segment.

Fracture of a Vertebra

Fracture of a cervical vertebra, the so-called "broken neck," may or may not be a critical injury, depending on whether there is spinal cord or cervical nerve root involvement.

Simple wedge compression fractures of the vertebral bodies without dislocation, fracture of the transverse and spinous processes,

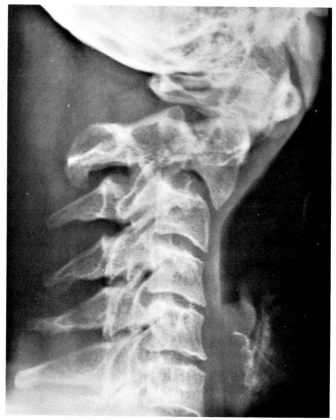

Figure 134. Lateral x-ray of cervical spine, illustrating fracture through posterior elements of C2, with forward and downward displacement of body of C2 on C3.

and fracture of the laminae and pedicles without displacement are almost never complicated by spinal cord or nerve root damage. The injury can be readily diagnosed by adequate x-ray examination and usually heals uneventfully following immobilization in plaster or brace.

On the other hand, displaced fractures of the cervical vertebrae with bone fragments encroaching upon the spinal canal and fracture-dislocations of the cervical vertebrae are grave injuries that may be associated with varying degrees of temporary or permanent paralysis or even death. Patients so afflicted require specialized, experienced care in regard to first aid measures, transportation, and definitive treatment. Casual, inexpert care at any stage carries the grave implication of increasing the degree of paralysis or even causing death of the patient.

THE THORAX

The thoracic cage is conical in shape and exhibits elements of both rigidity and mobility. Rigidity is supplied by the sternum, ribs, and thoracic vertebrae. Mobility is supplied by the muscles of respiration. In addition to housing and protecting the cardiopulmonary apparatus, the thorax acts as a point of fixation for the upper extremities. The thorax may be affected or deformed directly, or it may be involved secondarily by malformations or curvatures of the spine.

The orthopaedic surgeon's interest in the thorax centers about certain developmental and acquired lesions, fractures of the ribs and sternum, and occasionally tumors involving the ribs.

FUNNEL CHEST (PECTUS EXCAVATUM)

This is a developmental deformity of the chest wall characterized by a funnel-shaped depression of the lower end of the sternum that is associated with shortening of the central tendon of the diaphragm, posterior angulation of the costal cartilage, and an outward flare of the lower ribs. As a rule there is little to no alteration of cardiopulmonary function. The condition is mainly a cosmetic liability and is best treated by a thoracic surgeon.

PIGEON BREAST (PECTUS CARINATUM)

This is a developmental or acquired deformity in which overgrowth of the costal cartilages buckles the sternum forward, causing it to project outward as a cosmetically objectionable ridge. Corrective surgery is best managed by a thoracic surgeon.

KYPHOSCOLIOSIS

The term kyphoscoliosis refers to a severe cosmetic deformity of the spine consisting of two components, kyphosis and scoliosis. It is most serious when it involves the thoracic spine because it frequently causes pulmonary and cardiac disability. It may be produced by tuberculosis of the spine, poliomyelitis involving the trunk and chest muscles, or congenital scoliosis.

Treatment involves management of the cause in addition to obtaining cosmetic correction. Mechanical treatment of the deformity is similar to that described for scoliosis (p. 303).

TIETZE'S SYNDROME

This is an ill-defined painful condition of unknown cause involving the anterior chest wall, and of importance mainly because it may be confused with a tumor. It is thought to represent inflammatory, traumatic or degenerative changes involving the costochondral and chondrosternal junctions and occasionally the sternoclavicular joint. The condition causes pain, tenderness, and some enlargement of the affected part. It is most frequently seen affecting the second and third costochondral junctions. The condition usually subsides with supportive treatment and requires no definitive measures.

FRACTURE OF RIBS AND STERNUM

Trauma to the chest wall may cause fracture of one or more ribs or the sternum. All fractures in this area cause pain with movement of the thoracic cage and are associated with some degree of respiratory embarrassment. With no displacement of fragments, these fragments

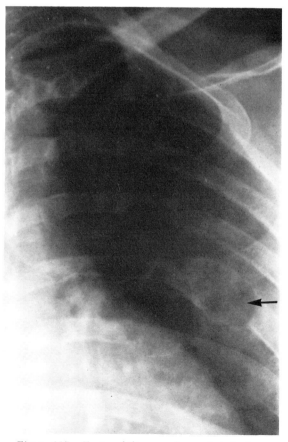

Figure 135.   Eosinophilic granuloma of sixth rib.

usually heal uneventfully if the chest is strapped or a rib belt is used for immobilization. Intercostal nerve block is a helpful adjunct.

With displacement, bone fragments may penetrate the pleural cavity to pierce the lung or an intercostal artery. If this occurs the fracture will be complicated by pneumothorax or hemothorax.

Severe trauma to the chest wall may cause multiple fractures of the ribs and sternum with the subsequent development of a flail chest. Unsatisfactory expansion of the lungs due to the flail chest causes distressing dyspnea. Skeletal traction to the chest wall gives stability to the thorax until sufficient bone healing has occurred.

BONE TUMORS

A variety of bone tumors may affect the bony thorax, particularly the ribs. In some cases the tumor may cause pain and, occasionally, a pathologic fracture of the rib. In other cases, the tumor may come to light when the patient first notices a lump on the rib cage (Fig. 135). The diagnosis rests upon the x-ray findings and histologic interpretation of tissue obtained at biopsy.

Among the benign tumors most commonly affecting the ribs are enchondroma and fibrous dysplasia.

Primary malignant bone tumors affecting the ribs include chondrosarcoma, osteosarcoma, and Ewing's tumor. Involvement of ribs with metastatic carcinoma is relatively common. The primary sites of these metastatic cancer deposits are usually breast, lung, kidney, thyroid, and prostate.

References

Bateman, J. E.: The Shoulder and Neck. Philadelphia: W. B. Saunders Co., 1972.

D'Abreu, A. L.: Thoracic injuries. J. Bone and Joint Surg., 46-B:581, 1964.

Fielding, J. W.: Normal and selected abnormal motions of the cervical spine from the second cervical vertebra to the seventh cervical vertebra based on cineroentgenography. J. Bone and Joint Surg., 46-A:1779, 1964.

Friedenberg, Z. B., and Miller, W. T.: Degenerative disc disease of the cervical spine: A comparative study of asymptomatic and symptomatic patients. J. Bone and Joint Surg., 45-A:1171, 1963.

Hohl, M., and Baker, H. R.: The atlanto-axial joint. Roentgenographic and anatomical study of normal and abnormal motion. J. Bone and Joint Surg., 46-A:1739, 1964.

Robinson, R. A., Kahn, E. A., White, J. C., and Bosworth, D. M.: The cervical spine. Editorial, J. Bone and Joint Surg., 41-A:1, 1959.

Southwick, W. O., and Keggy, K.: The normal cervical spine. J. Bone and Joint Surg., 46-A:1767, 1964.

Chapter Thirteen

The Spine, the Low Back, and the Pelvis

THE SPINE

For our purposes, the spine may be defined as a series of articulated vertebrae acting together to support the weight of the trunk and to protect the spinal cord and nerve roots from damage. It may be subjected to congenital, acquired, or traumatic deformities.

The thoracic segment of the spine usually consists of twelve vertebrae and the lumbar segment of five vertebrae. The sacral and coccygeal vertebrae are fused together in the adult and are considered clinically as single bones. Except for the sacrum and coccyx, the articulated vertebrae are separated by intervertebral discs, which act as shock absorbers and greatly enhance the flexibility of the back. The spine is held erect by the paravertebral muscle masses, which act as lateral supports or guy wires. Their normal stimulus for postural tone is the upright position. These muscles are completely flaccid in the prone or supine position.

The back is an extremely important segment of the body from an orthopaedic point of view. Clinical problems referable to the back, particularly to the low back area, are common in orthopaedic practice. Congenital and mechanical deformities may cause symptoms at any period of life. Trauma to the back takes on added significance because of the proximity of the spinal cord. Infections, metabolic diseases, and tumors frequently implicate the spine (Fig. 136).

294

with herniated intervertebral disc. The principal structural cause is true spinal scoliosis.

When the back is examined in the lateral view, it is seen that the spine is not straight but rather consists of four gentle curves. Curvature exists with the convexity forward in the cervical and lumbar regions and with the concavity forward in the thoracic and sacral regions. These are normal physiologic curves varying in magnitude from one person to another. In normal health or in normal mechanical alignment, however, the amplitude of the concave curves should just about balance the amplitude of the convex ones. In certain abnormal conditions, these curves may be either greatly accentuated or almost entirely obliterated.

The term "round back" refers to accentuation of the thoracic curvature—the deformity brought on by an increase beyond the normal physiologic curve of the thoracic segment of the spine. This may be the result of poor posture, particularly in tall, thin individuals. It may also be caused by the effects of Scheuermann's disease (p. 89), or it may be secondary to anterior wedging of the vertebral bodies as a result of osteoporosis of the thoracic spine in elderly people (p. 175).

When the thoracic spinal curvature passes beyond the "round back" stage and becomes a sharp, angular deformity, it is referred to as a *kyphosis,* meaning knuckle. This is always a serious deformity because the sharp, bony curvature may produce an angular kinking of the spinal cord with resultant neurologic damage. This type of deformity may be caused by compression fracture of a vertebral body or by tuberculosis of the spine.

The term *lordosis* refers to accentuation of the cervical or lumbar curvature beyond physiologic levels. In the lumbar region, the forward curve can be accentuated by lumbar vertebral deformities, such as spondylolisthesis, forward tilt of the pelvis, obesity, paralysis of the abdominal muscles, congenital dislocation of the hips, or hip flexion contractures. In both the cervical and lumbar regions, spasm of the paravertebral muscles may be associated with loss or flattening of the normal forward curve.

In general, the spine makes every effort to keep the head and trunk in balance. Deformity of one part of the spine is usually balanced by deformity in the opposite direction in another region of the spine, in order to maintain the trunk erect and the head centered over the pelvis. For example, a thoracic round back would be accompanied by relative cervical and lumbar lordosis, while flattening of the lumbar spine would be associated with flattening of the thoracic spine. Lateral scoliotic curves are similarly associated with compensatory curves above and below the primary or main curve.

In some disease states, the portion of the spine that should compensate for a deformity may be too damaged or rigid to respond. In these instances the trunk and head are forced out of line and out of balance, resulting in a severe disabling deformity for the patient.

Congenital Deformities

Congenital deformities of the spine are very common. It has been estimated that not more than one of five persons has a completely normal vertebral column by x-ray examination. Fortunately, only a few of these deformities usually cause symptoms.

The congenital anomalies most frequently seen on x-ray examination are variations in the structure of the lumbosacral joint, including spina bifida, variations in the number of lumbar vertebrae, and abnormalities of the lateral articulations. Some of these are occasionally associated with lumbosacral instability (Fig. 138). Hemivertebra and spondylolisthesis are important congenital deformities of the spine that frequently manifest symptoms.

HEMIVERTEBRA

Hemivertebra is a developmental error in the spine brought about by lack of formation of a vertebral body growth center. It may affect any area of the spine and produces a wedge-shaped vertebra or one-half of a vertebra. The adjacent vertebrae tilt to fill the gap, and this mechanism usually results in the development of a structural scoliosis (Fig. 136).

SPONDYLOLISTHESIS

The term spondylolisthesis means gliding of a vertebra and is used to describe a deformity of the spine in which a vertebral body with the vertebral column above it subluxes or glides forward on the vertebral body below. The body and pedicles of the affected vertebra tend to slip forward, while the laminae and spinous process remain behind with the vertebra below (Fig. 139).

Spondylolisthesis arises from a defect or break in the bony continuity between the anterior and posterior halves of the neural arch. Although most authorities believe that the cause of this defect is a congenital developmental error, there is some support for an ischemic or traumatic basis. The defect is found most frequently at the lower end of the spine, with the fourth lumbar vertebra displaced forward on the fifth, or the fifth lumbar vertebra displaced forward on the sacrum. Patients are sometimes seen in whom the defect is visible on oblique x-ray views, but in whom little to no displacement of the vertebral body has occurred. If there is no displacement of the vertebral body, the condition is called *spondylolysis*.

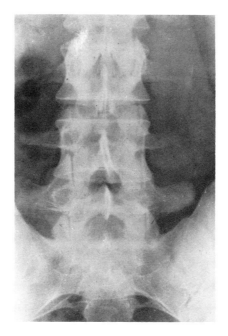

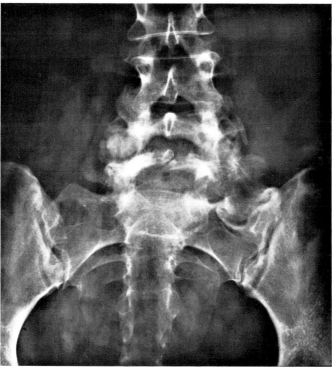

Figure 138. A, normal-appearing lumbosacral joint. B, congenital anomaly involving the lumbosacral joint, including spina bifida occulta and sacralization of the fifth lumbar body.

299

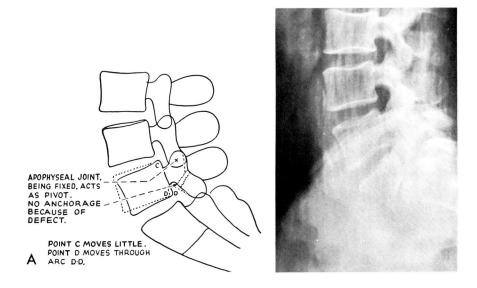

APOPHYSEAL JOINT,
BEING FIXED, ACTS
AS PIVOT.
NO ANCHORAGE
BECAUSE OF
DEFECT.

  POINT C MOVES LITTLE.
  POINT D MOVES THROUGH
A ARC D·D.

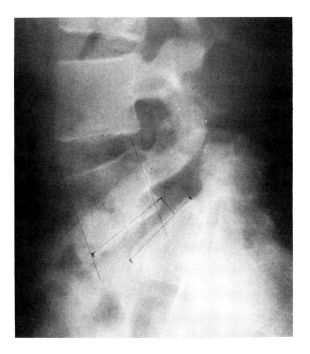

Figure 139. A, diagram and roentgenogram illustrating the usual mechanism of spondylolisthesis. (Diagram from Meschan, I.: Analysis of Roentgen Signs, Vol. 1. Philadelphia: W. B. Saunders Co., 1973.) *B*, lateral view of spine showing moderate forward slipping of body of fifth lumbar vertebra on sacrum.

The chief complaint with spondylolisthesis, especially in young adults, is back pain. Occasionally, fibrocartilage piles up along the bone defect, causing pressure on the adjacent lumbosacral nerve roots. If this occurs, the patient develops the signs and symptoms of lumbosacral nerve root compression syndrome (p. 312) in addition to back pain. Sciatica can also complicate spondylolisthesis when an intervertebral disc is herniated at a vertebral level just above the level of the spondylolisthesis.

Frequently back pain in this condition can be controlled by the use of a back support, such as a corset or brace. Surgery is reserved for those who fail to respond to conservative measures or who are disabled by the pain of nerve root compression. If the back pain cannot be adequately controlled by bracing, spinal fusion of the involved area is indicated.

If the major problem is sciatic pain, the loose laminae and spinous process or an associated herniated disc could be the cause. If surgery is contemplated in this instance, correction of the cause of the sciatica must be accomplished along with spinal fusion.

Acquired Deformities

SCOLIOSIS

The term scoliosis refers to a lateral curvature of a segment of the spine from the normally straight midline position. The term actually describes only a physical deformity, not a diagnosis. The known causes of scoliosis are many and include intrinsic deformity of the vertebrae, involvement of the muscle and nerve elements that support the spine and, occasionally, causes arising outside the spine itself. The deformity affects females much more frequently than males, occurring, according to estimates, in about 2 per cent of the juvenile female population.

In general, two types of scoliosis are recognized: functional and structural.

Functional scoliosis is caused by postural influences on the spine and is not associated with any structural spinal changes. Functional curves are flexible and disappear when the patient lies recumbent. The cause may be poor posture, leg length inequality, pelvic tilt, hip joint contractures, or paravertebral muscle spasm. As a rule, functional scoliosis poses no real orthopaedic problem.

Structural scoliosis is a spinal deformity that begins during childhood and results in a fixed curvature of varying rigidity, associated with wedge-shaped vertebral bodies and rotation of the vertebrae to the convex side of the curve. A structural scoliotic curve, unlike a functional curve, does not disappear when the patient lies recumbent.

Structural scoliosis may have congenital origins similar to those of hemivertebra. It may also accompany some disease process affecting the vertebral bodies, such as neurofibromatosis, or result from paralysis of the spinal musculature secondary to poliomyelitis. In about 80 per cent of patients with structural scoliosis, however, the cause remains unknown. This form is called *idiopathic scoliosis* and is the type for which the orthopaedist is usually consulted.

Clinical Picture. Several types of curvatures are recognized clinically and are classified by location. The most common is a primary or major curve that arises in the thoracic segment with the convexity to the right, associated with a compensatory curve above in the cervical segment and one below in the lumbar segment, both with the convexity to the left. The parent's or patient's attention is usually first drawn to the deformity by the postural asymmetry caused by this combination of curves or by poorly fitting clothes.

Idiopathic structural scoliosis is associated with the growth period of the spine. It is thought to begin insidiously and, because of the concealing effect of clothing, may reach considerable proportions before being noticed. The deformity caused by the curvature may worsen appreciably during the child's periods of rapid growth, but the curvatures are not thought to increase much in magnitude once spinal growth has been completed.

Curvature due to structural scoliosis does not disappear when the child lies recumbent. Although the spinal column may seem flexible in early stages of this disorder, a structural scoliosis generally becomes more rigid as the curvature increases, making correction more difficult. Generally, the younger the patient at the time the curve is discovered, the worse is the prognosis.

The postural asymmetry resulting from a typical right thoracic, left lumbar scoliosis forces the child to stand with the right shoulder elevated and the left iliac crest prominently tilted upward. Rotation of the vertebral bodies to the right in the thoracic segment causes an increase in the posterior angulation of the rib cage on the same side and also prominence of the right scapula. The opposite side of the posterior thorax appears flattened. The asymmetry of the posterior thorax is accentuated when the spine is flexed (Fig. 140).

As a rule, a child with scoliosis does not have back pain despite the appearance of the deformity. Some older children complain of back fatigue and pain, these being on a muscular basis secondary to the long-standing imbalance. Constant back pain usually signals the complication of degenerative arthritis within the affected vertebral segment. This complication is seen most frequently in adults, in whom degenerative arthritis develops in the curved segment secondary to the bony malalignment of uncorrected scoliosis.

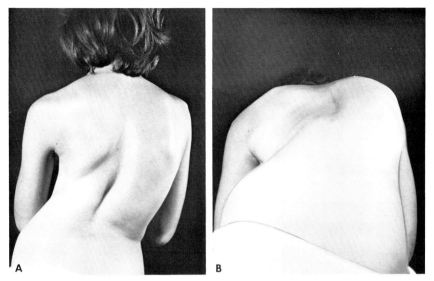

Figure 140. A, postural deformity caused by idiopathic thoracolumbar scoliosis. B, asymmetry of posterior thorax accentuated with patient flexed.

In patients with severe curvature, the organs of the chest and abdomen may be compressed by the resulting skeletal deformity. Marked thoracic scoliosis may result in cardiorespiratory distress. Almost all patients with thoracic deformity show some decrease in pulmonary vital capacity. Severe scoliosis may produce a restrictive ventilation abnormality. Chronically inadequate ventilation of the alveolar capillary bed may lead to pulmonary hypertension and kyphoscoliotic heart disease.

A complete x-ray study of the spine is needed to establish the diagnosis and to identify the characteristics of the curvature in regard to flexibility and correctibility.

Treatment.   Idiopathic structural scoliosis is thought to be a self-limiting process. Progression of the curvature slows as the child grows older, essentially stopping with the cessation of spinal bone growth. The aim of treatment, therefore, is to keep the child as straight and as free from postural deformity as possible until this occurs. Regardless of the method of treatment chosen, the child must be observed carefully and the status of the vertebral deformity checked by x-ray examination every several months.

If the curve is of relatively mild degree and if the spine is flexible, a heel lift of sufficient thickness to level the pelvis might be prescribed. This should be combined with spinal stretching exercises designed to increase the flexibility of the vertebral column.

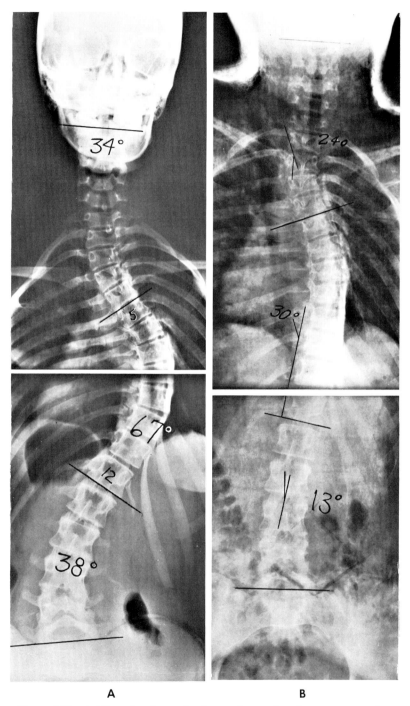

Figure 141. A, idiopathic thoracolumbar scoliosis of moderate severity. B, same patient. Spine is being straightened in plaster localizer jacket.

If the curve is progressive and of substantial degree, however, definitive treatment must be considered. The only brace that has been successfully used in the nonoperative treatment of scoliosis is the Milwaukee brace. This is a specially designed scoliosis brace with occiput and chin pieces, a molded pelvic girdle, lateral pads, and upright spinal bars. The brace is used in conjunction with exercises and affords comfortable, passive support by distraction and the holding force of lateral pads. Use of the Milwaukee brace is indicated in most adolescent patients with idiopathic curves of moderate severity and in all young children, no matter what the etiology or magnitude of the deformity. In many instances prolonged use of the brace results in permanent correction of the scoliosis. In others it may diminish the severity of the curve sufficiently to make subsequent surgery less extensive and formidable.

The indications for surgical treatment of structural scoliosis are: (1) the presence of a rapidly progressing curve, (2) the presence of an objectionable cosmetic deformity, and (3) the presence of a curvature that causes the patient's spine to be out of balance. The definitive operation for scoliosis is spinal fusion of the involved segment. However, before fusion is performed, the spine should be straightened as much as possible. Usually this consists of correcting or straightening the major or primary curve with a large body cast that makes use of a turnbuckle or traction device. Once satisfactory correction has been obtained, surgical fusion of the primary curve is performed, and another cast is applied during the postoperative period to aid in maintaining the correction until the fusion is solidly healed (Fig. 141).

In some centers, metallic internal fixation devices called Harrington rods are used as the time of surgery both to obtain and maintain correction of the spinal curvature. Their use is combined with spinal fusion (Fig. 142).

ARTHRITIS

The spine is a common site for the development of arthritic changes of various types.

Degenerative arthritis, or osteoarthritis, frequently involves the spine, particularly in older age groups. The lumbar spine is a favorite location (p. 323). In young individuals, degenerative arthritis may involve the thoracic or lumbar spine, particularly as a complication of some primary problem that causes malalignment of the vertebrae, such as Scheuermann's disease (p. 89) or scoliosis.

Ankylosing spondylitis is a systemic collagen disease that tends to begin in the sacroiliac joints but often progresses from the lumbar area to involve the entire vertebral column (p. 103). It is seen most frequently in men between the ages of 20 and 40.

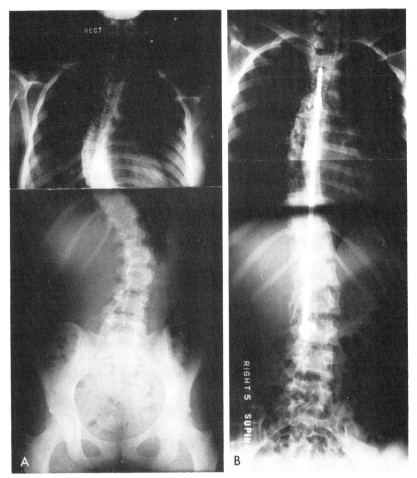

Figure 142. A, idiopathic thoracolumbar scoliosis of moderate severity. *B*, same patient after Harrington rod correction and spinal fusion.

INFECTION

Pyogenic infection of the spine is called *vertebral osteomyelitis* or *pyogenic spondylitis*. The infecting organism is usually blood-borne to the spine from some primary focus of infection elsewhere in the body. Rarely infection may develop following spinal surgery or spinal puncture. Not infrequently it may appear to commence as a disc space infection.

The patient notices back pain that may or may not be associated with systemic signs of infection. The back pain is frequently quite severe and is associated with functional disability. X-ray examination eventually discloses evidence of bone destruction involving one or more vertebral bodies, accompanied by characteristic narrowing or loss of the intervertebral disc space (Fig. 143). In contrast to its inability to resist the tubercle bacillus, bone tissue exhibits a positive host response to invading pyogenic organisms. Eventually the x-ray film shows the presence of reactive bone formation around the destructive lesion, illustrating a walling-off process.

Treatment is rest to the spine and adequate antibiotic therapy. In some instances it may be possible to obtain material for culture from needle biopsy of the involved area. Rest to the spine may be obtained in bed, or by the use of a plaster body cast or brace.

As healing occurs, serial x-ray examinations will show filling or healing of the destructive lesions in the vertebrae. Frequently, the involved vertebrae may progress to spontaneous bony fusion. On rare occasions it may be necessary to operate in order to drain the abscess, particularly if neurologic complications appear.

In years past, tuberculous infection of the spine, known as *Pott's disease*, was one of the commonest causes of vertebral kyphosis or "hunchback" deformity. The spine, particularly the dorsolumbar junction, is the skeletal area most frequently involved with tuberculosis (p. 142).

Radiostrontium bone-scanning techniques may be useful when the diagnosis of vertebral infection is not clear. The scanning method is based on the observation that strontium is deposited in the bones in the same way as calcium. In local skeletal lesions, such as infection,

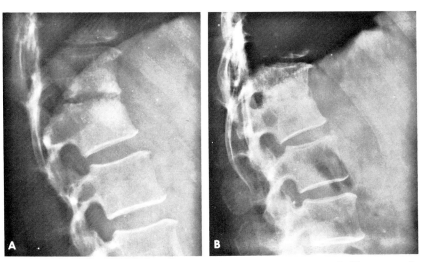

Figure 143. A, pyogenic infection of the T12-L1 interspace. B, fifteen months later solid bony fusion existed.

fractures, or tumors, the rate of mineral metabolism in the area of the lesion is increased. Intravenously injected radiostrontium accumulates at the site of the lesion, with resultant increased radioactivity over the area involved. The method is useful in the early diagnosis of dubious primary lesions and recurrences, but it cannot differentiate between pyogenic spondylitis and tuberculosis.

Tumors of the Vertebral Column

Benign tumors involving the vertebrae are unusual.

Hemangioma, a benign blood vessel tumor, may appear in the substance of a vertebral body, giving rise to characteristic vertically striped trabeculation within the vertebral body, as seen on x-ray examination. The tumor may weaken the structure of the bone, leading to pathologic fracture with collapse of the vertebral body.

Aneurysmal bone cyst is an expanded balloon of bone protruding from the cortical surface of a bone and containing a mass of vascular tissue. It is a benign bone tumor that may arise in the vertebrae (p. 199).

Except for plasma cell myeloma, primary malignant bone tumors arising in the vertebral column are quite rare. Much more frequently the spine is the site of metastatic cancer deposits from primary tumors in the breast, prostate, thyroid, kidney, and lung. Secondary involvement of the vertebral column may also accompany leukemia, Hodgkin's disease, and malignant lymphoma.

Chordoma. Chordoma is an uncommon tumor that occurs in bone primarily at either end of the vertebral column. It develops from remnants of the embryonic notochord, such as nucleus pulposus or abnormal "rests" of notochordal tissue. More than half the tumors occur in the bone of the sacrococcygeal region. The tumor is slow-growing, affects mostly patients in the middle years of life, and is considered malignant because it is locally invasive.

Treatment is surgical excision, which is frequently incomplete because of the tumor's capacity for extensive growth.

Intraspinal Tumors. Although their treatment is not within the scope of orthopaedic surgery, intraspinal tumors may give rise to back and leg pain and should thus be considered in differential diagnosis of back pain, and particularly of radiculitis. Approximately 1 per cent of patients operated upon for herniated lumbar disc are found to have an intraspinal tumor.

In general, two types of intraspinal tumors are described: extradural and intradural. A careful history and physical examination, coupled with a close review of the x-ray findings and myelographic pattern, help one to differentiate tumor from other causes of nerve root compression.

Usually, extradural tumors are secondary, representing metastatic carcinoma or spreading from lymphatic system tumors, such as Hodgkin's disease, lymphosarcoma, and reticulum cell sarcoma.

Intradural tumors are most often primary and include meningioma, neurofibroma, glioma, medulloblastoma, and ependymoma.

Traumatic Deformities

Fracture or dislocation involving the thoracic or lumbar segment of the spine is not accompanied by severe cord involvement as frequently as are similar injuries occurring in the cervical segment. Severe spinal cord involvement is the exception in the thoracic and lumbar regions, and consequently most patients who "break their backs" suffer no cord or nerve root injury.

The most common fracture in the thoracic and lumbar spine is a compression fracture of a vertebral body (Fig. 144). Next in frequency

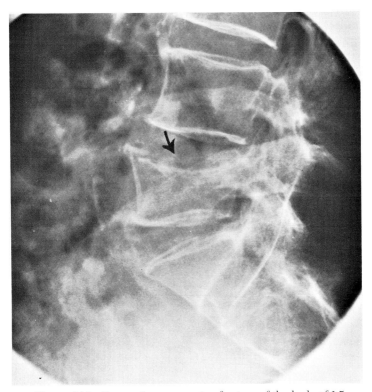

Figure 144. Traumatic compression fracture of the body of L5.

are fractures of the transverse processes and fractures of the spinous processes. These fractures are almost never complicated by cord or nerve root involvement and usually heal uneventfully.

Severely displaced fractures or fracture-dislocations in the thoracic and lumbar regions may encroach upon the spinal canal and cause neurologic damage (see Traumatic Paraplegia, p. 157). Paralysis following trauma to the thoracic spine is usually permanent. The spinal cord ends, as a rule, at the level of the first or second lumbar vertebra as the conus medullaris. Fractures at the thoracolumbar junction causing injury to the conus are associated with saddle anesthesia, loss of sphincter control and, usually, loss of ankle reflexes. Injuries to the lumbar spine below the first lumbar vertebra have a better prognosis from a neurologic standpoint because the cauda equina, having mobility, is less vulnerable to trauma.

LOW BACK PAIN

Low back pain is one of the commonest patient complaints heard by physicians. There are no accurate frequency studies available from the United States, but a study in Sweden concluded that 65 per cent of the adult Swedish population had at one time or another sought medical attention for back pain. It is well understood that the basic causes of low back pain are myriad and can be medical, obstetric, gynecologic, urologic, metabolic, and psychosomatic as well as orthopaedic. Most low back pain, however, has an orthopaedic basis. Some conditions of the spine that can cause low back pain have already been discussed in this chapter. The most frequent orthopaedic causes of low back pain are now considered in this section and include acute lumbosacral strain, unstable lumbosacral mechanism, osteoarthritis of the lumbar spine, and problems involving the intervertebral disc.

General Considerations

Regardless of the underlying orthopaedic cause of low back pain, patients frequently have certain signs and symptoms in common. They may exhibit paravertebral muscle spasm of varying degree and severity. Their pain may be localized to the small of the back, or it may radiate up along the spinal column toward the neck and head or down into the pelvis, buttocks, or thighs. Low back pain may be associated with sciatica, which is a symptom of nerve root irritation and causes pain along the anatomic distribution of the sciatic nerve.

Paravertebral Muscle Spasm

The paravertebral muscles play a dual role in body mechanics (Fig. 145). Normally they act as physiologic guy wires, helping to hold the trunk erect. Their normal stimulus for postural tone is the upright position. These muscles are completely flaccid in the prone or supine position.

Their second role in body mechanics is that of a protective mechanism. A painful stimulus arising from the low back area may trigger

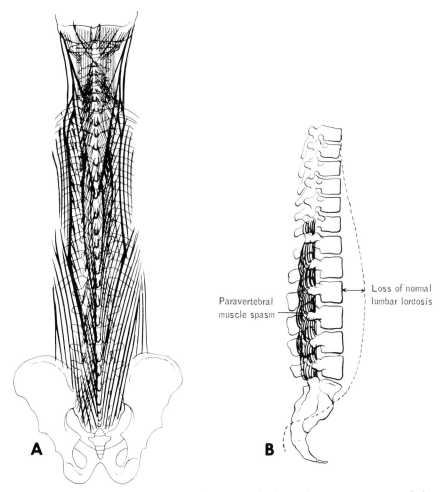

Paravertebral
muscle spasm

Loss of normal
lumbar lordosis

A   **B**

Figure 145. *A*, in normal health the paravertebral muscles act as guy wires to help hold the spine erect. *B*, following a painful stimulus, the paravertebral muscles may go into spasm as part of the body's defense mechanism.

paravertebral muscle spasm, which is defined as markedly exaggerated muscle tone, initiated by a stimulus of trauma or pain and maintained by the upright position. It is, in effect, a warning to the patient to protect his back from movement and from possible further damage. The occurrence and effects of paravertebral muscle spasm can be aborted by removing the stimulus of the upright position through absolute bed rest. If the patient is allowed to remain ambulatory, the low back area is progressively splinted by the muscle spasm. If unchecked, the clinical symptoms produced by paravertebral muscle spasm are often completely disabling.

SCIATICA

Patients may present with low back pain with posterior leg radiation representing an associated sciatica. This type of leg pain must be carefully differentiated from the diffuse muscular and ligamentous radiation pattern associated with tight hamstring muscles or accompanying some of the mechanical and degenerative lesions of the low back.

Sciatica attendant upon low back pain represents the peripheral manifestations of compression of the lumbosacral spinal nerve roots (Fig. 146). The most frequent causes of this compression are herniated intervertebral disc, compression of a spinal root by an osteoarthritic spur, and intraspinal tumors. The symptoms and signs accompanying nerve root compression in this area, regardless of cause, are similar and constitute the so-called *lumbosacral nerve root compression syndrome*. A physician can uncover the presence of an associated nerve root compression syndrome by a thorough history and physical examination. Further tests are necessary to pinpoint the exact cause of the nerve root compression.

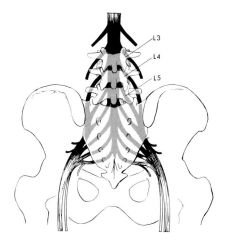

Figure 146. Relationship of lumbosacral nerve roots to lumbar vertebrae.

The predominant symptom of lumbosacral nerve root compression is leg pain that follows the sciatic distribution (buttock, posterior thigh, popliteal space, and calf), and which may then divide to involve either the medial or lateral border of the foot. The pain is aggravated by spinal movements and by anything that raises the intrathecal pressure, such as lifting, coughing, sneezing, or straining. The pain is characteristically sharp and severe, and may be associated with a tingling sensation or hypesthesia over the foot and toes. There is usually tenderness to palpation over the sciatic nerve trunk in the posterior thigh and buttock. If the pain is due to sciatica, it will be reproduced or aggravated by the straight leg raising test and the sitting root test.

The positive neurologic signs produced by lumbosacral spinal nerve root compression are those of a lower motor neuron lesion. The Achilles reflex, and occasionally the patellar reflex, depending on the level of involvement, may be normal, depressed, or absent, but never hyperactive. The muscles most frequently affected by compression at the lower lumbar levels are the anterior tibial and toe extensors. The motor power of these muscles may be normal, weak, or absent, but never increased or spastic. Sensation over the dermatome supplied by the compressed spinal nerve root may be normal, diminished, or absent, but not increased.

Examination of the Low Back

HISTORY

Once the examiner has ascertained that the patient's chief complaint is low back pain, he should, by direct questioning, determine its specific location, duration, and character, and whether or not it radiates to another part of the body. Location is best determined by asking the patient to point to the place that hurts.

The character of the pain is discovered by asking about its severity, constancy, and intensity. Acute low back pain is generally more severe and of shorter duration. Chronic low back pain is frequently described as an ache and tends to be present intermittently. Since most causes of orthopaedic low back pain are mechanical, it is important to discover if the pain is influenced by movement of the spine. Often low back pain is aggravated by bending and lifting and relieved by resting the back. Frequently, particularly in degenerative lesions of the lumbar joints, an element of stiffness is noted by the patient following periods of relative immobility, as on arising from bed in the morning or after a long automobile trip.

It is important to determine whether the pain radiates to another part of the body. Most commonly the pain may radiate up the back toward the neck and head, down into the muscles of the buttocks and thighs, or down the posterior aspect of either leg. It is unusual for pain originating in the low back area to radiate to the abdominal or genital area.

Physical Examination

The patient should be undressed and draped so that the entire back, pelvis, and legs are visible to the examiner. A satisfactory low back examination procedure is outlined in Table 3.

Inspection. The patient is first examined while standing erect

---

TABLE 3. Outline for Examination of the Low Back

History

1. Chief complaint and duration
2. Location of pain
3. Character of pain
    a. What aggravates pain?
    b. What relieves pain?
4. Radiation of pain
    a. Location
    b. Type

Physical Examination

1. Inspection—standing
    a. General contour of back
    b. Status of pelvis
    c. Status of paravertebral muscles
    d. Lumbar lordosis—present or absent
    e. Spinal motions
2. Palpation—standing
    a. General contour of back
    b. Status of iliac crests
    c. Status of paravertebral muscles
3. Palpation—lying
    a. General contour of back
    b. Status of paravertebral muscles
    c. Determination of areas of local tenderness
4. Hip joint range of motion
5. Leg length determination
6. Leg tests
7. Neurologic examination
8. X-ray examination

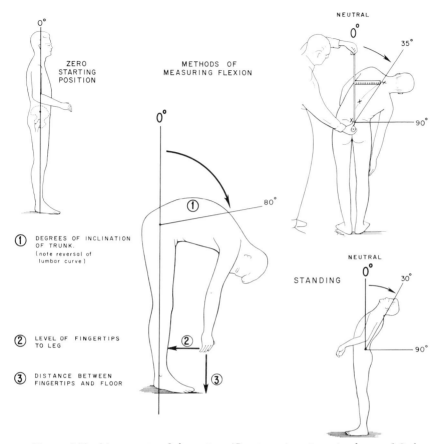

0°

ZERO
STARTING
POSITION

METHODS OF
MEASURING FLEXION

0°

80°

① DEGREES OF INCLINATION
OF TRUNK.
(note reversal of
lumbar curve)

② LEVEL OF FINGERTIPS
TO LEG

③ DISTANCE BETWEEN
FINGERTIPS AND FLOOR

NEUTRAL
0°
35°
90°

NEUTRAL
0°
STANDING
30°
90°

Figure 147. Movements of the spine. (Courtesy American Academy of Orthopaedic Surgeons.)

with his back to the examiner. The general contour of the spine in the
standing position is evaluated in terms of straightness, curvature, pelvic tilt, list or other visible deformity (p. 295). The presence or absence of the normal lumbar lordotic curve is noted, since this finding
is closely related to the presence or absence of paravertebral muscle
spasm.

Movements of the low back are then examined and any pain or restriction of motion noted. The patient is asked to bend forward as far
as possible *(flexion)*, and then to bend backwards as far as possible
(hyperextension). Left lateral bend and right lateral bend complete
the usual motions examined (Fig. 147).

Palpation (Standing). While the patient remains standing, the
examiner palpates the back to assess the general contour and to deter-

mine whether both iliac crests are level. The elevation of one iliac crest above the other indicates a pelvic tilt, which could be related to curvature of the spine, paravertebral muscle spasm, or an inequality in leg length.

The tone of the paravertebral muscles is determined by palpation with the patient erect.

Palpation (Lying).   The patient then lies completely prone on the examining table with the arms relaxed at the sides and the head comfortably turned.

The general contour of the back in this position is compared with that noted in the erect posture. The factors of spinal straightness, curvature, or pelvic tilt are compared between the erect and prone positions. All deformity directly related to paravertebral muscle spasm will disappear in the relaxed prone position. Deformity not directly related to paravertebral muscle spasm tends not to disappear in the prone position.

The paravertebral muscles should feel relaxed and flaccid when the patient is in the prone position. The examiner then notes the presence or absence of local tenderness about the lower lumbar spine and lumbosacral joint, sacroiliac joints, sciatic notch, and sciatic nerve trunk.

Hip Joints.   Both hip joints should be put through a full range of passive motion and any restriction noted. Degenerative diseases of the hip joint, early in their course, are associated with loss of rotation motions of the hip that may cause pain radiating to the low back area.

Leg Length.   The length of both lower extremities is obtained with a tape measure by measuring from the anterior superior iliac spine to the medial malleolus with the patient lying supine and the pelvis straight. Unequal leg length may be related to pelvic tilt, curvature of the spine, or low backache, and could be the cause of a gait abnormality.

Leg Tests.   Various tests involving passive bending of the low back or legs have been popularized in the past to demonstrate mechanical abnormalities of the low back region. These include the Gaenslen, Nacklas, Ober, Lasèque, and Patrick tests and are still performed routinely by some examiners.

Two leg tests should be done whenever lumbosacral nerve root compression is suspected. Both depend upon stretching the sciatic nerve and are positive if they reproduce or aggravate sciatica (Fig. 148).

1. *Straight leg raising test.* With patient lying supine, the extended leg is flexed on the trunk at the hip by the examiner.

2. *Sitting root test.* The patient sits erect on the edge of an examining table with the chin bent down on the chest. The examiner

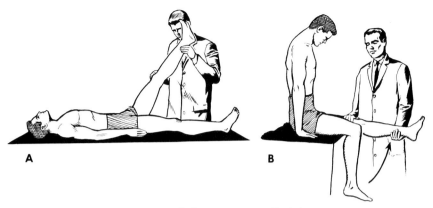

Figure 148. A, straight leg raising test. B, sitting root test.

fixes the thigh to the table with one hand while extending the leg on the flexed thigh with the other.

These tests are positive only if they reproduce or aggravate pain of a sciatic distribution. They are considered negative if they produce pure back pain or discomfort due to hamstring muscle tightness.

Neurologic Examination. The neurologic examination should be as complete as is warranted by the suspected condition. Routinely, the Achilles and patellar reflexes should be tested. Estimation is made of the relative strength of the anterior tibial, long toe extensor, and common toe extensor muscles. These muscles are routinely tested for weakness because they are involved in motor weakness pattern most commonly associated with lumbosacral nerve root compression. If present, the clinical findings associated with motor weakness of this dorsiflexor muscle group may vary from simple impairment of toe extension power to complete foot drop.

Tests for sensory deficit are made in the dermatome patterns of the toes and foot. Part of the dermatome pattern of the first sacral nerve root involves the fifth toe and lateral border of the foot. Nerve root compression at the lumbosacral interspace will implicate the first sacral nerve root. Loss of sensation, if present, will therefore be found over the fifth toe and lateral border of the foot.

Part of the dermatome pattern of the fifth lumbar nerve root involves the great toe and medial border of the foot. Nerve root compression at the L4-L5 interspace will implicate the fifth lumbar nerve root. Loss of sensation, if present, will therefore be found over the great toe and medial border of the foot.

X-ray Examination. Anteroposterior, lateral, and oblique views of the lumbar and lumbosacral spine area should be taken of every patient seeking attention because of low back pain.

Orthopaedic Causes of Low Back Pain

ACUTE LUMBOSACRAL STRAIN

Acute lumbosacral strain is the commonest cause of acute low back pain. The lumbosacral joint, because of its position in the skeleton, supports the body weight and acts as a fulcrum for this weight in activities involving bending and lifting. Mechanical damage to this joint is frequent because of the functional demands placed on the low back area by everyday activities. In this particular joint the traumatic force is usually a lifting load applied to a forward flexed spine with the lumbosacral joint as fulcrum; or a load applied to the spine while it is twisted or rotated, or less often, a sudden force applied unexpectedly before the back muscles brace themselves to meet it.

The resulting pathologic change is a partial tearing or stretching of the overlying paravertebral muscles, lumbar fascia, and interspinous ligaments. If the injury results in more serious damage to the spine, by definition it cannot be a lumbosacral strain. The injury to the soft parts initiates paravertebral muscle spasm, which accounts for the clinical picture seen with this entity.

Two facts are basic to the understanding of an acute lumbosacral strain. First, the stimulus for normal tone of the paravertebral muscles is the upright position. These muscles are in normal postural tone only in the standing or sitting positions and are completely flaccid in the prone or supine positions. Spasm of the paravertebral muscles is markedly exaggerated tone initiated by the stimulus of overload and maintained by the stimulus of the upright position. If the patient were put to bed immediately after sustaining the straining injury, it is doubtful whether the symptoms and signs associated with an acute lumbosacral strain could develop. It is this basic physiologic fact that accounts for the extreme duration of pain and disability in patients with paravertebral muscle spasm who are allowed to remain ambulatory. It also accounts for the rapid subsidence of symptoms that results from absolute bed rest.

Secondly, in patients with acute lumbosacral strain there is almost always a lag period between the time the low back damage was sustained and the onset of clinical symptoms. This lag period may vary from hours to days and is totally dependent upon the patient remaining upright. It is during this period that the paravertebral muscle spasm builds up to the point of clinical significance.

Clinical Features. The severity of the clinical features of acute lumbosacral strain depends directly upon the degree of paravertebral muscle spasm present. The patient gives a history of twisting or lifting injury to the low back area and states that the onset of symptoms oc-

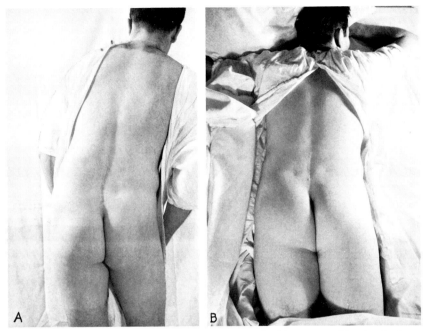

Figure 149. *A*, paravertebral muscle spasm with obliteration of lumbar lordosis, elevation of left side of pelvis, and list of spine to the right. *B*, the postural deformity disappears once the patient is relaxed in the prone position.

curred either immediately or, more commonly, following a lag period of hours or days. He walks slowly and guardedly because movement of the spine is painful. The back may be held in a forward flexed attitude or may exhibit a list to one side with a tilted pelvis (Fig. 149). The paravertebral muscles feel extremely taut and hard, and the normal lumbar lordotic curve is obliterated. Spinal movements are limited in direct proportion to the amount of spasm present and are associated with a sharp, diffuse, "catching" type of pain in the low back area, with possible radiation to the buttocks and thighs or up toward the neck.

It is painful for the patient to lie on the examining table and to turn from abdomen to back and vice versa. Once the patient is completely relaxed in the prone position, all the postural deformity caused by paravertebral muscle spasm seen in the upright position disappears, and the paravertebral muscles feel soft and flaccid. If the postural deformity of the spine noted in the upright position does not disappear in the prone position, the cause of the deformity is probably a structural disorder of the spine and not paravertebral muscle spasm.

Once the patient is able to lie flat and relaxed on the examining table, the physical findings are minimal because of the subsidence of the muscle spasm. Palpation will reveal diffuse tenderness over the low back area, particularly at the lumbosacral joint and along the paravertebral muscle masses. Coughing, straining, or turning over on the examining table aggravates the low back pain. The straight leg raising and sitting root tests produce low back pain, not sciatic radiation. Passive movement of the hip joints does not produce pain, and the neurologic examination is negative. X-ray examination of the spine is negative except for flattening of the normal lumbar curve, noted on the lateral view, indicative of paravertebral muscle spasm.

Treatment. The basic principle of treatment is to remove the stimulus for paravertebral muscle tone by means of absolute bed rest. Only patients with minimal spasm can recover rapidly under treatment on an ambulatory basis. The most effective treatment for almost all patients is absolute bed rest, except for bathroom privileges, continued until the patient can turn from side to side in bed without pain. This usually takes from three to ten days. In addition to bed rest, local heat to the back, analgesics, and muscle relaxant drugs may be helpful.

Once the patient is able to move freely in bed without pain, he may become ambulatory and is allowed gradually to resume full activity. A daily hot soaking tub bath is beneficial during this period. If considered necessary, muscle strengthening exercises can be added to the program.

Important Diagnostic Points. Some important considerations in arriving at a diagnosis are:

1. History of a lifting or twisting injury or sudden strain to the low back.
2. Usually a lag period between incident and onset of symptoms.
3. Severe paravertebral muscle spasm with all objective findings directly proportional to degree of spasm.
4. Degree of disability often out of proportion to severity of injury.
5. Negative x-ray examination; negative neurologic examination.
6. Rapid recovery with absolute bed rest and local heat.

UNSTABLE LUMBOSACRAL MECHANISM

The term unstable lumbosacral mechanism is used to describe a lumbosacral joint that is architecturally unable to meet the functional demands placed upon it. As long as the functional demands do not exceed the strength of the joint, the patient remains asymptomatic. Factors allowing the functional demands to exceed the strength of the joint are called precipitating factors and include pregnancy, gradual loss of muscle tone due to overweight or increasing age, sedentary occupations, and local trauma to the back. When the strength of the joint is exceeded, the patient becomes symptomatic and presents with chronic low back pain or repeated episodes of acute low back pain.

Some of these patients complain of pain radiating to the buttocks, anterior thigh and groin, or along the lateral aspect of the thigh to the knee, but this radiation is along a muscular and ligamentous distribution and not along nerve pathways. The patients with muscular leg radiation must be carefully differentiated from those with nerve root compression syndrome, in which the leg radiation is posterior and follows specific nerve root pathways.

X-ray examination may be negative or may reveal some potential mechanical abnormality, such as some congenital anomaly of the lumbosacral joint or the presence of an acute lumbosacral angle (Fig. 150).

Treatment. Treatment consists of first relieving the paravertebral muscle spasm, if present, and then strengthening the unstable joint.

Each acute episode of low back pain sustained by the patient is treated exactly as an acute lumbosacral strain. Once the paravertebral

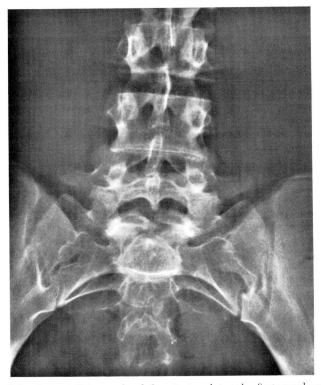

Figure 150. Spina bifida occulta deformity involving the first sacral segments.

muscle spasm has subsided, attention is directed to strengthening the low back area through spinal exercises.

Hyperextension spinal exercises can be used to increase the strength and tone of the paravertebral muscles until these muscles are strong enough to function as a physiologic brace for the spine (Fig. 151). In addition, many orthopaedists recommend mobilization by

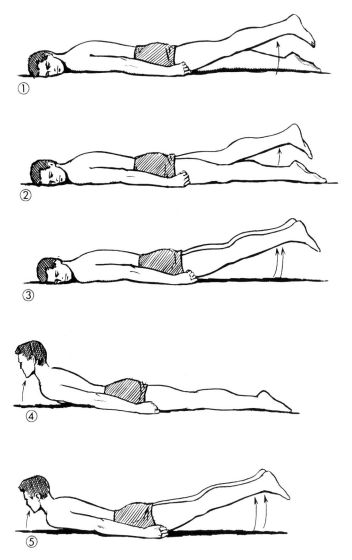

Figure 151. An exercise program designed to strengthen the paravertebral muscles.

postural, pelvic tilt, and flexion exercises, which should be done regularly for at least a three month period, then gradually decreased depending on symptoms. Between 50 and 75 per cent of patients can be maintained satisfactorily on exercises alone.

If exercises are not sufficient, or in patients who cannot exercise for one reason or another, the use of a firm lumbosacral belt or brace is indicated. It must be remembered that extrinsic support will further weaken the back muscles, and everyone who wears a support should also exercise if at all feasible.

If symptoms are not adequately controlled by exercises or support, lumbosacral fusion is indicated. It has been estimated that no more than 10 per cent of patients ever progress to the point of requiring a fusion operation for pain relief.

OSTEOARTHRITIS OF THE LUMBAR SPINE
(See also p. 106)

The lumbar spine is a common site for osteoarthritis in patients past the fifth decade of life. The disorder may be either a part of a generalized disease process or localized to one spinal segment as a result of trauma or repeated occupational stresses over a long period of time. Patients may remain pain-free for long periods, only to have symptoms triggered by trauma to the back. This is the condition usually referred to by the layman as "lumbago."

The disease attacks primarily the articular hyaline cartilage, causing degeneration and thinning of the cartilage, which results in narrowing and irregularity of the joint space. With narrowing of the joint space, bone sclerosis gradually appears at the subchondral joint margins, giving the joint its characteristic dense appearance on the x-ray film (Fig. 152). Spurs may form at both the anterior and posterior joint margins as a result of local pressure stresses and disease activity.

Clinical Features. The characteristic presenting complaint of patients with osteoarthritis of the lumbar spine, especially those over 50 years of age, is stiffness and ache in the low back area. Stiffness following periods of inactivity is typical. The patients note this stiffness particularly in the morning upon arising from bed, or after prolonged periods of sitting or car riding. The sensation of stiffness is relieved by motions of the spine and by activity, but prolonged activity will bring back the ache. Discomfort is usually aggravated by cold damp weather and is frequently relieved by rest and local heat. Many patients have associated muscular and ligamentous radiation of pain into the buttocks, anterior thigh area, pelvis, and along the tensor fascia lata to the lateral aspect of the knee. Often an associated trochanteric bursitis is noted.

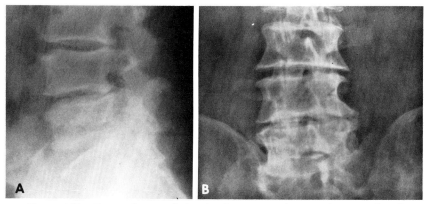

Figure 152. Osteoarthritis of the lumbar spine showing hypertrophic bone changes, spur formation, and narrowing of the intervertebral disc spaces. *A,* lateral view. *B,* AP view.

If osteoarthritic spurs impinge on the lower spinal nerve roots in the root canals, the clinical picture will be complicated by sciatica associated with the signs of a lumbosacral nerve root compression syndrome.

The patient with this condition presents a stiff, tight lumbar spine, with spinal mobility decreased in proportion to the stiffness. There is usually little or no paravertebral muscle spasm, but constant tenderness over the lumbar segment is noted on palpation. X-ray examination reveals narrowing of the involved lumbar interspaces, dense sclerotic vertebral body margins, and the hypertrophic spur formation that is characteristic of the condition. In older patients and in patients with severe disabling pain, a degree of osteoporosis is usually noted in the affected segment.

Treatment. Effective relief of symptomatic pain and stiffness in these patients is dependent upon recognizing and treating the underlying osteoarthritis. The drug of choice at the present time seems to be Butazolidin (phenylbutazone) when no medical contraindications, such as duodenal ulcer, blood dyscrasia, or the simultaneous use of anticoagulant medicine, exist. Butazolidin is given orally in 100 mg tablets or capsules. A usual starting dose would be 100 mg after each meal for a one to two week period. The dose is then gradually decreased to a maintenance level of 100 mg daily until the symptoms are brought under control.

Salicylates are also beneficial. Oral steroid therapy seems to have little consistent effect in alleviating osteoarthritis of the spine.

In addition to oral medication, treatment should include weight reduction if indicated, adequate rest, and the use of local heat in the form of hot tub baths. Exercise within toleration limits helps to maintain muscle tone and joint mobility.

Brace and corset support should be avoided if at all possible. It will be remembered that these joints tend to stiffen with immobility and generally benefit if kept flexible by exercise, with the symptoms controlled by the systemic medication. Various physical therapeutic measures, such as diathermy and massage, may be helpful in relieving symptoms.

Surgery plays a very limited role in this condition. Unless the process is limited to the lumbosacral joint, a fusion operation would have to be quite extensive to control symptoms, and the technical failure rate would be quite high. Surgical decompression of spinal nerve roots is occasionally necessary when osteoarthritic spurs impinge on the nerve roots to cause sciatica.

Important Diagnostic Points.   The following should be considered in making a diagnosis:

1.   Most patients are in the older age group.
2.   There is a characteristic history of low back pain and stiffness, noted particularly after periods of relative inactivity.
3.   There is little or no paravertebral muscle spasm.
4.   The condition may be part of a generalized osteoarthritis.
5.   There is a characteristic x-ray appearance.
6.   Neurologic examination may show evidence of lumbosacral nerve root compression, and the myelogram may be positive if osteoarthritic spurs impinge on nerve roots.

The Intervertebral Disc

An intervertebral disc functions as a shock absorber between two vertebral bodies and consists of several parts (Fig. 153). The center is a semi-liquid mucicartilaginous mass, the remnant of the embryonic notochord, called the *nucleus pulposus*. The nucleus is maintained in place by a thick fibrous band called the *annulus fibrosus*. The intervertebral disc is further stabilized by the superior and inferior cartilage end-plates that fix the structure to the vertebral bodies above and below. In addition, the anterior and posterior longitudinal spinal ligaments pass in front of and behind the disc, thus also acting as limiting membranes. The normal intervertebral disc serves a definite purpose in the physiology of the human spine. It is the structurally abnormal intervertebral disc that alters the physiology of the spine and results in clinical symptoms.

Structurally, the normal intervertebral disc consists of collagen and mucopolysaccharides. The central part of the disc, the nucleus pulposus, is a gelatinous substance with a high water content in which

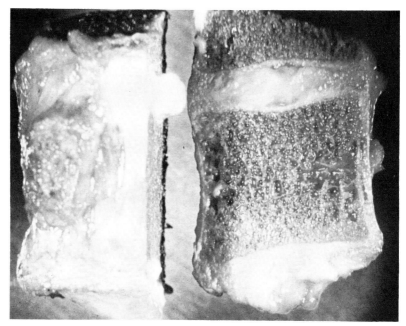

Figure 153.   Gross specimen illustrating a normal disc's role as an intervertebral shock absorber.

the collagen network is masked by a rich layer of chondroitin sulfate. The collagen fibers form a fine network resembling a porous system. The annulus fibrosus has a considerably denser and more regular collagenous pattern. The fibrils are grouped in bundles of varying thickness which pass in a spiral course from one vertebra to the next. They are attached to the hyaline cartilage end-plate, which divides the bony structure of the vertebra from the intervertebral disc itself (Fig. 154). The normal shock absorbing mechanism of the intervertebral disc depends upon the nucleus pulposus having the right amount of hydration, and upon the annulus fibrosus and vertebral end-plates being intact.

In some individuals, a structural disintegration of the disc occurs which resembles premature aging. Chemically, the protein in the disc increases while the mucopolysaccharide decreases. The water content of this protein polysaccharide complex gradually diminishes, and the nucleus pulposus loses its gelatinous properties. Once the nucleus pulposus has undergone degeneration and has lost its gelatinous properties, it becomes converted into a fibro-cartilaginous mass which no longer complies with the laws applicable to a fluid under a compressive force (Fig. 155). The forces once normally tolerated by an

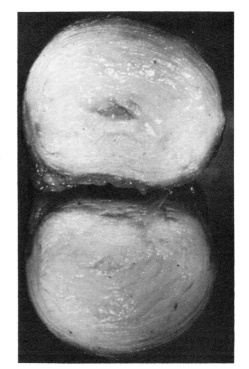

Figure 154. Cross section of normal intervertebral disc.

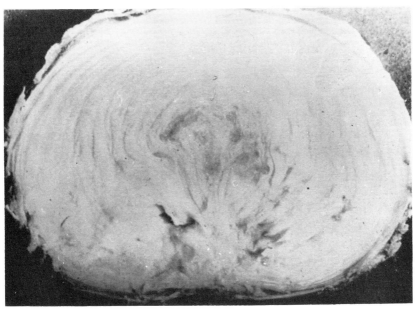

Figure 155. Cross section of degenerated intervertebral disc.

intact spine now place abnormal stress on the degenerated intervertebral disc, the apophyseal joints, and the annulus fibrosus. In a degenerated disc, the annulus fibrosus is subjected to a relatively higher stress than in a normal disc.

Once it has begun, degeneration of the intervertebral disc and annulus fibrosus is a progressive and irreversible process that may start as early as the second decade of life. This apparently natural biologic process, which has been observed in numerous other vertebrates, is probably a consequence of the special vascular conditions characterizing all adult cartilaginous tissue. Once growth has been completed, the intervertebral discs are totally avascular. Their normal metabolic balance presumably depends upon a nutrient diffusion mechanism, from the vascular spaces of the cancellous bone through the hyaline cartilage end-plates and nucleus pulposus gel to the notochordal cells. Interference with this nutrient diffusion mechanism may be the inciting factor in the onset of intervertebral disc degeneration.

The essential lesion, therefore, of intervertebral disc degeneration is a partial degradation of the protein-polysaccharide complex, with a loss of mechanical properties. Two clinical states may arise from the pathologic lesion of disc degeneration. If the annulus fibrosus remains intact, the abnormal mechanical stresses placed on a degenerated disc cause chronic low back pain and the condition is called *degenerative disc disease.* If the annulus ruptures, fragments of degenerated nuclear material bulge against the posterior longitudinal spinal ligament to compress the adjacent nerve root. This condition is called a *herniated disc.*

DEGENERATIVE DISC DISEASE

Degenerative disc disease characteristically involves the lumbosacral joint and is probably the most common cause of chronic low back pain. Advancing degeneration of the nucleus pulposus and annulus means lessening of the mechanical efficiency of the disc to act as a shock absorber or insulator between two vertebral bodies. Under these circumstances, the anterior margins of the involved vertebrae soon begin to show wear and tear changes characterized by sclerosis and osteophyte formation. A degenerated disc loses height, allowing the vertebral bodies to move closer together. An additional pathologic finding secondary to the compromise of an intervertebral disc as a functioning entity is the change in the apophyseal joints. An intact disc not only keeps two vertebral bodies separate but also serves as a center or axis for much of the spinal movement. With collapse of the intervertebral disc space, the axis of motion shifts posteriorly to the apophyseal joints. These joints cannot withstand the increased stress, and deteriorative changes soon follow to alter the smooth contour of the apophyseal joints.

Clinical Features.   The clinical picture presented by these patients is chronic low back pain. Age may range from the second to the sixth decade of life. The pain is characteristically worse upon arising from bed in the morning and after long periods of sitting or car riding. Prolonged standing, bending, lifting, coughing, and sneezing frequently aggravate the back pain. Many patients will have associated unilateral or bilateral leg pain. In all patients the leg pain will be along muscular and ligamentous pathways and will not represent sciatica. In this condition, therefore, the objective neurologic examination will be negative. Paravertebral muscle spasm may develop if the patient overstresses the defective joint.

Often the only positive physical finding will be tenderness on palpation of the lumbosacral joint.

X-ray examination characteristically reveals narrowing of the height of the intervertebral disc space and frequently shows degenerative changes in the apophyseal joints (Fig. 156).

Treatment.   The pain in degenerative disc disease is thought to arise from inflammation of the surrounding tissues induced by the chemical changes accompanying disc degeneration. Anti-inflamma-

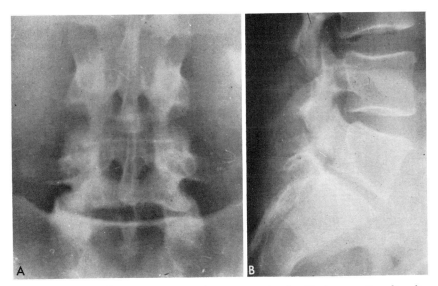

Figure 156.   Characteristic x-ray changes associated with degenerative disc disease involving the lumbosacral joint. A, AP view. Note degenerative changes involving the apophyseal joints. B, lateral view. Note narrowing of the height of the intervertebral disc space.

tory drugs are quite useful in controlling the symptoms of these patients. Butazolidin (phenylbutazone) can be given in the dosage range described for osteoarthritis of the lumbar spine.

Once the pain is controlled, hyperextension spinal strengthening exercises should be started to increase the strength of the paravertebral muscles. The patient should be taught to bend and lift properly to protect the lumbosacral joint from stress. Many orthopaedists favor the use of back braces and supports in the treatment of degenerative disc disease. In some patients, however, the wearing of a back brace increases the sensation of low back stiffness.

For the few patients whose low back pain is not adequately relieved by nonoperative treatment methods, lumbosacral spine fusion is indicated.

Herniated Intervertebral Disc

Abnormal physical stresses placed on a degenerated disc may exceed the mechanical strength of the degenerated disc and annulus, with resulting rupture of the annulus. Herniation or prolapse of nuclear material, either wholly or in fragments, into the spinal canal to cause either compression of or tension on a lumbar or sacral spinal nerve root as it prepares to exit from the spinal canal is the essential pathologic lesion of the condition known as herniated intervertebral disc (Fig. 157). The nuclear material may push the posterior longitudinal spinal ligament ahead of it like a hernial sac, or the material may rupture through the posterior longitudinal spinal ligament to extrude directly into the spinal canal.

The general process of intervertebral disc degeneration may extend over a period of years, but the clinical picture characteristic of herniated intervertebral disc does not arise until some of the nuclear material herniates or ruptures the posterior longitudinal spinal ligament to cause pressure on the adjacent spinal nerve root as it passes by on its way to exit from the spine. The actual contact between disc material and nerve root may be quite sudden and commonly follows an acute rise in intrathecal pressure triggered, for instance, by sneezing, lifting, or straining at stool.

Clinical Features. Herniated intervertebral disc occurs most often between the ages of 20 and 45 years and is more common in males. Approximately 90 per cent of intervertebral disc herniations occur at either the L4-L5 interspace or lumbosacral interspace, involving the fifth lumbar or first sacral nerve roots. Back pain is usually associated with the disc degeneration, but the predominant symptom is sciatic pain, beginning when the nuclear material protrudes posterolaterally into the spinal canal and compresses a nerve root. In most in-

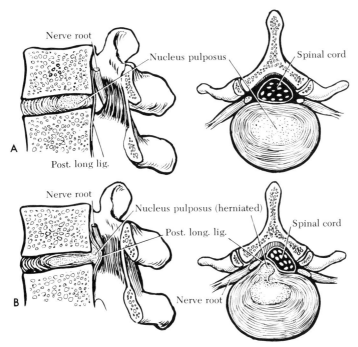

Figure 157. *A,* normal relationship of nucleus pulposus to intervertebral disc and spine. *B,* course taken by herniated nuclear material.

stances a diagnosis of a herniated disc is untenable in the absence of sciatic leg pain. The point to remember is that many back conditions may be associated with leg pain, but only nerve root irritation at this level gives pain along the distribution of the sciatic nerve associated with signs of a lumbosacral nerve root compression syndrome.

The patient with herniated intervertebral disc presents with low back pain accompanied by radiation into the posterior buttock and leg, or with just leg pain alone. When viewed standing, the patient may exhibit a list of the pelvis or the so-called "sciatic scoliosis." Anything that increases irritation of the affected nerve root (bending, lifting, coughing, sneezing) will aggravate the leg pain. There is usually tenderness to deep palpation over the affected vertebral interspace and over the course of the sciatic nerve. The straight leg raising and sitting root tests are positive if pain over the distribution of the sciatic nerve is reproduced. These tests do not indicate nerve root irritation if the pain produced occurs only in the back or if it is due to hamstring muscle tightness.

If the nerve pressure is severe enough, the Achilles reflex may be depressed or absent. The strength of the long toe extensors and anterior tibial muscle may be lessened, even to the point of a complete foot drop. The patient may complain of a sensation of numbness and tingling in the toes and feet, associated with an objective sensory loss in the affected dermatome.

Routine x-ray films are usually negative but may show narrowing of the affected interspace. Electromyographic examination and the myelogram are extremely helpful in localizing the site of the lesion, but the best guide to diagnosis is the clinical picture presented by the patient (Fig. 158).

Treatment.   Treatment is conservative for the most part, with some patients requiring surgery. Adequate conservative treatment should include a minimum of 10 days of absolute bed rest combined with local heat and appropriate analgesics. Putting the patient to bed reduces intradiscal pressure. This frequently allows the disc "bulge" to subside and drop away from the irritated nerve root. Scar tissue may then form over the rent in the annulus, thus accounting for the "cures" that follow successful conservative therapy.

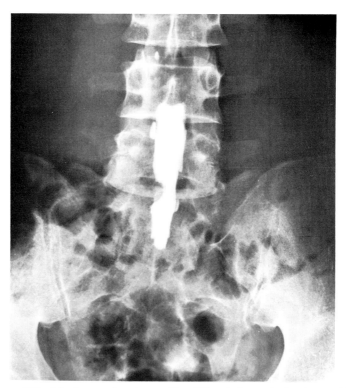

Figure 158.   Myelogram showing positive filling defect at the lumbosacral joint on the right side.

Traction is often used, although it has been shown to have no specific influence on a herniated disc and is probably justified only as a measure to keep the patient in bed.

The success of conservative therapy is measured by the gradual subsidence of the signs and symptoms of nerve root irritation. Once the nerve pressure subsides and the symptoms disappear, the patient is started on back strengthening exercises. Some orthopaedists favor the use of a back brace after the acute symptoms have receded.

Bed rest, or any form of conservative therapy, will usually be unsuccessful if the nuclear material has ruptured through the posterior longitudinal spinal ligament to extrude directly into the spinal canal. Most of these patients require surgical decompression of the affected nerve root for relief of sciatic pain. Surgical treatment consists of excision of the protruding disc material. Most orthopaedists favor the combined operation of disc removal and fusion of the interspace if the protrusion is at the lumbosacral interspace. The indications for surgery are:

1. Failure of conservative treatment.
2. Repeated disabling attacks.
3. The presence of severe or progressive abnormal neurologic signs.

Important Diagnostic Points.   The presence of a herniated intervertebral disc is suspected when:

1. The patient is between 20 and 45 years of age, with signs and symptoms of lumbosacral nerve root compression syndrome.
2. Leg pain follows the distribution of the sciatic nerve and is aggravated by raising the intrathecal pressure.
3. Paravertebral muscle spasm is not a predominant feature.
4. Straight leg raising and sitting root tests are positive.
5. Routine x-ray films are insignificant.
6. Neurologic examination, electromyographic examination, and myelogram are positive.

THE PELVIS

The term pelvis is derived from the Latin and means basin. The bony pelvis or pelvic ring is formed by the right and left ilium, ischium, and pubis, which articulate in front at the symphysis pubis and behind with the first three sacral vertebrae at the sacro-iliac joints. The pelvic ring is built for the stability of the trunk and the protection of its contents. It is united to the vertebral column through the sacrum and lumbosacral joint. Contained within the pelvis are important visceral structures that may be torn or lacerated by pelvic trauma or secondarily compromised by disease involving the pelvis.

Ankylosing spondylitis or Marie-Strumpell disease characteristically begins in the sacro-iliac joints (p. 103). Paget's disease is frequently found to involve the pelvis (p. 184). Benign and malignant tumors may arise in the component bones of the pelvic girdle. Not infrequently metastatic carcinoma may seed through the bony pelvis. Metastatic deposits in the sacrum may involve the lumbosacral plexus to cause sciatic pain that might mimic the clinical picture of a herniated disc in the lower lumbar spine.

The pelvis is most often at risk from trauma. The incidence of pelvic fracture, with or without associated dislocation of the sacro-iliac joints or symphysis pubis, appears to be increasing. A high proportion of pelvic fractures are caused by vehicular accidents or falls from a height. A pelvic fracture may occur as an isolated injury or as an associated injury in a patient with multiple injuries.

Pelvic fractures may be accompanied by severe intrapelvic hemorrhage, rupture of the membranous urethra or bladder, and paralytic ileus. Published studies relating to this injury have pointed out that too frequently in the past, preoccupation with associated injuries has resulted in total neglect of the pelvic injury. Hypovolemic shock is combatted by blood transfusion to restore blood volume. Valuable information about the integrity of the membranous urethra and bladder can be obtained by inserting an indwelling catheter and performing a cystogram. Paralytic ileus should be treated by gastric suction.

Fractures of the pelvis can be classified as stable fractures of the pelvic ring and unstable fractures of the pelvic ring.

Stable fractures of the pelvis include fractures of one to three of the four pubic rami, fractures of the iliac ala, and fractures of the sacrum. Involvement of one to three of the four pubic rami is by far the most commonly encountered stable pelvic fracture. Visceral complications are rare with these injuries. Bed rest for a few days up to six weeks is the only treatment required for stable pelvic fractures.

Unstable pelvic fractures disrupt the pelvic ring and are frequently associated with severe intrapelvic hemorrhage or rupture of the bladder or urethra. Unstable fractures include hemipelvic displacement with dislocation of the sacro-iliac joint, displaced fracture of all four pubic rami with involvement of the symphysis pubis, opening of the pelvic ring with disruption of the symphysis pubis and sacro-iliac joints, and combinations of these injuries.

Depending on the particular fracture, treatment methods include bed rest, manipulation, pelvic slings, spica casts, and skeletal traction. Open reduction, with or without internal fixation, is rarely employed in the treatment of unstable pelvic fractures.

References

American Academy of Orthopaedic Surgeons: Symposium on the Spine. St. Louis: C. V. Mosby Co., 1969.

DaRoza, A. C.: Primary intraspinal tumours: Their clinical presentation and diagnosis. J. Bone and Joint Surg., *46-B*:8, 1964.

Dunn, A. W., and Morris, A. D.: Fractures and dislocations of the pelvis. J. Bone and Joint Surg., *50-A*:1639, 1968.

Goldstein, L. A.: The surgical management of scoliosis. Clin. Orth. and Rel. Res., 77:32, 1971.

Harrington, P. R.: Treatment of scoliosis: Correction and internal fixation by spine instrumentation. J. Bone and Joint Surg., *44-A*:591, 1962.

Moe, J. H.: The Milwaukee brace in the treatment of scoliosis. Clin. Orth. and Rel. Res., 77:18, 1971.

Moe, J. H., Tambornino, J. M., and Armbrust, E. N.: Harrington instrumentation in correction of scoliosis. J. Bone and Joint Surg., *46-A*:313, 1964.

Nicholas, J. A., Wilson, P. D., and Freiberger, R.: Pathological fractures of the spine. Etiology and diagnosis. J. Bone and Joint Surg., *42-A*:127, 1960.

Peltier, L. F.: Complications associated with fractures of the pelvis. J. Bone and Joint Surg., *47-A*:1060, 1965.

Rothman, R. R. (Ed.): Symposium on disease of the intervertebral disc. Orthop. Clin. North Am., 2:2, July, 1971.

Willis, T. A.: Lumbosacral anomalies. J. Bone and Joint Surg., *41-A*:935, 1959.

Chapter Fourteen

The Lower Extremity

GENERAL CONSIDERATIONS

Weight bearing and locomotion are the principal activities required of the lower extremities in man. Proper performance of these functions requires strength and stability of the part, coupled with sufficient mobility to allow walking, running, and leaping. The stability demanded of the lower extremity is obtained at the price of mobility. As a consequence, the joints of the lower extremity do not have as great a range of mobility as those of the upper extremity.

As seen with the upper extremity, the functions performed by the lower extremity influence, to a great extent, the type of musculoskeletal disorders encountered. The addition of weight bearing adds further stress to the joints and helps explain the marked increase in the incidence of degenerative joint disease in the lower extremity. The ability to walk, run, and jump carries with it the increased likelihood of injury. It is not surprising, therefore, that trauma produces a great proportion of the orthopaedic problems involving the lower extremity.

Before discussing localized problems of the lower extremity, we must appreciate that many general disorders exist that include deformities of the lower extremity in their clinical picture. As mentioned in Chapter 7, disorders of neuromuscular origin, such as cerebral palsy, anterior poliomyelitis, and Friedreich's ataxia, frequently are accompanied by lower extremity complaints and deformities. Rheumatoid arthritis, hemophilic arthritis, neuropathic joint disease, gout, and Paget's disease all may involve the lower extremity in the disease process. As mentioned in Chapter 9, the distal end of the femur and the proximal end of the tibia are sites commonly afflicted with benign and malignant bone tumors.

For descriptive purposes, local problems involving the lower extremity are presented in discussions of the hip joint, thigh, knee joint, leg, ankle joint, and foot.

THE HIP JOINT

The hip joint is the pivotal joint of the lower extremity, and its functional demands require great stability coupled with a wide range of motion. To meet these demands, the hip is built to be a close fitting, deeply set ball and socket arrangement between the femoral head and the acetabulum. It is further supported by a strong capsule that runs from the acetabular rim to the intertrochanteric line of the femur. The hip joint is inherently stable by virtue of its construction and, unlike the shoulder and knee joints, needs no particular supporting ligaments.

Normally, the femoral neck makes an angle of approximately 135 degrees with the femoral shaft. Increase in this *angle of inclination* is called *coxa valga* and decrease in the angle is *coxa vara* (Fig. 159). The angle of inclination is not to be confused with the angle of anteversion (see p. 57).

The muscles that flex the hip joint are massed anteriorly, while the extensors lie posteriorly. The adductor muscles are grouped medially and extend into the groin. The hip abductor muscles are placed laterally and insert on and about the greater trochanter of the femur.

Disorders affecting the hip joint in children and adults are important and frequently serious orthopaedic problems.

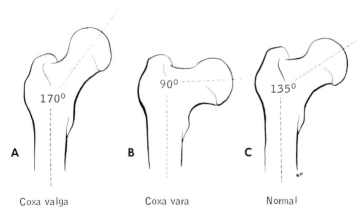

Figure 159. Angle of inclination of the femoral neck. *A*, coxa valga. *B*, coxa vara. *C*, normal.

Clinical Aspects of Hip Disorders

The majority of patients presenting because of a hip joint problem may do so because of pain, stiffness, limp, or deformity.

Pain of hip joint origin may be localized to the groin and from there may radiate down the medial or anterior aspect of the thigh; it may also arise in the region of the greater trochanter and radiate laterally along the course of the fascia lata toward the knee. Hip joint pain may present posteriorly in the region of the ischial tuberosity and must be carefully differentiated from the complaint of sciatica (see p. 312). Frequently, the pain is referred to the low back area or knee and can be reproduced or accentuated by movements of the hip joint.

Subjective stiffness of the hip joint may be noted by the patient following periods of immobility, such as after prolonged sitting or upon arising from bed in the morning. In more advanced degenerative states affecting the hip joint, objective stiffness may be noted by the examiner. In degenerative arthritis of the hip joint, for example, the patient will lose hip joint motion sequentially, with the ability to rotate the hip being lost first, followed by abduction and adduction, and hip flexion being maintained to the last. For this reason, many patients with degenerative arthritis of the hip describe difficulty in putting a shoe and stocking on the affected leg, since this action usually requires the ability to rotate the hip joint externally.

Limp is a pathologic asymmetrical gait, and several mechanisms may be operating about a hip joint either singly or in combination to produce it. Shortening of the lower extremity and marked stiffness about the hip joint may be sufficient to alter gait pattern significantly. The limp may be protective because of weight bearing pain. This type of abnormal gait, called an *antalgic* gait, is characterized by a very short stance phase. The gait most characteristic of hip joint disease, however, is called a *gluteal lurch* and relates directly to a structural or functional weakness of the gluteus medius muscle on the affected side. Any abnormality of the pelvic-femoral lever arm may weaken the gluteus medius muscle. If this occurs, the muscle can no longer support the pelvis and trunk on the lower extremity. As a consequence, the patient's trunk lurches to the affected side with weight bearing (*positive Trendelenburg test*).

Visible deformity of the lower extremity is frequently associated with injuries or disease affecting the hip joint. A patient with a fracture of the hip joint usually presents with the lower extremity held in marked external rotation. A patient who has sustained a traumatic dislocation of the hip joint usually presents with the lower extremity held in internal rotation. Degenerative arthritis of the hip joint is frequently associated with flexion-adduction-external rotation contractures. Flexion and adduction contractures about the hip, external rotation position of the lower extremity, shortening of the leg, and limp are characteristic deformities that may be produced by hip joint disorders.

Examination of the Hip Joint

The patient must be suitably draped so that both lower extremities, the pelvis, and the spine are visible to the examiner.

INSPECTION

The examiner notes the appearance of the patient in the standing position, whether weight is borne equally on both feet with the legs in a normal position, and any increase in lumbar lordosis or pelvic tilt.

If the patient is able to walk, any limp or abnormal gait pattern is noted.

With the patient lying supine, the legs are inspected for visible deformity.

PALPATION

The joint is palpated to detect evidence of swelling or local heat. The presence of tenderness over the joint anteriorly or posteriorly or over the greater trochanter is noted. The position of the greater trochanter relative to the anterior superior iliac spine is compared on both sides.

RANGE OF MOTION

With the patient lying supine on an examining table, the examiner puts both hip joints through a full range of passive motion, testing the motions of flexion, abduction, adduction, internal rotation, and external rotation (Fig. 160). When testing abduction and adduction of the hip joint, the examiner steadies the pelvis by placing a hand on the iliac crest.

Extension of the hip joint is tested with the patient lying prone.

In the absence of joint stiffness, the range of active joint motion is tested to determine the presence or absence of muscle weakness about the hip joint.

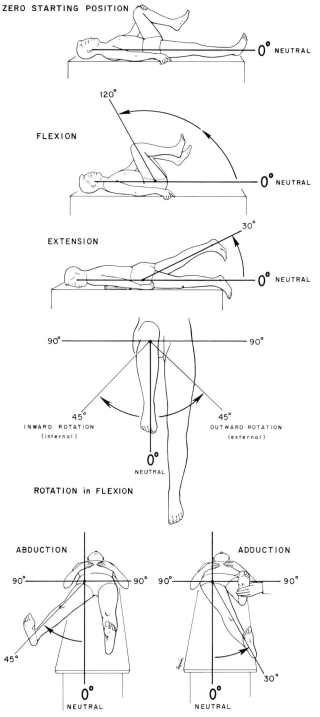

Figure 160. Motions of the hip. (Courtesy American Academy of Orthopaedic Surgeons.)

340

SPECIAL MANEUVERS

Test for Hip Flexion Contracture. A hip flexion contracture can be hidden so well by an increased lumbar lordosis that its presence may be missed by the examiner unless it is revealed by a special maneuver.

With the patient lying supine, the normal hip is acutely flexed on the abdomen to flatten the lumbar spine and obliterate the lordosis, permitting a hip flexion contracture to become apparent and its degree noted (Fig. 161).

Leg Length Measurement. Shortening of a leg may be caused by hip joint disorders. The amount of shortening is determined by accurate tape measurement. The patient lies supine on an examining table with the body straight and both legs in the same position. The distance from the anterior superior iliac spine to the tip of the medial malleolus is measured on each leg, and the results are compared.

Trendelenburg's Test. Normally, when all the body weight is borne on one foot and the opposite leg is raised from the ground, the pelvis on the raised side rises slightly with the leg. When the gluteal muscles on the affected side are unable to support the pelvis properly, the pelvis on the raised side does not rise but falls, and the test is said to be positive (Fig. 162).

A positive Trendelenburg test indicates some abnormality in the musculoskeletal mechanism between the pelvis and the femur. The test is positive in many deformities involving the femoral neck, dislocation of the hip, and weakness or paralysis of the gluteus medius muscle. This is the biomechanical mechanism operating to produce the so-called gluteal lurch in patients with various disorders of the hip joint.

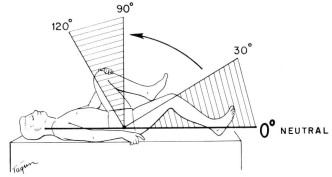

LIMITED MOTION in FLEXION

Figure 161. Test for hip flexion contracture. (Courtesy American Academy of Orthopaedic Surgeons.)

DISTURBANCES OF
GLUTEUS MEDIUS
MECHANISM

1. Bony
   a. Ankylosis (fibrous or bony)
   b. Deformity of the neck of the femur
      1) Coxa vara (congenital or acquired)
      2) Shortening of the neck of the femur
   c. Loss of continuity
      1) Fractures about the hip (intra- and extracapsular)
      2) Pseudoarthrosis
   d. Instability
      1) Dislocation of the hip
      2) Subluxation of the hip
2. Muscular
   a. Weakness or paralysis of the gluteus medius muscle
   b. Spasticity of the gluteus medius muscle

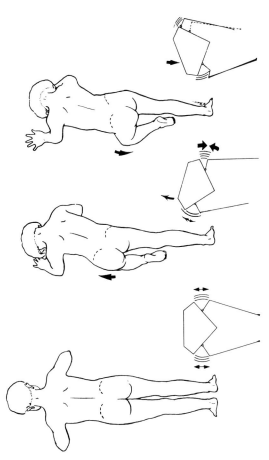

STANDING ERECT (Glut. med. relaxed)

LEFT LEG RAISED. PELVIS LIFTED ON LEFT (Rt. glut. med. contracts): Negative test

LEFT LEG RAISED. PELVIS "FALLS" ON LEFT (Rt. glut. med. mechanism disturbed): Positive test

Figure 162.   Trendelenburg's test. (From Manual of Orthopaedic Surgery, American Orthopaedic Association.)

X-RAY EXAMINATION

Proper evaluation of a problem affecting the hip joint cannot be made without x-ray examination. Anteroposterior and lateral views are standard for the hip joints.

Disorders of the Hip Joint in Children

CONGENITAL DISLOCATION OF THE HIP (See p. 55)

TRAUMATIC DISLOCATION OF THE HIP

Traumatic dislocation of the hip is an uncommon lesion in the child, but it has been seen following difficult deliveries, athletic injuries, and vehicular accidents. The majority of the patients are male. The femoral head is usually dislocated posteriorly, so that the leg assumes the characteristic positional deformity of shortening and internal rotation.

The less common anterior dislocation of the femoral head carries with it the threat of impingement against the femoral artery.

Reduction of the dislocation should be carried out promptly, certainly within the first 24 hours following injury. The dislocation can usually be corrected by closed reduction, followed by a period of rest to the joint by means of traction or a plaster cast. Weight bearing can be resumed three months following reduction. If there is no associated injury about the hip joint, the majority of patients make a full recovery from the injury.

The prognosis for future hip function is not as good if the dislocation is associated with fracture about the femoral head or acetabulum, since this implies more severe violence to the joint at the time of injury. Open reduction of the fracture fragments may be required.

Some children sustaining fracture-dislocation of the hip joint may develop the complications of avascular necrosis of the femoral head (see p. 356) or of degenerative arthritis of the hip (see p. 352). Both of these complications may severely compromise the function of the involved hip joint for the remainder of the patient's life.

In general, however, traumatic dislocation of the hip in a child is a more benign injury in regard to future hip function than a similar hip injury in the adult.

SYNOVITIS OF THE HIP (OBSERVATION HIP)

A twisting strain applied to the hip joint may cause a traumatic irritation of the synovial membrane, with the formation of a synovial effusion within the joint. Some authorities believe that an irritative synovitis may also be caused by viral inflammation of the synovial membrane.

The child may develop a painful limp, muscle spasm about the hip, and limited joint motion. X-ray examination is negative except for evidence of capsular distention.

The differential diagnosis between nonpyogenic synovitis of the hip and pyogenic arthritis, Legg-Calvé-Perthes disease, and tuberculosis of the hip is based upon an afebrile clinical course, negative x-ray examination, and the recovery of sterile fluid from the hip joint on needle aspiration.

Synovitis of the hip joint responds rapidly to rest, local heat, and close observation of the patient. Severe hip pain can be alleviated by traction applied to the leg in the form of Buck's extension.

An occasional patient thought to have synovitis of the hip will eventually develop Perthes disease.

PYOGENIC ARTHRITIS OF THE HIP (See p. 138)

TUBERCULOSIS OF THE HIP (See p. 145)

LEGG-CALVÉ-PERTHES DISEASE (See p. 85)

SLIPPED CAPITAL FEMORAL EPIPHYSIS

In the adolescent, it is not uncommon for the epiphysis of the femoral head to slip from the neck of the femur (Fig. 163). Unlike other epiphyses (Chap. 4), the capital femoral epiphysis may displace downward and backward from the femoral neck in the absence of specific trauma, for reasons that are still poorly understood. If this condition is not recognized early and treated rapidly, severe structural deformity of the head and neck of the femur may result. The problem assumes great functional significance because of the importance of the joint involved.

The condition occurs most frequently in boys 10 to 16 years of age. It may be bilateral.

Etiology. The cause of slipping of the capital femoral epiphysis is unknown. Many authorities favor an underlying endocrine imbalance because the condition frequently occurs in two types of children: (1) the overweight child with underdeveloped genitalia (*Fröhlich's adiposogenital syndrome*), and (2) the tall thin child showing a rapid adolescent growth spurt. Proof for this hypothesis has not been forthcoming.

Other authorities have suggested trauma, low grade infection, nutritional defects, and weakening of the periosteum as causes, but these too have not been proved.

Pathology. It has been reported that the basic pathologic change

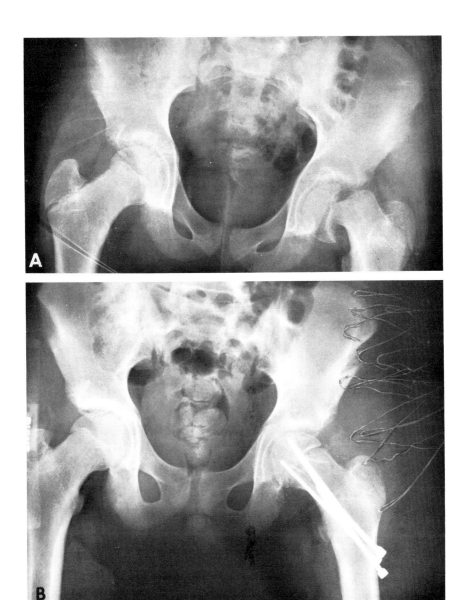

Figure 163. A, Complete slip of capital femoral epiphysis of left hip. *B*, same patient after operative replacement of the epiphysis, bone pegging of the growth line, and fixation with metallic pins. (Courtesy Dr. John Dowling, Lankenau Hospital, Philadelphia, Pa.)

associated with slipped capital femoral epiphysis occurs in the cartilage of the growth plate. The growth plate, instead of producing endochondral bone, becomes transformed into fibrous tissue, which weakens the attachment of the capital epiphysis to the femoral neck and may allow it to slip off following minimal trauma.

The epiphysis gradually slips downward and backward on the neck of the femur, but because of periosteal attachment, the two structures never become completely separated. Callus tissue gradually forms in the angle between the head and neck of the femur, and in time, the femoral neck becomes rounded.

The articular hyaline cartilage of the femoral head and acetabulum is unaffected.

Clinical Features. The onset of symptoms is gradual in the majority of patients, and a history of some trauma may be obtained. The patient, frequently overweight, may complain of vague discomfort about the hip with pain that radiates to the anterior thigh and knee. Often the pain will appear to be confined totally to the anterior aspect of the lower thigh and the knee. An antalgic limp may be present, frequently associated with a sensation of stiffness. As the deformity progresses, the affected extremity may develop shortening and an externally rotated appearance, and the limp becomes a gluteal lurch.

The telltale physical sign is the externally rotated position assumed by the thigh as the hip is flexed. Internal rotation of the hip is markedly limited.

In an occasional patient, acute and sudden displacement of the epiphysis may follow a specific trauma to the hip. In this instance, the physical signs produced will resemble those produced by fracture through the neck of the femur.

X-ray Findings. The presence of this condition may be discovered on an x-ray film before actual slipping of the epiphysis occurs. This is known as the preslipped stage, and is characterized by an abnormally widened and irregular growth plate associated with some rarefaction in the metaphysis of the femur, but no actual displacement of the epiphysis.

Actual slipping of the capital epiphysis can be first detected on lateral x-ray view. The epiphysis tends to displace downward and backward in relation to the femoral neck. As the condition progresses, rounding of the femoral neck becomes apparent.

Treatment. To prevent further displacement, weight bearing should be prohibited as soon as the diagnosis is made. Active definitive treatment should be undertaken as soon as possible.

The goal of treatment is to correct whatever deformity exists between the head and neck of the femur, and to bring about premature closure of the growth plate, so that the capital epiphysis cannot slip again. The attainment of this goal is most often sought by surgical means.

No significant amount of deformity between the head and neck of the femur exists in the preslipped stage or in those patients in whom the capital epiphysis has slipped less than one centimeter. In these instances, the surgeon proceeds directly to operative closure of the growth plate. This can be accomplished by driving a metal nail or multiple metal pins across the growth plate or by the use of bone grafts. Weight bearing is prohibited until closure of the growth plate has occurred. Because this condition usually occurs toward the end of the growth cycle of the child, and because the proximal femoral growth plate contributes less than 30 per cent to the total length of the femoral shaft, no significant shortening of the leg follows premature closure of the growth plate in these patients.

In addition to inducing early premature closure of the growth plate, the surgeon may also have to correct structural deformity or malalignment between the femoral head and neck. Deformity between the head and neck can be corrected by careful surgical osteotomy through the neck of the femur or the subtrochanteric region. The bone fragments are held in the corrected position by some metallic internal fixation device.

Complications. If the diagnosis of slipped capital femoral epiphysis is made early before significant deformity occurs, and if proper treatment is carried out promptly, the final result is excellent in the majority of patients. Delay in diagnosis and the presence of significant structural deformity increase, proportionately, the percentage of poor results.

A few patients, following surgical treatment, may develop acute cartilage necrosis of the femoral head, or avascular necrosis of the femoral head because of damage to the blood supply (see p. 356). These complications usually result in a painful, stiff hip.

Residual deformity of the head and neck of the femur may cause mechanical malalignment of the hip joint. Weight bearing stresses on a mechanically imperfect joint may lead to the complication of degenerative arthritis in later years (see p. 352).

Disorders of the Hip in Adults

FRACTURE OF THE HIP

Fracture of the hip refers specifically to fractures occurring through the neck of the femur and through the intertrochanteric region of the femur. This is a serious injury that occurs mostly in older patients. Although fracture of the hip may occur in the child, this is relatively rare. Management of the problem is complicated by the fact that about one-third of the adult patients have an associated medical disease of some significance, such as diabetes, renal deficiency, or a disorder of the cardiovascular system.

The fracture may occur following a twisting injury to the leg or a fall directly on the hip. In patients with osteoporosis, fracture of the hip may occur in the seeming absence of specific trauma. Metastatic tumors to the neck or intertrochanteric region of the femur may result in pathologic fractures. The patient may note severe pain and inability to move the leg or bear weight upon it. Following fracture of the hip, the affected leg assumes a characteristic position of shortening, adduction, and external rotation.

Fracture through the Neck of the Femur (Transcervical, Intracapsular). Fractures occurring through the neck of the femur are more difficult to treat and slower to heal than fractures occurring through the intertrochanteric region, mainly because the proximal fragment is small, contains a high proportion of cortical bone, and has a relatively poor blood supply. Even under optimum conditions, about 25 per cent of patients with transcervical fractures will develop nonunion.

The treatment of this fracture consists of accurate reduction of the two fragments by either closed or open methods, followed by operative insertion of some metallic internal fixation device, such as a three-flanged Smith-Petersen nail or multiple Hagie pins, to fasten the broken fragments together until healing occurs (Fig. 164). Effective internal fixation allows the patient to be out of bed, but weight bearing is prohibited until subsequent x-ray examination reveals complete healing. This may take as long as six months.

In selected frail or aged patients, or in those few patients in whom the head fragment cannot be reduced, the femoral head can be removed and a metallic femoral head prosthesis inserted (Fig. 165). All things considered, however, it is better for the patient to obtain healing of the fracture by means of internal fixation than to have prosthetic replacement of the femoral head.

Fracture through the Intertrochanteric Region of the Femur (Extracapsular). Intertrochanteric fracture of the femur occurs most commonly in women. As a general rule, these patients are older than those breaking the neck of the femur. Healing is more favorable at this location, however, because of the blood-rich cancellous bone found here.

Treatment of this fracture is operative, and consists of open reduction and internal fixation of the fragments in the reduced position by means of a metallic nail plate device (Fig. 166). Effective internal fixa-

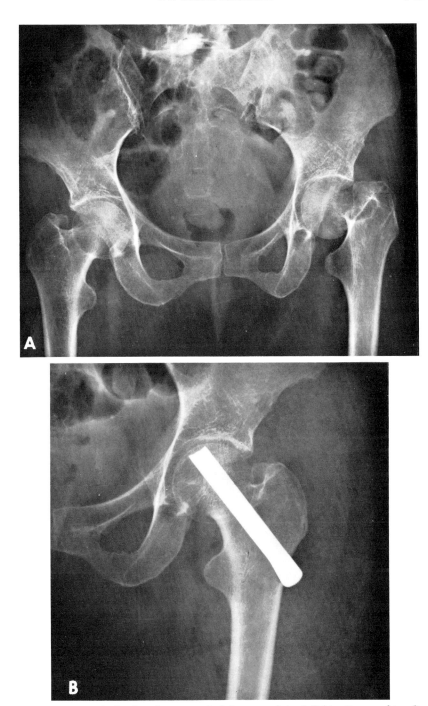

Figure 164. A, displaced transcervical fracture of the left hip. B, same hip after open reduction and internal fixation with Smith-Petersen nail.

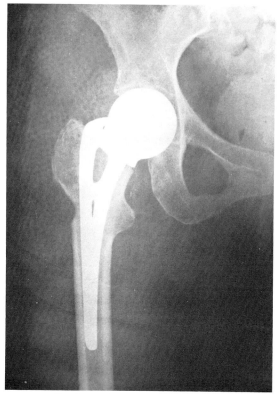

Figure 165. Metallic femoral head prosthesis replacing head of femur.

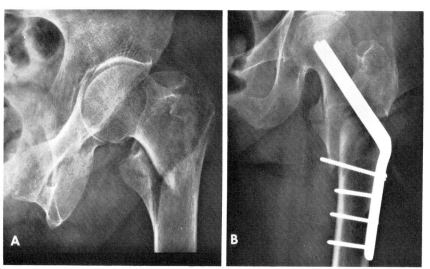

Figure 166. A, intertrochanteric fracture of hip. B, same hip following open reduction and metallic nail fixation.

tion allows the patient to be out of bed, but weight bearing is prohibited until subsequent x-ray examination reveals complete bone healing. This may take from four to six months.

Complications of Hip Fracture. It has been estimated that one patient of every four sustaining a fracture through the neck of the femur fails to obtain successful healing and develops nonunion of the fracture. The main reasons for nonunion at this site are: inadequate reduction of the fracture, inefficient internal fixation, and damage to the blood supply to the femoral head fragment. This complication is usually painful and requires another operative procedure for its correction, usually the insertion of a metallic femoral head prosthesis (Fig. 165).

Two complications of fracture through the neck of the femur that may occur after the fracture has healed are avascular necrosis of the femoral head (see p. 356) and degenerative arthritis of the hip (see p. 352). Both complications are usually painful and may require another operative procedure for correction.

Nonunion, avascular necrosis, and degenerative arthritis of the hip joint are rarely encountered following intertrochanteric fractures of the hip because of the relative abundance of the blood supply in this essentially cancellous segment of the femur.

DISLOCATION OF THE HIP JOINT

Traumatic dislocation of the hip joint in the adult occurs most commonly as the result of automobile accidents, in which the patient's flexed knee strikes the dashboard and the transmitted force dislodges the femoral head posteriorly. The characteristic attitude assumed by the affected leg is shortening, flexion, and marked internal rotation.

Anterior dislocation of the hip joint is uncommon.

Other injuries that may accompany posterior dislocation of the hip, particularly if sustained in automobile trauma, are fractures of the patella, fractures of the posterior rim of the acetabulum, and stretch injury of the sciatic nerve sustained as the femoral head is displaced posteriorly.

Prompt reduction of the dislocation is essential to the preservation of good function in the hip joint, and in the majority of patients, reduction can be achieved by closed manipulation. If this is unsuccessful, open reduction is carried out. Weight bearing is usually prohibited for three months following reduction. Large bone fragments broken from the rim of the acetabulum have to be replaced at operation and secured in position with metallic screws, or the joint will be unstable and dislocation may recur (Fig. 28).

Traumatic dislocation of the hip in the adult results from severe violence, since it takes a large force applied to the hip joint to effect dislocation. It takes much less force to effect traumatic dislocation of the hip in the child. For this reason, traumatic dislocation of the adult hip has more serious prognostic implications for future function than a similar lesion in the child.

It has been estimated that approximately 50 per cent of adult patients sustaining traumatic dislocation, or fracture dislocation, of the hip develop traumatic degenerative arthritis of the hip joint or avascular necrosis of the femoral head as later complications of the injury. Both of these complications may require major reconstructive hip surgery for their relief.

DEGENERATIVE ARTHRITIS OF THE HIP (OSTEOARTHRITIS)

Osteoarthritis involving the hip joint is a common, progressive disorder characterized, pathologically, by deterioration of articular cartilage and overgrowth of juxta-articular bone. It is a disease mainly of middle and old age, and affects females more frequently than males.

In general, osteoarthritis is a degenerative disease process of joints, affecting mostly weight bearing joints. The hip joint, therefore, may become involved as part of the generalized disease process (see p. 106). Primary osteoarthritis of the hip may also occur in the apparent absence of predisposing factors. In a third situation, the condition may be secondary, arising in a previously abnormal hip.

A long-standing mechanical malalignment within the hip joint may be a predisposing factor in osteoarthritis. In this instance, the stress of daily wear and tear gradually erodes the articular hyaline cartilage and induces the secondary effects characterized by the hypertrophic bone changes. Mechanical malalignment of the hip joint may be caused by primary hip disorders occurring in childhood, such as congenital dislocation of the hip, pyogenic arthritis of the hip, Legg-Calvé-Perthes disease, slipped capital femoral epiphysis, or traumatic dislocation of the hip.

Osteoarthritis of the hip may occur as a complication of other primary hip disorders in adults, such as fractures and fracture-dislocations involving the femoral neck, femoral head, or acetabulum.

Clinical Features.   Whether osteoarthritis of the hip develops as a primary disease process or as a secondary effect of long-standing mechanical malalignment, its clinical characteristics are the same. The problems of management are compounded if both hips are involved.

Osteoarthritis of the hip produces pain, limp, limited joint motion, and deformity of the affected leg. Pain is felt in the region of the groin and may be referred along the anterior surface of the thigh to the knee, along the lateral aspect of the thigh, or posteriorly to the buttock or low back area. Pain is invariably associated with a sensation of stiffness. In severe hip joint involvement, the affected leg tends to shorten and turn in the direction of external rotation. The leg is usually flexed and adducted at the hip joint.

Limp may be due to pain, stiffness, shortening of the leg, or a disturbance in gluteus medius function. Often, several of these factors operate to produce an abnormal gait in a patient with an externally rotated extremity.

Flexion contracture of the hip, if present, can be detected by performing the maneuver illustrated in Figure 161. The presence of limited joint motion is detected by comparing the passive range of motion obtained in both hips. As mentioned previously, patients with osteoarthritis involving the hip joint will lose hip joint motion sequentially. The ability to rotate the hip joint internally or externally is always lost first. The motions of abduction and adduction are lost next, with hip flexion being maintained to the last.

X-ray Findings.   X-ray examination reveals the characteristic deformity of the hip joint. Loss of articular hyaline cartilage results in a corresponding reduction in the joint space. Hypertrophic bone changes are evident about the femoral head and the acetabulum, which reflect a dense appearance on the x-ray films. Bone spurs appear as irregular projections extending outward from the joint margin around the femoral head and the edges of the acetabulum. Cysts may be noted within the bone substance of the femoral head and the acetabulm (Fig. 167).

Treatment.   The symptoms in some patients with osteoarthritis of the hip may be controlled by nonoperative measures, such as the use of a cane in the opposite hand to "unload" the hip joint in order to relieve pain, or the use of a heel lift on the affected side to compensate for shortening. The anti-inflammatory drugs may also be useful in relieving pain.

A great many patients with symptomatic degenerative arthritis of the hip, however, eventually require some type of operative treatment. Three operative procedures have the greatest general usefulness:

TOTAL HIP REPLACEMENT.   Since 1961 in Europe, and 1971 in the United States, a new surgical procedure has become available for the surgical reconstruction of the arthritic hip that produces excellent results more frequently, more readily, and more routinely in more difficult problems than any other method. The operation is called total hip replacement. In this procedure, the femoral head and neck are replaced by a metallic prosthesis, and the acetabulum is replaced by a

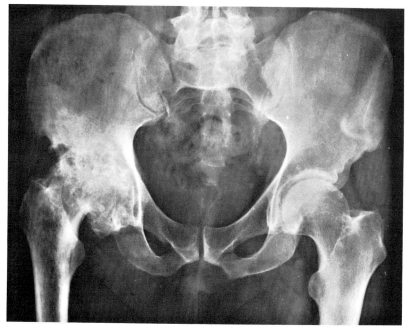

Figure 167.   Severe degenerative arthritis of the right hip.

plastic cup, both components being fixed to bone by methyl methacrylate or "bone cement" (Fig. 168).

Polymerization of the methyl methacrylate commences when the
methacrylate powder and the liquid methacrylate monomer are mixed
together. Once doughy in consistency, the "cement" can be applied to
the prepared bone surfaces. Although it does not adhere to bone in the
nature of a glue or cement, it gains fixation by extruding into the rami-
fications of the bone trabeculae and into special holes made in the
bone to receive projections of the methacrylate bolus as anchoring
sites. Once polymerized (a process usually taking from eight to 12
minutes), the methacrylate holds the component rigidly in place.

Because of the procedure's relative newness, long-term end result
studies are not yet available. The United States Food and Drug Administration did not release methacrylate for use in the hip joint until
1971. Short-term studies indicate an expected excellent result in
about 90 per cent of patients in whom total hip replacement was performed for osteoarthritis of the hip. This operation has replaced other
forms of arthroplasty of the hip, such as cup arthroplasty and metallic
femoral head prosthesis (Fig. 165), as the surgical procedure of choice
for osteoarthritis of the hip. Cup arthroplasty is still a valuable procedure in the patient 50 years of age or younger with rheumatoid arthri-

tis of the hip (Fig. 14). Until total hip replacement can be evaluated over a long period of time, it is considered wise to limit its use in unilateral hip disease to patients 60 years of age and older, and in bilateral hip disease to patients 50 years of age and older. An absolute contraindication to total hip replacement is a history of prior hip infection.

DISPLACEMENT OSTEOTOMY. Osteotomy means the surgical cutting of a bone. When applied to osteoarthritis, displacement osteotomy refers to cutting through the shaft of the femur about the trochanteric level and displacing the fragments to change the line of weight bearing thrust on the hip joint, and rolling the femoral head up or down to bring a more normal area of articular cartilage in contact with the acetabulum. This operation is designed for those patients who are early in the course of their disease and exhibit minimal deformity and loss of motion. Its chief benefit is pain relief. It usually does not result in any increase in hip joint motion.

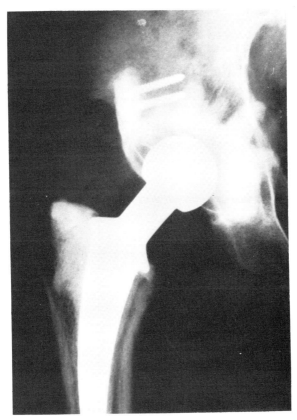

Figure 168. Total hip replacement unit in right hip. Opaque material represents methacrylate "cement."

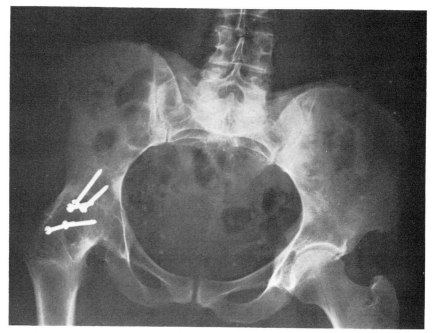

Figure 169. Arthrodesis of right hip by a technique that involved use of a large iliac bone graft fixed with screws, bone chips along superior margin of the joint, and subtrochanteric osteotomy.

ARTHRODESIS. This term refers to the operative procedure designed to stiffen a joint permanently by fusing the apposing joint surfaces together, usually with a bone graft (Fig. 169). This results in a painless and stable hip joint. The obvious disadvantage is that there is no motion in the joint.

Many patients refuse to consider arthrodesis at the present time in light of the interest in joint replacement with the retention of joint motion. Nevertheless, arthrodesis appears to continue to have a place in treatment for the patient with prior or present hip joint infection. The young male planning to do heavy work in his career, and with one hip severely involved, would be well advised to accept hip arthrodesis.

AVASCULAR NECROSIS OF THE FEMORAL HEAD (OSTEONECROSIS)

The term "avascular necrosis" is used to describe the changes that occur in bone tissue after interruption of its blood supply by trauma or disease. This condition may affect any living bone, but it is encountered most frequently in the head of the femur.

When avascular necrosis of the femoral head complicates fractures or dislocations about the hip joint, the mechanism of physical interference with the extraosseous and intraosseous blood supply is usually obvious; but when avascular necrosis of the femoral head occurs in systemic conditions without associated trauma, such as decompression syndromes, hypercortisonism, and alcoholism, the mechanism is less well understood. It has generally been assumed that some degree of vascular insufficiency is common to all of these conditions, but the precise mechanism of osseous ischemia, resulting in infarction, remains obscure.

Avascular necrosis of the femoral head may complicate the treatment of a congenital dislocated hip or a slipped capital femoral epiphysis in a child, or a fracture or fracture-dislocation of the hip in an adult. Avascular necrosis is the underlying pathologic process encountered in the osteochondroses (see p. 84). Osteochondritis dissecans is thought to represent localized bone necrosis (see p. 376).

The known systemic conditions associated with nontraumatic avascular necrosis of the femoral head in adults include decompression syndromes (*Caisson disease*), sickle cell hemoglobinopathies, hypercortisonism, alcoholism, pancreatitis, and Gaucher's disease.

In a large group of patients, the cause of the femoral head avascular necrosis cannot be positively identified. The condition is then termed *idiopathic femoral head necrosis* or *Chandler's disease.*

Pathologic Features. Interruption of the circulation to an area of bone results in death for that segment of bone tissue. The affected bone softens and dies. The pathogenesis of the necrosis produced by systemic nontraumatic causes is a matter of considerable controversy. There seems little doubt, however, that the bone end-stage following both traumatic and nontraumatic causes is remarkably similar. Necrotic bone is removed and replaced by viable bone through a process called "creeping substitution." This is the method bone tissue uses to repair the effects of avascular necrosis.

Highly vascularized fibrous tissue from the adjacent viable bone tissue invades the interstices of the dead bone, generates osteoblasts to resurface the dead trabeculae, and resorbs necrotic bone and marrow debris with the aid of osteoclasts and histiocytes.

The final stage of avascular necrosis is that of reossification. Areas where dead bone has been resorbed are filled with new bone; other areas have appositional new bone deposited on the surfaces of dead bone trabeculae. Cellular death, removal of dead bone, and reossification occur simultaneously in different parts of the affected bone.

X-ray Findings. X-ray examination of an area of avascular necrosis in bone reveals intermingled irregular areas of decreased bone density and increased bone density (Fig. 170). The areas of decreased bone density represent living bone that has undergone atrophy with decalcification; those of increased density represent zones of hypertrophic living bone, necrotic bone with reactive bone around it, and dead bone. The resorptive activity of the granulation tissue is usually focal, resulting in an x-ray appearance of irregular islands of mottled radiolucent spaces in the dead bone.

Necrotic bone is unable to stand the stress of weight bearing, and secondary subchondral fractures may occur through the necrotic segment. The necrotic segment may thus appear flattened and depressed on the x-ray films because of compaction of dead cancellous bone fragments into a smaller volume (Fig. 171).

Treatment. In the child, treatment of avascular necrosis of the femoral head is the prevention of weight bearing for a period of time long enough to allow "creeping substitution" to revitalize the affected portion of the head. Weight bearing must be prohibited to prevent the soft necrotic femoral head from becoming flattened and deformed.

In the adult, "creeping substitution" does not appear to be the effective repair mechanism that it is in the child, possibly because weight bearing is rarely prohibited early. Flattening and collapse of the necrotic segment are seen more frequently in the adult patient. Fragmentation and collapse represent an advanced and probably irreversible stage of avascular necrosis. For this reason, most adult

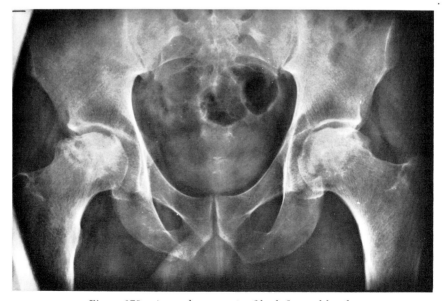

Figure 170. Avascular necrosis of both femoral heads.

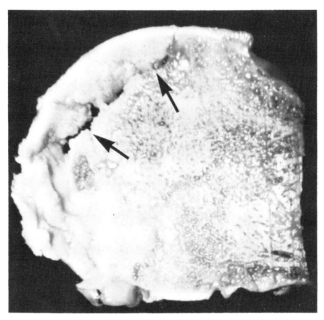

Figure 171. Section through femoral head with avascular necrosis secondary to sickle cell disease. Arrows point to necrotic segments showing collapse and fragmentation.

patients with avascular necrosis of the femoral head require reconstructive surgery of the hip joint for pain relief. Depending upon the stage of hip joint destruction, cup arthroplasty, metallic femoral head prosthesis, or total hip replacement is the procedure of choice.

THE THIGH

FRACTURE OF THE FEMORAL SHAFT

Fracture through the femoral shaft is a relatively common injury that may occur in children or adults. It is usually produced by severe trauma. The line of pull and the great strength of the muscles of the hip and thigh produce, as a rule, marked displacement of the bone fragments (Fig. 172A). This fracture is typically accompanied by extensive hemorrhage into the soft parts of the thigh, sometimes severe enough to precipitate shock. Generally, in civilian medical practice, this fracture is closed rather than open.

The affected leg appears shortened, and the thigh may present an anterior and lateral angulation. The lower part of the limb usually lies

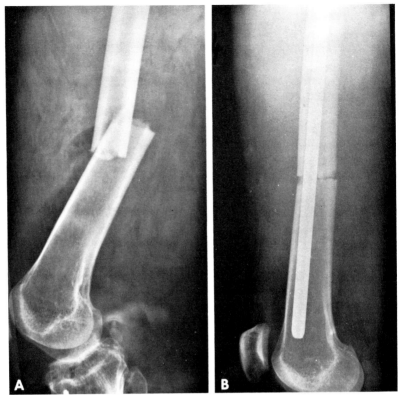

Figure 172.   A, transverse fracture through the lower shaft of the femur in an adult. B, same patient after open reduction of fracture and fixation with intramedullary rod.

in abnormal rotation. The patient is unable to move the leg, and attempts to do so cause severe pain. Damage to the sciatic nerve may accompany this fracture.

In children, fractures of the femoral shaft may be treated by closed reduction followed by immobilization in a plaster hip spica cast or by the use of traction. It is generally agreed that open reduction of these fractures is not required in children.

Fractures of the femoral shaft in adults may be treated in skeletal traction, by the use of ambulatory cast braces, by open reduction and internal fixation with a long metal rod driven down the intramedullary cavity (Fig. 172B), or by the use of dual compression plates placed along the shaft of the bone at right angles to each other.

Myositis Ossificans

Myositis ossificans has been discussed previously in relation to the elbow joint (see p. 241).

The condition may also occur in the anterior aspect of the thigh in response to hemorrhage in quadriceps muscle. The cause is trauma to the front of the thigh. Contusion and tearing of muscle fibers with resulting hematoma in the muscle, a common sports injury, is called "charleyhorse." If this muscle hematoma becomes converted to bone, the condition is then called myositis ossificans.

OSTEOMYELITIS OF THE FEMUR

Open fracture involving the femur may be complicated by the development of infection that may progress to osteomyelitis. Closed fractures treated by open reduction with internal fixation may develop wound sepsis that also may progress to osteomyelitis.

The treatment of this disease in the femur follows the general principles outlined in Chapter 6 (see p. 127).

THE KNEE

General Considerations

The knee is the largest joint in the body, but it is far from the strongest. Because of its exposed position in the limb and the great functional demands imposed by weight bearing stresses—such as walking, running, and jumping—the knee suffers derangement of its function and stability more frequently than any other joint.

The knee is basically a hinge joint between the femur and tibia; it permits the motions of flexion and extension. A slight amount of rotation and lateral motion is allowed when the knee is flexed. Since the knee lacks the inherent bony stability of the hip joint, it must depend upon muscles and strong ligaments to bind the component bones together (Fig. 173).

The hinge effect of the knee joint is formed between the rounded femoral condyles and the shallow depressions on the tibial plateaus. The tibial spine is a twin peaked projection that lies between and separates the two tibial plateaus. Lying on top of the tibia are two semilunar-shaped pieces of fibrocartilage known as the medial and lateral menisci. The menisci move forward and backward with the tibia, and act to promote a snugger fit between the femur and tibia when the knee joint is in extension.

Medial stability of the knee joint is maintained by the medial collateral ligament, which runs from the medial femoral condyle to the medial tibial condyle. The deeper layer of the medial collateral ligament is attached to the outer border of the medial meniscus.

Lateral stability of the knee is maintained by the lateral collateral

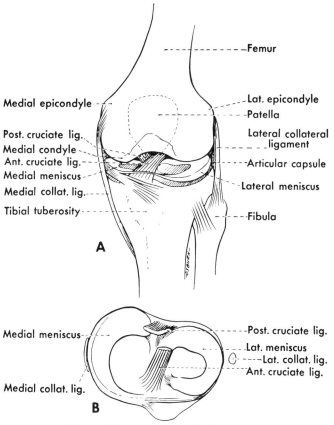

Medial epicondyle

Post. cruciate lig.
Medial condyle
Ant. cruciate lig.
Medial meniscus
Medial collat. lig.

Tibial tuberosity

Femur

Lat. epicondyle
Patella

Lateral collateral
ligament

Articular capsule

Lateral meniscus

Fibula

A

Medial meniscus

Medial collat. lig.

Post. cruciate lig.

Lat. meniscus
Lat. collat. lig.
Ant. cruciate lig.

B

Figure 173.   Anatomy of the knee joint.

ligament, which runs from the lateral femoral condyle to the fibular head, but has no attachment to the lateral meniscus.

Within the joint itself are found the cruciate ligaments, two binding ligaments so named because they run in a criss-cross fashion. The anterior cruciate ligament runs from the anterior surface of the tibia to the posterior aspect of the femur and acts to prevent forward displacement of the tibia on the femur. The posterior cruciate ligament runs from the posterior surface of the tibia to the anterior aspect of the femur, and acts to prevent backward displacement of the tibia on the femur.

The knee joint is lined with a relatively thick synovial membrane containing many folds and villi that secrete lubricating fluid. The synovial membrane of the knee joint is continuous with the suprapatellar bursa lying just above the knee on the anterior aspect of the thigh.

The knee joint is braced and stabilized by the quadriceps muscle to support the body weight. It has been claimed that the action of the quadriceps extensor apparatus is the most important factor in maintaining the erect position in man.

Normal knee function is possible, therefore, only in the presence of muscular control, intact supporting ligaments, and smooth, well-aligned joint surfaces.

Clinical Aspects of Knee Disorders

The majority of patients presenting with a knee joint problem do so because of pain, joint swelling, limited joint motion, or joint instability.

PAIN

Pain of knee joint origin may be noted anteriorly or posteriorly, or it may be localized to either the medial or lateral side of the knee. The pain is characteristically aggravated by use of the joint, and may be referred to the muscles of the thigh or calf.

SWELLING

Joint swelling may indicate synovial effusion or hemarthrosis.

Synovial effusion is an outpouring of essentially normal-appearing synovial fluid in response to irritation of the synovial membrane. Synovial irritation may arise as a result of trauma, mechanical disorder, or disease. The excess fluid distends and swells the joint, resulting in pain and limitation of joint motion.

Hemarthrosis is extravasation of blood within the joint, where it is mixed with synovial fluid. The presence of blood within the joint may occur with hemophilia, or it may follow major injury to the knee.

JOINT MOTION

In reference to the knee, limited joint motion means a decrease in the arc of motion between complete flexion and full extension. Motion may be limited because of pain, stiffness, fluid, or locking.

Following trauma to the joint, the knee may be held firmly in the position of semiflexion by hamstring muscle spasm, and the patient may voluntarily resist all efforts to extend the knee because of pain.

Stiffness is synonymous with limited joint motion and may indicate degenerative or mechanical malalignment of the articular surfaces, or flexion contracture of the joint.

Fluid within the joint limits motion because of the pain of capsular distension and the hydraulic effect of intra-articular liquid.

Locking is the situation that arises when a loose piece of tissue interposes itself between the femur and tibia and effectively blocks full extension of the joint. A joint that is locked presents in flexion and cannot be extended until the lock is released. True mechanical locking must be differentiated from other causes that limit knee extension, such as knee pain with hamstring muscle spasm, joint effusion, and flexion contracture.

INSTABILITY

Joint instability may occur with rupture of one or more of the supporting ligaments of the knee. The sensation of the joint "giving way" may be associated with quadriceps muscle weakness or a torn meniscus.

Examination of the Knee Joint

The patient must be draped so that both lower extremities are visible for examination. Male patients must remove their trousers. Both knee joints are examined for comparison purposes.

VISUAL EXAMINATION

The physical appearance of both knee joints is compared, and any deformity, malalignment, or swelling is noted.

PALPATION

The knees are palpated for evidence of swelling or deformity. The patellae are compared for contour and mobility, and areas of palpable tenderness over the lower femur, upper tibia, articular margins, or in relation to the patella are noted. The presence of quadriceps muscle wasting can be confirmed by comparing the circumference measurement of both thighs, the measurements taken at corresponding locations three inches above each patella.

RANGE OF MOTION

The average range of motion in the normal knee joint begins at the zero starting position in full extension and moves through a 135 degree arc of motion in the direction of flexion (Fig. 174).

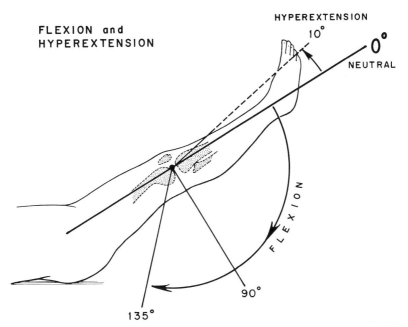

Figure 174. Range of motion allowed by knee joint. (Courtesy American Academy of Orthopaedic Surgeons.)

SPECIAL MANEUVERS

Test for Collateral Ligament Rupture. An abnormal opening of the medial aspect of the knee joint, noted when the medial collateral ligament is stretched with the knee partially flexed, indicates damage to the medial collateral ligament. When the opening is noted on the lateral aspect of the knee joint, the lateral collateral ligament has been damaged (Fig. 178).

Test for Cruciate Ligament Rupture. With the patient's knee flexed, the examiner grasps the leg just below the knee with both hands and pulls the tibia forward. Abnormal forward mobility of the tibia on the femur suggests rupture of the anterior cruciate ligament (drawer forward test). Abnormal backward mobility of the tibia on the femur suggests rupture of the posterior cruciate ligament (drawer backward test).

McMurray's Test for Torn Meniscus. With the patient lying supine, the knee is fully flexed and the foot is forcibly rotated outward to its full capability. With the foot held in the outwardly rotated position, the knee is slowly extended. A painful "click" indicates tear of the medial meniscus. If the painful "click" is felt when the foot is rotated inward, the tear is in the lateral meniscus.

ASPIRATION OF THE KNEE JOINT

The knee joint may be aspirated of fluid, blood, or pus as an aid to diagnosis, for the purpose of treatment, or to relieve the pain of joint distension. For this procedure, aseptic precautions and local anesthesia are recommended. Aspiration can be carried out through the suprapatellar pouch or through the anterior approach to the joint (see p. 12).

ARTHROSCOPIC EXAMINATION

It is possible to examine the inside of the knee joint with a special instrument called an arthroscope. Training is required to become familiar with its use. With the arthroscope, it is possible to visualize the synovia, the menisci, the cruciate ligaments, the articular cartilage of the joint, and the undersurface of the patella.

X-RAY EXAMINATION

Routine x-ray examination of the knee joints includes anteroposterior and lateral views. Special views may be taken as indicated.

ARTHROGRAM OF THE KNEE

An arthrogram of the knee is a special x-ray study performed after a mixture of air and radiopaque dye has been injected into the knee joint cavity. This allows roentgenographic visualization of some of the structures inside the knee joint, such as the menisci and the cruciate ligamen s. Depending upon the contour of the dye on the x-ray film, it is possible to get useful information about the menisci, many of the ligamentous structures, the integrity of the capsule, and presence or absence of cysts arising from the knee joint.

Disorders of the Knee Joint

PREPATELLAR BURSITIS (See p. 121)

TRAUMATIC SYNOVITIS

A jarring or twisting injury to the knee joint may irritate the synovial membrane and cause, some hours later, an outpouring of normal-appearing synovial fluid. Fluid distension of the joint may cause pain, limitation of motion, and a limping gait.

A diagnosis of traumatic synovitis may be entertained if injury to the joint surfaces, supporting ligaments, or menisci has been ruled out. X-ray examination of the knee joint will be negative except for possible capsular swelling due to the accumulation of fluid.

Treatment of traumatic synovitis consists of rest and support to the joint. Joint distension may be relieved by aspiration of the excess joint fluid.

HEMARTHROSIS

Extravasation of blood within the knee joint is rarely produced by trivial injury. It may be seen following severe sprain of the joint accompanied by a tear of the synovial membrane and joint capsule, rupture of the anterior cruciate ligament, fracture through the articular surface of the tibia, or fracture of the patella. Swelling of the knee joint appears much more rapidly with hemarthrosis than with traumatic synovitis.

Blood should be aspirated from the joint, because its continued presence may cause irritation to the joint and may contribute to the formation of adhesions. The presence of fat globules in the aspirated blood alerts the examiner to the possibility of an intra-articular fracture.

FRACTURE OF THE PATELLA

The patella may be broken by a direct blow, such as a fall on the knee or a dashboard injury, or it may be broken in two by a sudden and violent contraction of the quadriceps muscle.

Direct blows and sudden violent contraction of the quadriceps muscle, such as may occur when a person attempts to prevent himself from slipping or falling, may snap the patella in two. Usually, tears of the quadriceps expansion to the medial and lateral sides of the fracture site accompany this injury and allow marked displacement of the fragments. When this occurs, the patient loses the ability to extend the knee actively (Fig. 175).

If there is little or no displacement of the two fragments, the fracture may be treated by immobilizing the knee in a plaster cast in the position of extension. If the fragments are displaced, open reduction is performed. The fragments may be wired together and the torn quadriceps expansion repaired. Many orthopaedic surgeons, in addition to repairing the rent in the quadriceps expansion, simply excise the inferior patellar fragment, allowing the remaining fragment to function as the patella.

A direct blow to the patella may cause a crushing injury, resulting in a severely comminuted fracture. If immobilized and allowed to heal, a severely comminuted patellar fracture may heal with a de-

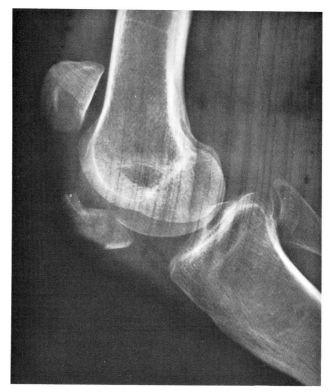

Figure 175. Lateral view of knee, showing displaced fracture of patella.

formed and irregular articular surface, and the patient may have a painful knee. For this reason, severely comminuted fractures of the patella may be treated by total excision of the knee cap with repair of the quadriceps expansion.

Rupture of the Quadriceps Tendon

In an older person, a sudden violent contraction of the quadriceps tendon may cause the tendon to rupture instead of snapping the patella in two. If this occurs, a sulcus may be palpated in the thigh just above the knee, and if rupture is complete, the patient will lose the ability to extend the knee actively.

Treatment is operative repair of the defect.

Chondromalacia Patellae

The word chondromalacia means softening of cartilage and is applied most frequently to a poorly understood disorder affecting the undersurface of the patella. This condition is seen most commonly in young adults and is associated with softening and degeneration of the articular hyaline cartilage lining the undersurface of the patella. The biochemical changes causing the softening are believed similar to the articular cartilage changes seen in osteoarthritis. The earliest biochemical change in both conditions is loss of chondroitin sulphate from the matrix. Chondromalacia may follow trauma to the knee cap, but in many patients the cause is not apparent. When examined grossly, the cartilage surface of the patella may appear yellowish and opaque in color, and may be soft and pitted. The remainder of the knee joint is usually normal.

The patient may complain of pain in the region of the patella, usually aggravated by bending the knee or stair climbing. Motions of the knee are often accompanied by a grating sensation beneath the patella, which is due to rubbing of the irregular articular surfaces. The patient may complain of a "giving way" sensation. There may be an associated irritation of the synovial membrane with a synovial effusion.

The grating sensation beneath the patella can usually be felt by the examiner when the knee is flexed and extended. Tenderness may be elicited by pressing the undersurface of the patella.

X-ray examination frequently shows a normal knee, since articular cartilage casts no shadow. Occasionally, an irregularity of the undersurface of the patella may be noted on the lateral x-ray view.

In later life, some of these patients progress to develop all the signs and symptoms of osteoarthritis of the knee and some do not. Symptoms of chondromalacia of the patellae may be relieved by use of the anti-inflammatory drugs combined with support to the knee. Frequently quadriceps exercises are helpful. More severe cases may require operation, in which the soft cartilage is scraped from the undersurface of the bone to aid in restoring a smooth articulating surface. If all else fails and the symptoms are severe enough, patellectomy may be performed.

RECURRENT DISLOCATION OF THE PATELLA

The patella may be dislocated forcibly by an injury or repeatedly as a result of congenital and postural factors. The second situation is more common and is known as recurrent dislocation of the patella.

This condition occurs most frequently in adolescent girls who often have an accompanying knock knee deformity and a congenitally flattened and small lateral femoral condyle. It is thought that the insertion of the patellar tendon is more laterally placed in these children. Contraction of the quadriceps muscle allows the patella to be pulled to the outside, where it slips over the flattened lateral femoral condyle and dislocates to the lateral side of the knee.

Children so afflicted may suffer frequent or infrequent dislocations accompanied by pain, joint swelling, and marked disability. Dislocations may become so frequent that they seriously curtail the child's physical activity.

Reduction of the dislocated patella is usually accomplished quite easily by fully extending the knee and manipulating the bone back into location. However, this does not cure the underlying defect, which requires more extensive treatment. In some patients, increasing the strength of the quadriceps muscle by resistance exercises may be sufficient to stabilize the patella. If this procedure is not successful, surgical repair is carried out. Many operative repairs have been advocated for the condition. A popular one involves transplanting the insertion of the patellar tendon to a more distal and medial location on the tibia.

INTERNAL DERANGEMENTS OF THE KNEE JOINT

The term "internal derangement" is used to group together a variety of joint conditions, usually of traumatic origin, in which the internal structure of the joint is affected to such an extent that its function and mechanics are compromised.

Meniscus Lesions. A rotatory force applied to the knee joint may trap a meniscus between the femur and tibia to produce the familiar "torn cartilage" lesion. A meniscus cannot be torn while the knee is in extension. To produce a tear, the knee joint must be first rotated in the flexed position to trap the meniscus, and then extended to produce the tearing force on the tissue. This combination of motions is frequently encountered on the football field or basketball court.

MEDIAL MENISCUS. Tears of the medial meniscus are encountered about nine times more frequently than tears of the lateral meniscus. This is believed to be so because the medial meniscus is attached to the deep layer of the medial collateral ligament, and because the mechanisms that cause tearing are more frequently applied to the medial aspect of the joint. Usually the patient sustaining this injury is a healthy young male who is hurt while engaging in some athletic activity.

A tear of the medial meniscus is associated with pain referred to the medial side of the joint and with synovial effusion. The pain caused by a torn meniscus is frequently aggravated by forced rotation of the foot and leg. Pain or a "click" may be produced by the McMurray test. Locking of the joint may or may not be present, depending upon the location of the tear.

Two types of tears occur most frequently:

1. The punch-press effect of the femoral condyle on the trapped meniscus may cause splitting of the meniscus along its longitudinal axis, producing the so-called "bucket-handle" tear (Fig. 176). In this instance, the inner portion of the torn cartilage may displace into the joint to cause locking. The joint may be unlocked by manipulation, but healing of the tear does not occur, since the meniscus lacks the capacity for total regeneration. This type of tear causes repeated locking of the joint and is the lesion usually present in the athlete with a "trick knee."

Treatment of a longitudinally torn meniscus is operative removal of the meniscus.

2. Under certain circumstances, the meniscus may be torn along its transverse axis. This type of tear usually does not cause locking of the joint. Pain is produced by momentary impingement of the irregular meniscus between the femur and the tibia on motions of the joint.

The symptoms caused by a transverse tear of the meniscus can frequently be relieved by the use of the anti-inflammatory drugs combined with rest of the joint. If symptoms persist, operative excision of the meniscus is indicated.

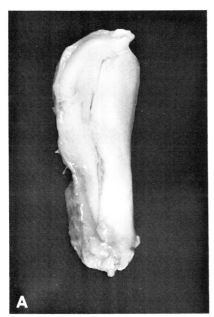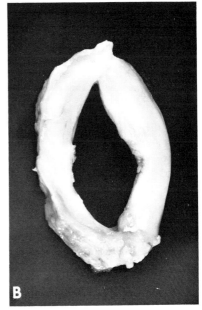

Figure 176. A, excised medial meniscus exhibiting tear along longitudinal axis. B, the bucket handle is opened when the inner portion of the meniscus is displaced into the joint. This may cause the knee to lock.

LATERAL MENISCUS. Lesions of the lateral meniscus include tears, cystic degeneration, and discoid meniscus.

Tears similar to those seen in the medial meniscus may involve the lateral meniscus, but they are less common.

Cystic degeneration, on the other hand, is much more common in the lateral meniscus than in the medial meniscus. In this condition, multiple cysts containing gelatinous material appear within the peripheral border of the meniscus. It is thought that repeated trauma causes their appearance. Once developed, cartilage cysts may cause pain and often can be seen and palpated along the lateral border of the knee joint.

Treatment consists of operative removal of the entire cystic meniscus.

A *discoid* meniscus is a congenitally abnormal lateral meniscus in which the structure assumes a thickened and rounded shape. Because of its thickness, the meniscus does not glide smoothly between the femur and tibia but must force its way through. As a result, a loud clicking noise is heard when the knee flexes or extends, but locking does not occur. The patient is usually a child who is brought for examination because of the loud snap. If symptoms are present, the entire meniscus should be surgically excised.

In the absence of locking, a tear of a meniscus can be difficult to diagnose. Before surgical treatment is undertaken, confirmatory evidence should be sought by careful evaluation of x-ray changes, by the performance of McMurray's test, and by an arthrogram or arthroscopic examination of the knee joint (Fig. 177).

Injury to Knee Ligaments. The medial and lateral collateral ligaments, the anterior and posterior cruciate ligaments, and the joint capsule all work together to maintain the integrity and stability of the knee joint. Twisting injuries, particularly those sustained in athletics, may sprain or rupture these ligaments to produce painful and often disabling conditions of the joint.

MEDIAL COLLATERAL LIGAMENT. A rotatory twist of the leg with the knee in flexion, such as may occur in skiing or football, may sprain or stretch the medial collateral ligament. Pain and tenderness are noted along the course of the ligament, but there is no instability, since the continuity of the ligament remains intact. X-ray examination is negative in the presence of sprain of a collateral ligament. This injury usually responds rapidly to rest and support to the joint.

Much more serious and disabling to the patient is complete rupture of the medial collateral ligament. The mechanism for this fairly common injury is usually a force applied to the lateral aspect of the knee joint when it is partially flexed or extended, as might be produced by a football block or "clip."

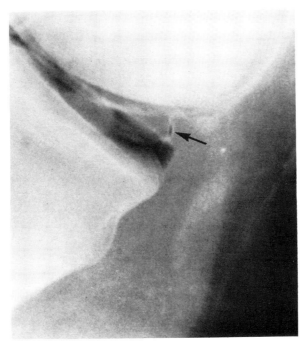

Figure 177. Arthrogram of knee. Arrow points to dark cleft indicating transverse tear in meniscus.

The ligament may be torn loose from its femoral or tibial attachment, or it may rupture through its mid-portion. Tears of the anterior cruciate ligament frequently accompany rupture of the medial collateral ligament. Severe trauma may cause simultaneous tearing of the medial collateral ligament, anterior cruciate ligament, and medial meniscus. This combination is known as the "terrible triad."

Rupture of the medial collateral ligament produces instability of the medial side of the joint. The diagnosis may be confirmed by taking an anteroposterior x-ray view of the partially flexed knee while an abduction force is being applied to the joint. This is known as a stress x-ray (Fig. 178). Opening of the medial side of the joint indicates rupture of the medial collateral ligament.

Treatment is immediate operative repair of the torn ligament.

LATERAL COLLATERAL LIGAMENT. Rupture of the lateral collateral ligament is relatively uncommon but may be produced by a force applied to the medial aspect of a partially flexed knee joint. The diagnosis may be confirmed by taking an anteroposterior x-ray view of the partially flexed knee while an adduction force is being applied to the joint. An opening in the lateral side of the joint indicates rupture of the lateral collateral ligament (stress x-ray).

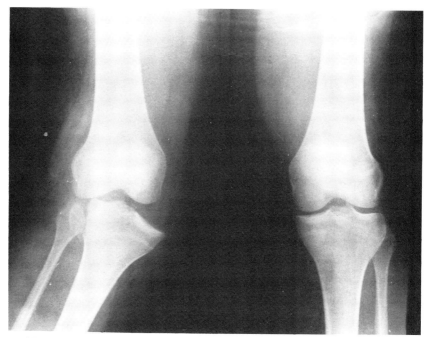

Figure 178. Positive stress x-ray indicating rupture of medial collateral ligament of right knee.

Treatment is immediate operative repair of the torn ligament.

ANTERIOR CRUCIATE LIGAMENT. The anterior cruciate ligament is frequently ruptured in association with tears of the medial meniscus or rupture of the medial collateral ligament. Isolated ruptures of this ligament may occur if the femur is forcibly driven backward when the knee is flexed. This may cause an avulsion fracture of the tibial spine, which pulls off and carries with it the inferior insertion of the anterior cruciate ligament.

The patient with a torn anterior cruciate ligament may exhibit a positive drawer forward test (see p. 365).

Treatment is operative repair of the torn ligament.

If the patient sustains a fracture of the tibial spine, reduction of the fracture may be carried out successfully by immobilizing the knee in the extended position. If this is unsuccessful, open reduction of the tibial spine fragment is indicated.

POSTERIOR CRUCIATE LIGAMENT. Rupture of the posterior cruciate ligament is relatively uncommon. It may occur with an injury that forces the tibia backward when the knee is flexed.

The patient with a torn posterior cruciate ligament may exhibit a positive drawer backward test (see p. 365).

Treatment is operative repair of the torn ligament.

Loose Bodies. Loose bodies are fragments of cartilage, bone, or calcified tissue that lie free within joints, causing pain, joint irritation, and locking (see p. 364). Loose bodies have been discovered in practically every joint in the body but occur most frequently in the knee. Locking occurs if the loose body becomes wedged between the bones, thereby forming a mechanical obstruction to complete extension.

The fragments may be pieces of bone broken from the articular surface — such as a piece of tibial spine, a detached bone spur in an osteoarthritic knee joint, or a torn portion of a meniscus — or they may result from osteochondritis dissecans or osteochondromatosis.

Loose bodies containing bone or calcified cartilage are visible on x-ray examination (Fig. 179). They are removed from the joint by

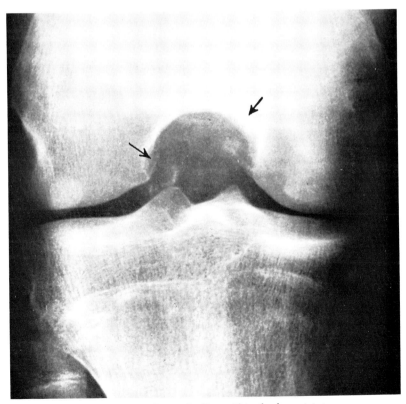

Figure 179. Loose bodies within the knee joint.

operation to relieve the symptoms produced and to protect the joint surfaces from further damage.

OSTEOCHONDRITIS DISSECANS. Osteochondritis dissecans is a relatively uncommon joint condition primarily affecting children and young adults. The process consists of a localized segmental area of avascular necrosis in the end of a long bone. This ultimately results in the formation of a button-shaped piece of dead subchondral bone covered with articular hyaline cartilage. If the overlying cartilage degenerates around the edges of the defect, the entire piece may separate from the rest of the normal bone and drop into the joint as a "loose body."

The exact cause of the localized avascular necrosis is unknown, but trauma, thrombosis of an end-artery, or an underlying metabolic defect have all been suggested. The condition occurs most commonly in the knee joint, but it may also be seen in the elbow, ankle, and hip joints.

The usual area of involvement in the knee joint is the medial femoral condyle close to the intercondylar notch. The presence of the defect may cause pain and joint irritation with synovial effusion and a "giving way" sensation. If the involved piece of condyle becomes detached, it may drop into the joint cavity to act as a loose body and cause locking.

The area of involvement on the medial femoral condyle may be visible on the x-ray film (Fig. 180).

If the diagnosis of osteochondritis dissecans of the knee joint is made before the fragment completely separates, healing of the defect by "creeping substitution" may occur if the joint is put at rest and protected from weight bearing. This process may take months. If healing does not occur, or if the fragment becomes detached, the knee joint should be operated on and the lesion excised.

OSTEOCHONDROMATOSIS. Osteochondromatosis is an unusual condition in which the synovial villi undergo metaplasia into bone and cartilage tumors. The disorder may arise in any joint, but it is most often seen in the knee joint. When these small hard masses become detached from the synovial membrane, they may drop into the joint cavity to act as loose bodies.

X-ray examination is quite dramatic, in that the joint may be flooded with literally hundreds of these small bodies.

Treatment is excision of the synovial membrane and all the loose bodies.

BAKER'S CYST (POPLITEAL CYST)

Baker's cyst is the name given to a firm, tense cystic mass occasionally found along the medial border of the popliteal space in

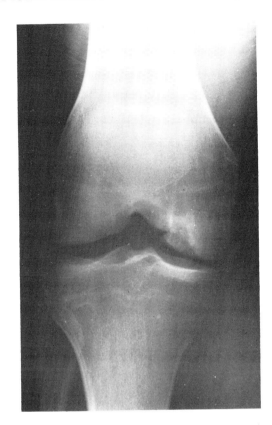

Figure 180. Osteochondritis dissecans of medial femoral condyle.

children. Although the condition may represent herniation through the posterior capsule of the knee joint, most popliteal cysts are believed to represent fluid distension of the bursal sac that is associated with the gastrocnemius and semimembranosus muscles.

The patient is usually a child, but popliteal cysts may also be seen in adults, particularly in patients with rheumatoid arthritis. Some cysts communicate directly with the joint cavity. No symptoms other than swelling may be noted. In some patients, however, the cyst may cause vague pain and discomfort associated with a sensation of weakness and "giving way."

If the cyst produces symptoms, it may be removed surgically.

KNOCK KNEE (GENU VALGUM)

A knock knee deformity is one in which the legs deviate outward from the long axis of the femur, with the apex at the knee joint. When normally straight legs are placed together in the extended position,

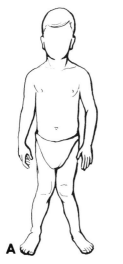 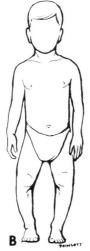

Figure 181. A, knock knee deformity. B, bowleg deformity.

the medial femoral condyles and the medial malleoli touch. In knock knee deformity, the medial malleoli are separated (Fig. 181a).

Knock knee may be caused by strain placed on the knee by severely pronated feet, or it may arise secondary to growth plate injury at the knee. Knock knee may also be produced by rickets in the child or arthritis of the knee in the adult.

Treatment depends on the cause. Shoe corrections for pronation may relieve the valgus strain on the knee. Leg braces may be necessary in certain cases. Severe deformity may require surgical osteotomy through the femur or tibia in order to realign the leg.

Bowleg (Genu Varum)

Bowleg deformity is a lateral curvature at the knee joint involving either one bone or both. In bowleg deformity, the medial femoral condyles are widely separated when the legs are placed together in the extended position (Fig. 181b).

The causes of bowleg are essentially the same as those of knock knee. Bowleg may be treated with shoe corrections, bracing, or surgical osteotomy.

Degenerative Arthritis of the Knee Joint (Osteoarthritis)

Osteoarthritis involving the knee joint is a common and frequently progressive disorder seen mainly in middle-aged and older patients. As discussed in Chapter 5, osteoarthritis is characterized by deterioration of articular cartilage with narrowing of the joint space and overgrowth of juxta-articular bone. The disease tends to strike females more frequently than males and affects mainly weight bearing joints.

The knee joint, as a major weight bearing joint, may become involved as part of the generalized disease process. It is not uncommon to see both knees involved. On occasion, osteoarthritis may affect one side of the knee joint more severely than the opposite side, resulting in the development of an angular deformity. Narrowing of the medial side of the joint may cause a genu varum deformity. A genu valgum deformity may result from narrowing of the lateral side of the joint (Fig. 63).

Osteoarthritis of the knee may follow as a later complication of an intra-articular fracture of the joint. Removal of a torn meniscus may be followed in later life by the development of osteoarthritis in that compartment of the joint.

This very common condition will cause the patient to complain of pain, grating, and stiffness in the joint. Pain may be referred to the thigh and calf muscles. Synovial effusion is frequently present, and the patient may complain of a tightness in the back of the joint. The joint outlines may be distorted by the effusion or by thickening of the synovial membrane. Some limitation of the joint motion usually occurs, and a flexion contracture may develop.

X-ray examination of the knee joint may disclose narrowing of the joint space associated with sclerotic changes in the subchondral bone. Bone spurs may arise along the joint margins and at the pole of the patella. The changes may be more marked on one side of the joint than the other (Fig. 182).

Symptoms produced by degenerative arthritis in the knee joint frequently may be relieved by the use of intra-articular hydrocortisone following aspiration of the effusion, if present. The systemic use of the anti-inflammatory drugs is usually helpful in relieving symptoms of pain and stiffness.

Some of these patients may require surgical treatment. In a patient with disease confined primarily to one side of the joint, the development of an angular deformity usually aggravates the pain. This deformity can be corrected by an osteotomy through the proximal tibia, which realigns the weight bearing stresses on the osteoarthritic joint and relieves pain (Fig. 183).

Severe, painful osteoarthritic changes in one knee following infection or trauma can be treated by fusion of the joint, provided the patient has a normal knee on the opposite side (Fig. 13).

Although not yet as well studied as a similar procedure in the hip

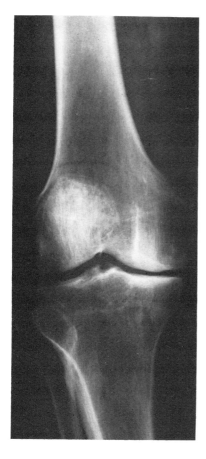

Figure 182. Narrowing of the medial joint space seen 10 years after excision of medial meniscus.

joint, total knee replacement is possible, using metal and plastic implants fixed to bone with methyl methacrylate (see p. 353) (Fig. 184). Until extended follow-up data are available, it is considered advisable to restrict total knee replacement to those patients with severe functional disability and for whom nothing else can be offered.

PYOGENIC ARTHRITIS OF THE KNEE JOINT
(See p. 138)

TUBERCULOSIS OF THE KNEE JOINT (See p. 146)

FRACTURES INVOLVING THE KNEE JOINT

Tibia. Fracture through the tibial condyles is the most common fracture involving the knee joint. This injury may be produced by direct compression, such as might occur when one jumps from a high place, or by a force applied to the outer or inner side of the leg, producing abduction or adduction at the knee joint.

Fracture of the lateral tibial condyle occurs more frequently than fracture of the medial condyle, because the outer side of the knee is unprotected and more exposed to trauma. All degrees of displacement and comminution may be seen on the x-ray films.

A force applied to the outer side of the leg to produce an abduction strain on the knee joint may cause a fracture through the lateral tibial condyle and, simultaneously, a rupture of the medial collateral ligament.

Some displaced tibial condyle fractures may be reduced by

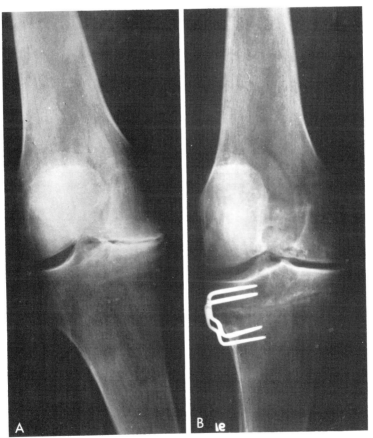

Figure 183. A, AP x-ray of knee, showing degenerative arthritis of medial joint compartment and angular deformity. B, same knee after correction of angular deformity by proximal tibial osteotomy. Note widening of medial joint space and staples used for internal fixation of the osteotomy site.

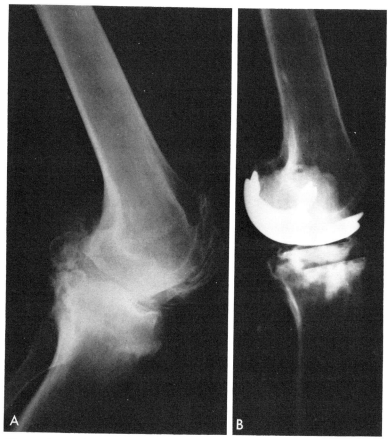

Figure 184. A, lateral x-ray of knee, showing advanced degenerative arthritis. *B*, same knee after insertion of total knee unit. Femoral component is metal and tibial component is plastic. Opaque material represents methacrylate "cement." (Courtesy Dr. Jerome Cotler, Thomas Jefferson University Hospital, Philadelphia, Pa.)

closed methods and held in a long leg cast. Others are best treated by skeletal traction. If these methods are not feasible, open reduction may be carried out and fragments held in position by some form of internal fixation.

Femur. IN CHILDREN. A hyperextension force applied to a child's knee may cause traumatic separation of the distal femoral epiphysis from the femoral shaft. The small distal epiphyseal fragment typically displaces to the front of the shaft and is tilted backward by pull of the gastrocnemius muscle.

The separated distal femoral epiphysis is usually reduced by closed manipulation, and is held in position by a plaster cast applied with the knee joint in a flexed position.

This is considered a serious joint injury in children. Complications are common and include residual shortening of the affected leg and subsequent development of angular deformity at the knee.

IN ADULTS.   Direct trauma to the knee in the adult may produce a fracture through the supracondylar region of the femur. The small distal bone fragment usually displaces to the front of the shaft and is tilted backward by pull of the gastrocnemius muscle. The popliteal artery may be damaged by projecting bone spikes on the end of the large femoral shaft fragment.

Theoretically, this fracture may be reduced by manipulation and immobilization in a hip spica cast or treated by skeletal traction. However, because the majority of adult patients sustaining supracondylar fractures of the femur are in the older age group, many orthopaedists elect open reduction and internal fixation in order to obtain early ambulation for the patient.

DISLOCATION OF THE KNEE

Dislocation of the knee joint is a rare injury, but it may occur as a result of extreme violence applied directly to the joint. The disrupting force usually damages all the supporting ligaments. Displacement of the joint may cause damage of the popliteal artery.

Immediate reduction is required, particularly if the circulation is affected.

Congenital dislocation of the knee is occasionally seen.

THE LEG

TIBIAL TORSION

The term "tibial torsion" refers to a deformity of the tibia seen in infancy in which the bone is twisted on its longitudinal axis in an inward or outward direction. With the patella pointing straight forward, the foot turns inward or outward, depending on the direction of the torsional deformity.

Tibial torsion is usually congenital and may be aggravated by allowing the baby to sleep on the abdomen. Internal tibial torsion is more common than external tibial torsion and, if not corrected, will produce an in-toe or pigeon-toe gait. Internal tibial torsion may accompany clubfoot deformity or may be associated with knock knees or bowlegs.

During infancy, tibial torsion may be corrected by manipulative exercises or by the use of plaster casts. More severe cases may require a Denis Browne splint. Older children may need surgical osteotomy to straighten the leg, but this is rare.

Congenital Pseudarthrosis of the Tibia
(See p. 67)

Fracture of the Tibia and Fibula

The exposed human shin is often the recipient of trauma sufficient to break simultaneously both bones of the lower leg. Industrial, highway, and athletic accidents all contribute to the incidence and severity of lower leg trauma, which frequently results in the fracture of both the tibia and the fibula. Open fractures are common, since the entire medial surface of the tibia is subcutaneous.

A direct blow to the shin delivered, for example, by the bumper of an automobile may cause a transverse fracture through the proximal, mid-shaft, or distal portions of the bones. The fracture frequently is comminuted. A torsional injury to the leg delivered, for example, while skiing may cause a spiral or long oblique fracture. In either instance, immediate pain and disability are noted by the patient. Usually the foot and ankle are rotated outward in relation to the knee. Treatment is directed toward restoring alignment and obtaining union of the tibial fracture, since this is the weight bearing bone of the leg. Reduction of the fibula usually accompanies reduction of the tibia.

Many of these fractures can be reduced by closed methods and held in alignment by a long leg cast (Fig. 185). Early weight bearing in a specially designed cast has been shown to be associated with rapid healing of the fracture in a high percentage of patients.

A severely comminuted fracture of the tibia and fibula may require treatment in skeletal traction, with the traction pin inserted through the os calcis.

A few fractures may require open reduction, with the bone fragments held in alignment by means of an intramedullary nail or compression plate.

Nonunion of fractures located in the middle or lower third of the shaft of the tibia is not uncommon. In a high proportion of patients, nonunion characterizes either open fractures or fractures associated with a high degree of soft tissue trauma (Fig. 26). This complication requires a bone graft for its correction.

Osteomyelitis of the Tibia

Open fractures involving the tibia may be complicated by the development of infection which may progress to osteomyelitis.

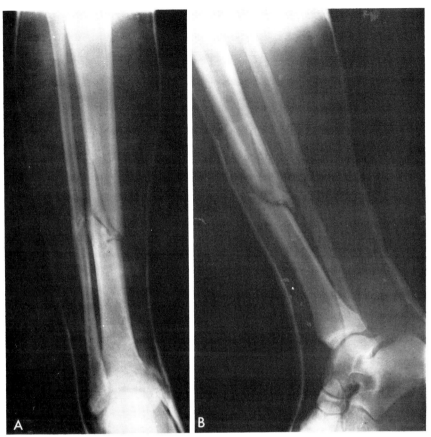

Figure 185. AP (*A*) and lateral (*B*) x-rays of patient with fracture of tibia and fibula, after closed reduction and application of cast.

Closed fractures treated by open reduction with internal fixation may also develop wound sepsis which may progress to an osteomyelitis.

The treatment of osteomyelitis in the tibia follows the general principles outlined in Chapter 6.

RUPTURE OF THE ACHILLES TENDON

Traumatic rupture of the Achilles tendon is not an uncommon occurrence, particularly in men during the prime of life. Sudden contraction of the calf muscle with the foot fixed to the floor may cause the Achilles tendon to pull apart suddenly. The tendon usually pulls apart within the sheath, leaving the sheath intact.

A patient so afflicted will immediately note sharp pain in the area, associated with inability to plantar flex the foot. On examination, a gap in the continuity of the tendon can be palpated.

Good results have been reported following the application of a walking cast with the foot held in marked plantar flexion. This position allows the ruptured tendon fragments to glide closer together within the intact sheath and ultimately heal. Healing by use of the plantar flexed cast usually takes between six and eight weeks. Operative repair of the Achilles tendon can be performed, but the operation is followed by a high incidence of skin necrosis and local wound infection.

RUPTURE OF THE PLANTARIS TENDON

The plantaris is a thin, inconstant muscle that lies between the gastrocnemius and soleus muscles. Rupture may occur with vigorous use of the legs, causing the patient to experience a sharp, stinging pain in the calf. Plantar flexion is unaffected.

Surgical treatment is not required. Rest, support to the calf, and the use of a heel lift are the only supportive measures needed.

THE ANKLE JOINT

The ankle joint is the hinge between the long lever arm of the leg and the presenting weight bearing surface of the foot. Because the body weight poised over this hinge joint may transmit abnormal forces along the tibial lever arm by means of running, jumping, twisting, or sliding motions, the ankle is one of the most frequently injured joints in the body.

General Considerations

Anatomically, the ankle is a hinge joint formed by the lower end of the tibia and the talus. The distal tibial supplies the medial malleolus, and the distal fibula supplies the lateral malleolus. The malleoli grasp the sides of the talus to form the ankle joint mortise. The bones are enclosed in a capsule, the anterior and posterior parts of which are loose to allow the hinge motions to occur. Strong ligaments add support to the medial and lateral joint margins (Fig. 186).

As in all hinge joints, the muscles that move the hinge are grouped in front and behind. The anterior tibial and toe extensor muscles lie in front of the joint and act as dorsiflexors of the ankle. The gastrocnemius and soleus muscles lie posteriorly and perform the motion of plantar flexion of the ankle joint.

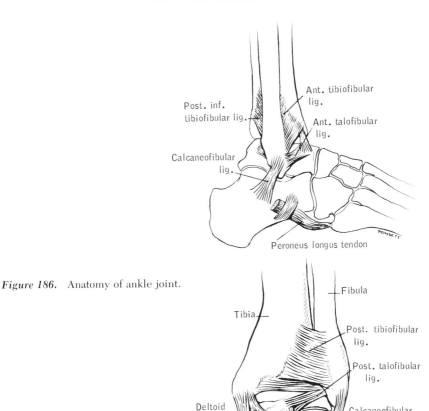

Figure 186. Anatomy of ankle joint.

The motions of eversion and inversion of the foot do not occur in the ankle joint proper, but rather through the joints below or distal to the ankle joint. These joints, frequently referred to as "the subtalar joints" by the orthopaedic surgeon, consist of the talocalcaneal joint, the talonavicular joint, and the calcaneocuboid joint. The posterior tibial muscle, acting through these joints, is the chief invertor muscle of the foot; the peroneals are the evertors.

Disorders of the Ankle Joint

A force applied to the ankle joint may cause a sprain, ligamentous rupture, fracture, dislocation, or a combination of injuries, depending on the amount of force applied, the duration of its application, and its direction. In all patients, details concerning the mechanism of injury, careful physical examination, and x-ray studies made in anteroposterior and lateral planes are prerequisites for correct diagnosis and proper treatment. Treatment should be carried out promptly because of the great tendency of the ankle joint area to swell rapidly following trauma.

SPRAIN

A sprain of the ankle joint is a stretch injury applied to the joint capsule and supporting ligaments by a twisting force. Rapid swelling, stiffness of the joint, and increased pain with walking are characteristic of joint sprain.

Examination frequently reveals the maximum swelling and tenderness to be localized to the tissues immediately below the lateral malleolus. X-ray examination is negative.

Ankle sprains respond favorably to rest and support. This may be obtained by strapping the joint or by supporting it in a plaster splint or cast. Crutches may be required. Immediate swelling may be controlled by ice packs. Later, soaking the ankle in hot water relieves residual edema and tenderness.

RUPTURED LIGAMENTS

Ruptures of the supporting ankle ligaments may occur as isolated injuries, but they more frequently occur in association with certain ankle fractures.

In the absence of joint fracture, x-ray evidence of displacement of the talus in relation to the tibia or fibula indicates rupture of supporting ligaments. In the absence of talar displacement, the diagnosis of ligament rupture is made by stress x-ray. Tilting of the talus on an anteroposterior x-ray with the foot forcibly inverted or everted confirms the diagnosis of ligament rupture (Fig. 5).

FRACTURES

Many complex mechanisms may be applied to the ankle joint by vehicular or athletic injuries, producing a variety of fracture combinations. Only the more commonly seen ankle fractures are discussed here (Fig. 187).

Ankle fractures require accurate repositioning of the fragments to restore normal weight bearing joint surfaces. This can frequently be accomplished by closed reduction. If closed reduction is not success-

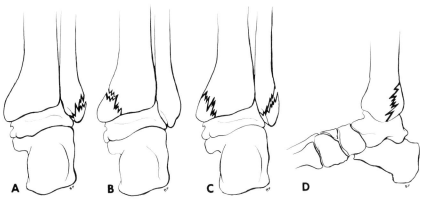

Figure 187.   Common types of ankle fractures.
A, fracture of lateral malleolus.
B, fracture of medial malleolus.
C, bimalleolar fracture (Pott's fracture).
D, fracture of posterior lip of tibia (trimalleolar fracture).

ful or feasible, open reduction is carried out, with the fragments held in position by internal fixation.

Fracture of the Lateral Malleolus.   Fracture of the lateral malleolus is the most common fracture of the ankle joint. It is frequently produced by the same type of force that might produce a joint sprain, but as a rule, pain and disability are greater.

X-ray examination will disclose the fracture and the position of the distal fibular fragment.

Closed reduction is carried out to reduce the fracture and restore the length of the fibula. If it is unsuccessful, open reduction with internal metallic fixation is performed.

Since the fibula is a non-weight bearing bone, fractures involving the lateral malleolus may be immobilized in walking casts.

Fracture of the Medial Malleolus.   An abduction force applied to the foot or a direct blow to the bone may cause fracture of the medial malleolus. This segment of bone frequently breaks off transversely at the level of the ankle joint and is displaced inward toward the talus by pull of the deltoid ligament.

X-ray examination will disclose the fracture and the position of the medial malleolar fragment.

With displacement of either malleolus, the talus may shift either medially or laterally, depending on the location of the fracture. A shift of the talus toward the side containing a fractured malleolus, in the face of an intact malleolus on the opposite side, indicates rupture of the supporting ligaments on the side of the intact malleolus.

Accurate replacement of the medial malleolar fragment is essential to stable, painless ankle function. This often can be achieved by closed manipulative reduction. If this is not possible, open reduction is carried out, with the fragments held in apposition with a metallic screw or pin.

Bimalleolar Fracture (Pott's Fracture).   Pott's fracture involves both malleoli and is an abduction injury caused either by a fall on the everted foot or by a direct blow on the outside of the ankle when the foot is in a fixed position. The force produces an oblique fracture of the lateral malleolus and a transverse fracture of the medial malleolus, usually at the level of the ankle joint. The talus shifts laterally and posteriorly whenever there is displacement of the malleoli.

X-ray examination will disclose the fracture and the position of the fragments.

Closed reduction is carried out to reduce the fractures and restore the integrity of the ankle mortise. If this is not successful or feasible, open reduction is carried out, with the fragments held in position by internal metallic fixation.

Trimalleolar Fracture.   A severe twisting injury applied to an ankle joint may cause both malleoli to fracture and may shift the talus posteriorly with such force that it breaks off the posterior lip of the tibia. Some authorities call this injury a trimalleolar fracture.

X-ray examination will disclose the fracture and the position of the fragments.

For a fracture of the posterior lip of the tibia, accurate reduction is necessary to restore the weight bearing surface of the tibia. It is imperative to obtain anatomic reduction if the posterior lip fragment amounts to one-third or more of the weight bearing surface. If this caliber of reduction cannot be achieved by closed methods, open reduction is carried out and the fragments held in position by internal fixation.

Fracture-Dislocation of the Ankle Joint.   A severe twisting force applied to the ankle may, in addition to causing fracture of the malleoli, dislocate the talus from its position beneath the tibia. Fracture-dislocation of the ankle joint is often an open injury because the malleoli lie just beneath the skin. The open wound is usually made when the tibia or fibula bursts through the skin as the foot is forcibly displaced to one side.

X-ray examination will disclose the fracture-dislocation and the position of the fragments.

Many fracture-dislocations of the ankle joint can be accurately placed into normal alignment by closed reduction. Any accompanying wound must be surgically debrided and closed.

Isolated dislocation of the ankle joint, without accompanying malleolar fracture, is a rare injury.

Recurrent Sprains of the Ankle Joint

Occasionally, a patient will complain of a weak ankle or an ankle that "gives way" or is repeatedly sprained. This condition can usually be traced to a specific injury in which the fibular collateral ligament ruptured and the proper diagnosis was not made. Invariably, the patient will tell of being treated for a bad ankle sprain in the past. When weight bearing is resumed, the talus may rock inward and forward on certain motions of the foot, giving rise to the sensation of instability.

The diagnosis may be confirmed by demonstrating tilt of the talus on a stress x-ray film taken with the foot forcibly inverted.

Treatment is surgical reconstruction of the fibular collateral ligament.

Recurrent Dislocation of the Peroneal Tendons

The peroneal tendons run through a bony groove behind the lateral malleolus at the ankle. In some patients, these tendons may be loosely attached in a shallow groove, allowing them to slip forward over the malleolus on active dorsiflexion of the foot. This abnormality may be associated with pain, weakness, and a "giving way" sensation about the ankle joint.

If symptoms warrant, the condition may be alleviated by surgical deepening of the peroneal groove.

Osteochondritis Dissecans

An area of osteochondritis dissecans may occasionally involve the weight bearing surface of the talus (see p. 376).

The defect should be visible on anteroposterior and lateral x-ray films.

The lesion may heal following a period of prolonged non-weight bearing. If this is unsuccessful, the fragment should be excised.

Degenerative Arthritis of the Ankle Joint

Degenerative arthritis may involve the ankle joint as part of a generalized disease process, but more commonly it involves the joint as a complication following ankle joint trauma (see p. 114). In this situation, the patient frequently gives a history of sustaining a fracture or fracture-dislocation of the ankle some years previously. Treatment of the original injury is typically followed by a period of relative calm, finally disturbed by the onset of symptoms of pain and stiffness in the ankle.

X-ray examination may disclose evidence of degenerative arthritis in the joint, usually superimposed on bone showing residual effects of trauma (Fig. 65).

Symptoms may be relieved by support to the joint in the form of an elastic bandage, Gibney boot, arch support, or brace. Intra-articular injections of hydrocortisone may be helpful. If pain and disability are severe, the operation of joint fusion may be performed for pain relief.

PYOGENIC ARTHRITIS OF THE ANKLE JOINT
(See p. 136)

TUBERCULOSIS OF THE ANKLE JOINT (See p. 139)

THE FOOT

The foot is the platform that supports the body weight during standing and moves the body during walking, running, and jumping. To bear this load most efficiently in the erect position, the foot has been constructed from a number of small bones aligned in the form of resilient arches (Fig. 188). The bones are lashed together by ligaments and supported to a certain extent by the surrounding musculature.

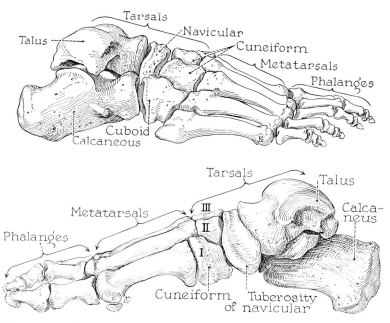

Figure 188. Skeletal anatomy of the foot. (From Hauser, E. D. W.: Diseases of the Foot.)

Structural weaknesses in the foot, imbalance between the bones and supporting musculature, or abnormal demands placed on the part may contribute to the production of symptoms referable to the feet.

The longitudinal arch of the foot spans the distance between the os calcis and the metatarsal heads. Its longer medial segment contains the os calcis, talus, navicular, three cuneiform bones, and first three metatarsal bones. Its shorter lateral border contains the os calcis, cuboid, and fourth and fifth metatarsal bones.

The anterior or metatarsal arch is formed by the heads of the five metatarsal bones. The presence of this arch can be appreciated only with the foot in a non-weight bearing position. In this posture, it can be noted that the first and fifth metatarsal heads are more prominent than the others. This arch flattens and disappears on weight bearing, as each of the five metatarsal heads bears a proportionate amount of weight.

Examination of the Feet

The feet are examined in both the non-weight bearing and the standing positions.

During the visual examination, notice is taken of any visible deformities of the feet or toes, including positional or structural abnormalities, edema, corns, calluses, or ulcerations. The status of the longitudinal arch is observed in the resting and standing positions.

The various motions allowed by the foot are checked by the examiner, and any decrease in flexibility is noted. Plantar flexion and dorsiflexion occur through the ankle joint. Eversion, or outward rotation of the foot and heel, and inversion, or inward rotation of the foot and heel, occur through the "subtalar" joints.

It is also possible to swing the forepart of the foot inward or outward in relation to the heel part of the foot, provided the heel part is firmly held by the examiner. This motion occurs through the talonavicular and calcaneocuboid joints. Outward swinging of the forepart of the foot is called forefoot abduction; inward swinging is forefoot adduction.

The muscles supplying activity to the foot are tested for strength and ability to perform. These include the anterior tibial, posterior tibial, peroneals, calf muscles, and the flexors and extensors of the toes.

The presence of any areas tender to palpation is noted. These areas are most likely to be found on the sole of the foot, in the region of the sinus tarsi, and between the metatarsal heads on the dorsum of the foot.

The toes are examined for evidence of structural deformity, joint stiffness, or callus formation.

An assessment of the circulation of the foot can be made by noting the dorsalis pedis and posterior tibial pulsations, and by evaluating the efficiency of the venous circulation.

The patient and his foot should be observed while he walks barefooted.

Congenital Disorders of the Foot

CONGENITAL CLUBFOOT (See p. 50)

CONGENITAL METATARSUS VARUS (See p. 53)

Disorders of the Arches

The arches of the foot may fail to function with full efficiency in children and adults for a variety of reasons. Breakdown of these important weight supporting structures may give rise to gait abnormalities, symptoms of pain and ache in the feet or legs, or pain referred to some distant segment of the body.

Abnormalities involving the longitudinal arch may be seen in children and adults, and are often lumped together under the descriptive term "flatfoot." Breakdown of the metatarsal arch occurs primarily in adults and, as a rule, poses no particular difficulty in diagnosis or treatment.

The descriptive term "flatfoot" is misleading and confusing when used to classify disorders associated with depression of the longitudinal arch. It is true that the foot assumes an appearance of flatness with weight bearing in all of these disorders, but the causes, and frequently the treatment, will vary. For that reason, "flatfoot," from an orthopaedic standpoint, can stand a more detailed dissection. The three most important types of flatfoot are pronation, structural flatfoot, and spastic flatfoot.

DISORDERS OF THE LONGITUDINAL ARCH IN CHILDREN

Pronation. The term "pronation" refers to the position assumed by some feet on weight bearing. Most feet called flat in children fall into this category. In this condition, the bone structure is normal, and the longitudinal arch appears unaffected in the non-weight bearing position. However, with weight bearing, congenital ligamentous laxity about the small bones of the feet allows the heel to evert and the forefoot to abduct, causing the foot to roll into a position of prona-

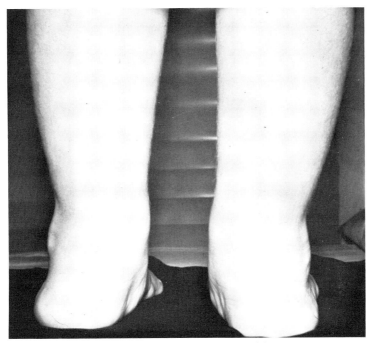

Figure 189.   Child with pronated feet.

tion (Fig. 189). The clinical impression received on viewing such feet is that of flatness of the arch.

As a rule, pronated feet are quite loose and flexible. The heel cord is usually slack, permitting extreme passive dorsiflexion of the foot. The synonym for this type of flatfoot is weak foot.

CLINICAL PICTURE.   Pronation may vary in degree and in the secondary effects produced. The most extreme degree of pronation may be noticed shortly after birth in an infant whose feet are held in a markedly everted and dorsiflexed position. This deformity is frequently called congenital calcaneovalgus, but in reality it represents the extreme degree of pronation.

At the other end of the scale is the child whose feet appear normal in the non-weight bearing attitude, but roll into slight pronation with standing. Moderate or severe pronation may delay the onset of standing or walking in an infant for several months, presumably because of the unsteadiness of the platform presented for weight bearing.

After walking begins, pronation may cause gait abnormalities. Parents may complain of an in-toe or out-toe gait in the child, or may simply describe the gait as awkward. Pronation may be a frequent cause of knock knee (see p. 377).

In later childhood, pronation may cause aching legs because of muscle fatigue due to postural strain of the leg muscles. The ache characteristically comes on at night while the child is in bed and may be relieved by massaging the affected leg.

As a rule, pronation in a child does not cause pain in the feet. However, it does cause a typical deformity of their shoes (Fig. 190).

TREATMENT. The child is placed in regular shank, hard sole, high top shoes with $1/8$-inch inner heel wedges as soon as standing position is assumed. The purpose of the wedge is to prevent the heel from everting in the standing position. The wear of the shoes is carefully watched. If treatment is effective, the shoe wear will appear balanced.

As the child's activity increases, the initial wedge usually loses its effectiveness, and the shoes may appear "undercorrected." This usually occurs between 14 and 18 months of age. At this time, the correction in the shoe may be raised to a $3/16$-inch inner heel wedge and a $1/8$-inch outer sole wedge.

At two years of age, the child may be placed in regular shank, low oxfords with a $3/16$-inch rubber longitudinal arch pad or scaphoid pad. Corrections continue until the arch tightens and tends to hold itself in the balanced position. When this occurs, the presence of the arch pad may cause a previously balanced shoe to appear "overcorrected."

Structural Flatfoot. Structural flatfoot is caused by skeletal deformities that allow depression of the longitudinal arch. Although much less common than pronation, structural flatfoot is a more serious and disabling condition.

The skeletal deformities usually found include congenital sagging or opening of the talonavicular joint, or the presence of a talus that is tilted down in a fixed plantar flexed position.

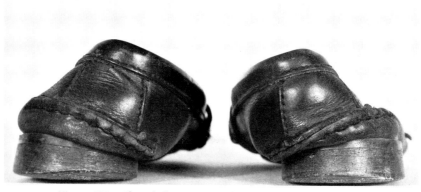

Figure 190. Shoe deformity caused by severely pronated feet.

A structural flatfoot soon assumes a flat appearance with or without weight bearing, but maintains good flexibility except for possible limitation of dorsiflexion. This type of flatfoot is frequently associated with pain in the feet.

X-ray examination confirms the diagnosis.

Treatment depends on the type of skeletal abnormality present. Some feet may be adequately supported by molded metal arch supports; others may require operative intervention for their correction.

Spastic Flatfoot. Spastic flatfoot is associated with a constant tightness or spasm of the peroneal tendons that pulls the foot into an everted or flat position. The peroneal spasm is usually associated with a tarsal abnormality, frequently a congenital bone bridge that locks the os calcis and navicular bones together.

A spastic flatfoot is usually very painful because of the peroneal spasm. The foot is held in rigid eversion by the tight peroneal tendons, thus maintaining a constant flat appearance.

The presence of tarsal abnormalities may be demonstrated on oblique x-ray views of the foot.

Some patients with spastic flatfoot may obtain relief of pain by the use of molded metal arch supports. A few patients may obtain pain relief by manipulation of the foot under anesthesia. Most patients, however, require surgical intervention for relief. If the diagnosis is made before secondary joint changes occur, resection of the bone bridge may be curative.

DISORDERS OF THE LONGITUDINAL ARCH IN ADULTS

Flatfoot in the adult is associated with painful feet and legs and has, as a rule, the same causes as flatfoot in children.

The most common cause of flatfoot in the adult is residual pronation. Some of these patients give a history of wearing shoe corrections since childhood. Others may deny having problems with their feet until the onset of foot pain. Some patients with pronation escape trouble during childhood only to develop painful feet as adults. In these instances, arch breakdown is usually aided by occupational demands for prolonged standing or walking, by obesity, by poor muscle tone, or by the use of shoes that do not give adequate support.

In some instances, severe pronation in the adult may be associated with excessive sweating of the feet, edema about the foot and ankle, and varicose veins.

The symptoms produced by pronated feet in the adult can usually be relieved by the use of resilient longitudinal arch supports.

Painful feet in the adult caused by structural or spastic flatfoot may require operative fusion of the "subtalar" joints for pain relief (triple arthrodesis).

DISORDERS OF THE METATARSAL ARCH

If the bones forming the metatarsal arch are asked to bear a disproportionate amount of weight, thick calluses may form on the ball of the foot, and the patient may experience a painful burning sensation in this area with weight bearing. This condition is known as *metatarsalgia*.

Metatarsalgia occurs primarily in the adult and is more common in the female. It may occur alone but is most frequently seen in association with pronation. In addition to the burning pain in the front of the foot and the callus formation, tenderness to palpation is usually noted between the metatarsal heads on the dorsum of the foot. Severe cases may be associated with clawing of the toes.

Symptoms can usually be relieved by the use of rubber metatarsal arch supports. These come in various sizes and are placed in the shoe to lie just behind the metatarsal heads.

Disorders of the Toes

HALLUX VALGUS (BUNION)

In general usage, the term "hallux valgus" or "bunion" refers to a deformity of the large toe consisting of three elements: lateral angulation of the large toe toward the second toe, bony enlargement of the medial side of the head of the first metatarsal bone at the metatarsophalangeal joint, and formation of a bursal sac over the point of the bony enlargement. In addition to being laterally deviated, the large toe frequently rotates medially on its long axis (Fig. 191). As the large toe progresses in a lateral direction, the long toe extensor tendon becomes displaced laterally and aids in maintaining the abnormal position. The deformity is frequently bilateral.

It has been stated that a congenitally short first metatarsal bone or a first metatarsal bone that is deviated medially is a factor in causing bunion. It is also believed that the wearing of pointed and poor fitting shoes or high heels is a contributing factor.

Bunions are found most frequently in women at or just past middle age. They may be painless and may give concern only because of a shoe fitting problem. Pressure of the shoe against the bursa may cause painful inflammation of the bursal sac. Extreme lateral deviation of

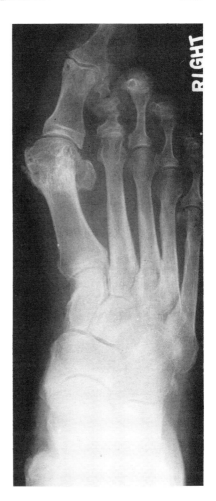

Figure 191. AP x-ray of foot with bunion.

the large toe may cause an overlapping of the second toe on the large toe. Bunion formation may be associated with hammer toe deformity of some of the remaining toes (Fig. 192).

Conservative treatment of bunion consists of wearing shoes that provide a wide forefoot or "bunion pocket," and the use of bunion pads to relieve shoe pressure on the bursal sac.

If the deformity is painful or extreme enough to make shoe fitting a problem, operative correction may be carried out. There are many operative techniques for removing the bursal sac and bony enlargement of the medial side of the first metatarsal head and correcting the lateral angulation of the large toe.

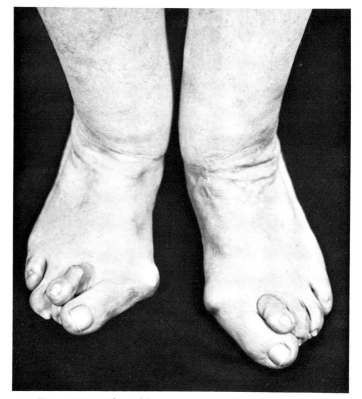

Figure 192. Bilateral bunions with overlapped second toes.

HALLUX RIGIDUS

The term "hallux rigidus" refers to a painful stiffness of the first metatarsophalangeal joint that is due to degenerative arthritis. The arthritic changes may accompany generalized degenerative arthritis or may follow local trauma to this joint.

Pain is usually first noted with walking when the joint stiffness prevents normal dorsiflexion of the large toe. The first metatarsophalangeal joint, in addition to being stiff, becomes enlarged and tender. X-ray examination reveals narrowing of the joint space with subchondral bone sclerosis and spur formation at the joint margins.

Conservative treatment consists of passive manual stretching of the first metatarsophalangeal joint combined with the use of intra-articular hydrocortisone. The sole of the shoe may be stiffened to decrease pain at the joint on walking.

If symptoms warrant, operation can be carried out and a joint fusion or an arthroplasty performed.

HAMMER TOE

The term "hammer toe" refers to a positional deformity of the toe consisting of a flexion contracture of the proximal interphalangeal joint and extension of the metatarsophalangeal joint. The end of the toe tends to point straight downward in the shoe, and painful calluses may develop on the tip of the toe and on the dorsum at the flexed interphalangeal joint (Fig. 193).

The deformity may be congenital in origin or may follow depression of the metatarsal arch with imbalance between the flexors and extensors of the toes.

Conservative treatment consists of passive, manual stretching of the tight proximal interphalangeal joint, and the use of a metatarsal arch support. If symptoms warrant, operation can be carried out and the flexed proximal interphalangeal joint fused in a straight position.

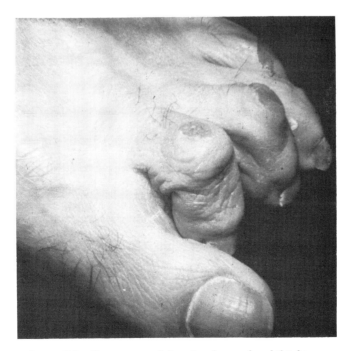

Figure 193.   Hammer toe deformity of second and third toes.

BUNIONETTE

Bunionette, or little bunion, is a bony enlargement of the lateral side of the head of the fifth metatarsal bone at the metatarsophalangeal joint. It is usually associated with an overlying bursal sac and a medial deviation of the fifth toe.

As in the case of bunion, treatment of a bunionette may be conservative or surgical.

INGROWN TOENAIL

The term "ingrown toenail" refers to a common and painful ailment usually affecting the outer margin of the large toenail. The nail margin grows into the soft lateral nail groove and surrounding skin. This is usually caused by the pressure of tight shoes or socks on a nail that has been cut too short. As a rule, the skin fold becomes infected and hypertrophied with granulation tissue.

Mild cases may respond to soaking the toe in hot water and tucking a small piece of cotton beneath the corners of the nail to raise it from the skin fold. If this is not successful, the involved margin of nail and a portion of the hypertrophied skin fold may be excised under local anesthesia.

PLANTAR NEUROMA (MORTON'S TOE)

The most lateral branch of the medial plantar nerve lies in the third webspace of the foot between the third and fourth metatarsal heads and supplies sensation to the third and fourth toes. Chronic impingement of this nerve between the metatarsal heads may lead to the formation of a neuroma or thickening of this branch of the nerve. Pressure on the neuroma with weight bearing may produce rather characteristic painful symptoms known as plantar neuroma or Morton's toe.

The condition is more common in women. The pain is usually localized to the metatarsal area of the foot, with radiation into the third and fourth toes. Most patients state they can relieve the pain by removing the shoe and massaging the ball of the foot. Occasionally, numbness and tingling are noted in the affected toes.

The pain can usually be reproduced by exerting downward pressure in the third webspace with a small object, such as the eraser end of a lead pencil, while maintaining upward pressure with the thumb on the sole of the foot between the third and fourth metatarsal heads.

The symptoms arising from pressure on a plantar neuroma are

often relieved by the use of a metatarsal arch support. If this is not successful, the enlarged segment of nerve may be excised at operation.

Local Foot Problems

CORNS

Corns are localized, painful, hard thickenings of skin due to continuous shoe pressure on bony prominences. They may be found associated with bunions and bunionettes, beneath the metatarsal heads on the sole of the foot, and on the dorsal surface of hammer toes at the flexed interphalangeal joint.

A corn may be softened with hot water or preparations containing salicylic acid, and then trimmed with a scalpel or razor blade. Steps must also be taken to relieve continuous shoe pressure on bony prominences.

SOFT CORNS

Soft corns are found between the toes and are produced when a small projecting bone spur on one toe presses into the skin of the adjacent toe. They are moist and painful.

A piece of cotton placed between the toes may separate them sufficiently to relieve pain. If symptoms warrant, surgical excision of the projecting bone spur may be carried out.

CALLUS

Callus is a circumscribed thickening of the skin similar to a corn, but generally larger in extent. Callus is found most frequently on the sole of the foot at the points bearing an abnormal amount of weight. Callus formation on the ball of the foot commonly accompanies depression of the metatarsal arch.

PLANTAR WART

A plantar wart is an extremely painful vascular papillomatous growth that may occur in any part of the skin on the sole of the foot. The surface of the wart is flat and continuous with the adjacent skin, and is pressed inward by weight bearing. Callus may form over the surface of the wart, increasing the degree of local tenderness.

Plantar wart may be removed by local excision with electrocoagulation or by surgical excision. Recurrence is not uncommon.

Traumatic Disorders

PAINFUL HEELS

The complaint of pain in the heel with weight bearing is frequently heard from children and adults. The most common cause in children is calcaneal apophysitis or Sever's disease (see p. 91). The most common cause in adults is plantar bursitis (see p. 123).

MARCH FRACTURE (FATIGUE FRACTURE)

Fracture of a metatarsal shaft, usually the second or third, may result from the stress associated with weight bearing after prolonged walking has exhausted the muscular and tendinous support of the foot. This type of stress or fatigue fracture is especially common in army recruits during their basic training.

Pain is usually noticed by the patient not at the moment of fracture, as in traumatic fractures, but a week or so later, after callus begins to appear. X-ray examination at that time typically reveals the fracture line surrounded by exuberant callus formation.

March fractures heal uneventfully with immobilization, which may be supplied by an adhesive strapping or plaster cast.

FRACTURES OF THE FOOT

Toe. Fracture of a toe may be caused by a weight falling on the toe or by stubbing the toe while barefoot. As a rule, these are painful but not serious injuries. The objective of treatment is to maintain the alignment of the toe so that overlapping or hammer toe does not result. This frequently can be accomplished by strapping the broken toe to its neighbor. If multiple toe fractures are present, a walking cast may be applied for immobilization.

Metatarsal. Fractures of the metatarsal bones are common and may be caused by twisting injuries to the forefoot or by heavy objects dropping on the foot. The objective of treatment of metatarsal shaft fractures is to maintain the alignment of the longitudinal arch.

A fracture through the neck of a metatarsal may allow the metatarsal head to displace toward the sole of the foot. Normal alignment must be restored to prevent the subsequent development of a painful plantar callus.

Many displaced metatarsal fractures can be treated by closed reduction and immobilization in a plaster cast. If this is unsuccessful, skeletal traction or open reduction with internal metallic fixation may be elected.

Heel.   The os calcis is the most frequently fractured of the tarsal bones. The injury may be relatively insignificant or very complex. The fracture may be caused by a powerful contraction of the gastrocnemius and soleus muscles, or by direct trauma to the heel. As a rule, two general types of fracture are seen: an avulsion fracture through the posterior portion of the bone, and comminuted or crush fractures of the bone involving the talocalcaneal joint. The objective of treatment is to restore contour of the bone, particularly the plantar surface and the talocalcaneal joint if possible.

Some os calcis fractures may be treated by closed reduction followed by plaster immobilization. Other fractures may require skeletal traction or open reduction.

The major complication after os calcis fracture is the development of traumatic arthritis in the talocalcaneal joint. If this occurs, the patient will have pain on weight bearing, particularly with motions requiring eversion and inversion of the foot (Fig. 186). If the pain arising from traumatic arthritis in the talocalcaneal joint cannot be controlled by nonoperative treatment methods, the operation of triple arthrodesis is carried out.

References

Adams, J. A.: Transient Synovitis of the hip joint in children. J. Bone and Joint Surg., *45-B*:471, 1963.

Alexander, C. J.: The etiology of femoral epiphyseal slipping. J. Bone and Joint Surg., *48-B*:299, 1966.

Anderson, L. D., Hamsa, W. R., Jr., and Waring, T. L.: Femoral head prosthesis. J. Bone and Joint Surg., *46-A*:1049, 1964.

Anderson, R. L.: Conservative treatment of fractures of the femur. J. Bone and Joint Surg., *46-A*:1371, 1967.

Barnes, R.: Fracture of the neck of the femur. J. Bone and Joint Surg., *49-B*:607, 1967.

Bianco, A. J.: Slipped capital femoral epiphysis. J. Bone and Joint Surg., *47-A*:432, 1965.

Bianco, A. J.: Treatment of mild slipping of the capital femoral epiphysis. J. Bone and Joint Surg., *47-A*:387, 1965.

Blount, W. P.: Osteotomy and the treatment of osteoarthritis of the hip. J. Bone and Joint Surg., *46-A*:1297, 1964.

Brahms, M. A.: Common foot problems. J. Bone and Joint Surg., *49-A*:1653, 1967.

Brown, E. W., and Urban, J. J.: Early weight bearing treatment in open fractures of the tibia: an end result study of 63 cases. J. Bone and Joint Surg., *51-A*:59, 1969.

Burrows, H. J.: Slipped upper femoral epiphysis — Characteristics of 100 cases. J. Bone and Joint Surg., *39-B*:641, 1957.

Charnley, J.: The bonding of prostheses to bone by cement. J. Bone and Joint Surg., *46-B*:518, 1964.

Charnley, J. (Ed.): Symposium on total hip replacement. Clin. Orth. and Rel. Res., *No. 72*, 1970.

Chung, S. M. K., and Ralston, E. L.: Necrosis of the femoral head associated with sickle-cell anemia and its genetic variant. J. Bone and Joint Surg., *51-A*:33, 1969.

D'Aubigne, R. M., et al.: Idiopathic necrosis of the femoral head in adults. J. Bone and Joint Surg., *47-B*:612, 1965.

Fahey, J. J.: Orthopaedic anatomy of the hip. Am. Academy of Orthopaedic Surgeons Instructional Course Lectures, Vol. IV. Ann Arbor: J. W. Edwards, 1947.

Fahey, J. J., and O'Brien, E. T.: Acute slipped capital femoral epiphysis. J. Bone and Joint Surg., 47-A:1105, 1965.

Ferguson, A. B., Jr.: The pathology of degenerative arthritis of the hip and the use of osteotomy in its treatment. Clin. Orth. and Rel. Res., No. 77, 1971.

Giannestras, N. J.: Foot Disorders: Medical and Surgical Management, 2nd Edition. Philadelphia: Lea and Febiger, 1973.

Helfet, A. J.: Diagnosis and management of internal derangement of the knee joint. Am. Academy of Orthopaedic Surgeons Instructional Course Lectures, Vol. XIX. St. Louis: C. V. Mosby Co., 1970.

Hinchey, J. J., and Day, P. L.: Primary prosthetic replacement in fresh femoral neck fractures. J. Bone and Joint Surg., 46-A:223, 1964.

Hirsch, C., and Frankel, V. H.: Analysis of forces producing fractures of the proximal end of the femur. J. Bone and Joint Surg., 42-B:633, 1960.

Jones, J. P., Jr., and Engelman, E. P.: Osseous avascular necrosis associated with systemic abnormalities. Arthritis Rheum., 9,5:728, 1966.

Kelikian, H.: Hallux Valgus, Allied Deformities of the Forefoot and Metatarsalgia. Philadelphia: W. B. Saunders Co., 1965.

Lipscomb, P. R., and McCaslin, F. E., Jr.: Arthrodesis of the hip. J. Bone and Joint Surg., 43-A:923, 1961.

Margo, M. K.: Surgical treatment of conditions of the forepart of the foot. J. Bone and Joint Surg., 49-A:1665, 1967.

Martin, A. F.: The pathomechanics of the knee joint. J. Bone and Joint Surg., 42-A:13, 1960.

Patterson, R. J., Bickel, W. H., and Dahlin, D. C.: Idiopathic avascular necrosis of the head of the femur. A study of fifty-two cases. J. Bone and Joint Surg., 46-A:267, 1964.

Robert, N.: Osteochondritis dissecans. J. Bone and Joint Surg., 39-B:219, 1957.

Smillie, I. S.: Injuries of the knee joint. Edinburgh and London: E. & S. Livingstone, 1970.

Stinchfield, F. E. (Ed.): Statistics on total hip replacement. Clin. Orth. and Rel. Res., No. 95, 1973.

Voshell, A. F.: Anatomy of the knee joint. Am. Academy of Orthopaedic Surgeons Instructional Course Lectures, Vol. XIII: 247. Ann Arbor: J. W. Edwards, 1956.

Chapter Fifteen

Orthopaedic Rehabilitation

*Phillip J. Marone, M.D.**

The reader is reminded that the definition of orthopaedics given in Chapter 1 contained the admonition that this discipline is concerned also with the restoration of the function of the skeletal system, its articulations, and associated structures. This means, of course, that the treating physician has a responsibility to restore his patient to normal living after illness or injury. Persons born with afflictions of the musculoskeletal system grow and develop with compensatory mechanisms that enable them to function within the scope of their disability. However, if a person is sound and then becomes disabled because of injury or disease, the return to full function frequently becomes a major effort.

The purpose of this chapter is to bring to your attention some of the methods utilized to return these patients to the point of being able to care for themselves.

TERMINOLOGY

It is essential that some of the terms used in orthopaedic rehabilitation be defined before the principles of orthopaedic rehabilitation can be discussed.

RANGE OF MOTION (R.O.M.)

The term range of motion refers to joint motion or the ability to move a part through its arc of motion at a joint. Many diseases of the

*Chief of Orthopaedic Surgery, Methodist Hospital, Philadelphia, Pa., and Clinical Associate Professor of Orthopaedic Surgery, Jefferson Medical College of Thomas Jefferson University, Philadelphia, Pa.

musculoskeletal system cause, or are associated with, impaired joint motion. In testing joint range, the physician must be aware of the normal range of motion for each specific joint (Fig. 160).

The instrument used for these determinations is called a *goniometer*, and the R.O.M. is conveniently expressed in degrees.

MUSCLE TESTING (M.T.)

This assessment is essential in determining the degree of impairment in affected muscles. The usual method of testing is manual and subjective. Various degrees of resistance are applied to the muscles, which are graded accordingly. The patient is placed in a test position that varies for each muscle or muscle group to be tested. The patient is then asked to move the muscles being tested through their full R.O.M. The muscle or muscle group is graded according to the response elicited. Three methods of recording these actions are in general use: (1) grade 0 through 5; (2) percentage of normal, 0 per cent to 100 per cent; (3) the Lovett scale, zero to normal. Although these methods of recording are interchangeable, an examiner should develop his skills in only one method. The Lovett scale is a very popular method of recording muscle strength. The definition of the terms used in the Lovett scale is as follows:

Zero — no contraction felt or seen.

Trace — muscle is felt to tighten, but cannot produce movement.

Poor — motion with gravity is eliminated, but muscle cannot function against gravity.

Fair — patient can raise the part against gravity, but without any outside resistance.

Good — patient can raise the part as in fair, but with resistance added.

Normal — muscle overcomes a greater resistance than a good muscle and, in actuality, is the same strength as its contralateral muscle when it is tested.

Muscle testing and its accompanying R.O.M. are fundamental in the diagnosis, evaluation, and programming of the disabled orthopaedic patient.

ACTIVITIES OF DAILY LIVING (A.D.L.)

The A.D.L. are the basic activities essential to carrying on daily life, including transportation and working where applicable. The goal to be reached in A.D.L. is to make the patient self-sufficient. A very close interrelationship exists between A.D.L. and exercise. The goals to be achieved depend upon whether one is dealing with bed patients, wheelchair patients, or ambulatory patients. Orthopaedics deals mostly with ambulatory patients, and the goal should be to return these patients to their environment as efficiently as possible.

OCCUPATIONAL THERAPY (O.T.)

Occupational therapy is the art and science of directing man's response to selected action to promote and maintain health, to prevent disability, and to treat or train patients with physical dysfunctions.

The occupational therapist, therefore, instructs and actively involves patients in a wide variety of purposeful activities common to their immediate environment or culture. They are thus stimulated to develop what is necessary to be productive and independent.

While it is usually the more seriously disabled patient who requires occupational therapy, it is necessary to be aware of its availability, as many times patients will achieve their goals more quickly with this service.

GAIT

Gait is defined as the manner or style of walking. No physical examination of the locomotor system is complete unless the gait pattern is analyzed. Limp is defined as a pathologic gait. To recognize a pathologic gait, one must be familiar with the normal gait pattern (p. 338).

The gait cycle consists of two phases: *stance phase* and *swing phase*. These phases repetitiously and rhythmically alternate to produce normal locomotion. When these motions become asymmetric, they are considered pathologic.

The stance or support phase starts with the foot in the forward position and the heel down. It ends with the toe pushing off and the foot leaving the ground, and measures longer than the swing phase. The swing phase, shorter in duration than the stance phase, begins when the foot leaves the ground and lasts through the next heel strike. There is a brief period when both legs are on the ground simultaneously. This is called the *period of double support.*

Gait is a three dimensional activity. When one moves forward or backward, several forces work to produce three dimensional displacement of the body. Even though the legs play the most conspicuous role in ambulation, other body elements, such as pelvis, trunk, and even the upper extremities, also play very important parts. All of these elements, consequently, must be carefully observed in a gait analysis.

ORTHOTICS

Orthotics deals with the application of exoskeletal devices to limit or to assist motion of any given segment of the human body. These exoskeletal devices are called *orthoses* when applied to patients suffering from neuromuscular or skeletal disorders. This, therefore, is a more inclusive term for devices than the old terms, such as brace or splint.

PROSTHETICS

Prosthetics is the addition or application to the body of an artificial device called a *prosthesis* to replace partially or totally missing extremities or organs.

The terms quadriplegia, paraplegia, and hemiplegia have already been defined in the chapter on neuromuscular disorders (p. 151).

PRINCIPLES OF PHYSICAL MEDICINE

THERMAL THERAPY

Heat is one of the measures most commonly employed in orthopaedic rehabilitation. It is frequently utilized before massage and exercise because it enhances the effects of the subsequent treatment measures. The physiologic effects of heat are to bring about an increase in tissue temperature, to produce vasodilatation, and to increase local circulation. These changes cause an increase in tissue metabolic activity, which leads to a further increase in tissue temperature and further vasodilatation, thus increasing transduction of tissue fluids. Excessive basal heat is controlled by blood flow away from the heated area to other parts of the body. Another well-known effect of heat therapy is mild sedation with relief of pain and muscular tension.

The methods of heat application are classified as *radiant, conductive,* or *conversive* heating. Each form of heat has its own effects and indications for use. Radiant heat is infrared. Conductive heating is the direct application of heat to the body in the form of hot water bottles, paraffin, or electrically heated pads. Conversive heating is an indirect form of heat resulting from the conversion of various forms of primary energies to heat in the body tissues. Radiant and conductive heating are superficial and readily available.

Superficial heating can be supplied by the infrared lamp, whirlpool bath, Hubbard tanks, hot packs, contrast baths (hot and cold), and paraffin baths. Any form of superficial heating takes between 20 and

30 minutes to produce the desired effect, and causes its maximal temperature increase in the skin and less in the deeper tissues. There is no significant rise in temperature beyond 1 to 2 cm. beneath the skin surface. The most commonly utilized means of applying superficial heat are the infrared lamp and the forms of hydrotherapy. Little danger of overdosage exists with superficial heating if local circulation and skin sensation are intact. The main contraindications to the use of superficial heating are the absence of skin sensation and a decrease in blood supply to the part to be heated. Superficial heat should never be applied to a part during the first four hours following an acute injury.

Deep or conversive heating is the result of high frequency alternating currents, and its margin of safety is lower than that of the superficial forms of heating. The deep heating devices in general use are short-wave diathermy, microwave, and ultrasound.

Short-wave diathermy has a maximum penetration of 2 to 3 cm. beneath the skin surface over a period of 30 minutes. The high frequency currents tend to spread as they enter the body and tend to heat a fairly large area. The large area heated and the margin of safety in its usage are advantages of short-wave diathermy over microwave and ultrasound. Although short-wave diathermy gives more equal heating than infrared, it possesses no other advantage over the superficial forms of heating.

Microwave is applied by means of radiated electromagnetic waves, which must go through a director or head focused several inches away from the skin surface. A layer of subcutaneous fat one-half inch thick will absorb 30 per cent of microwave energy, and part of microwave energy is lost by reflection from the body surface.

Ultrasound is energy that comes from a series of mechanical vibrations. Direct contact with skin is necessary for ultrasound treatment, since these waves do not travel through air. A coupling media, such as mineral oil, is a necessary part of its use. The subcutaneous fat must be at least 2 inches thick before 30 per cent of ultrasound energy is absorbed. No ultrasound energy is lost by reflection from the body surface.

In deep tissues of high water content, such as muscle, ultrasound has a greater penetration than microwave. The reverse is true if the tissue is of low water content, as is bone. Adequate deep heating effects can be obtained with either source of heat to a tissue depth of 5 to 6 cm. With proper application, an effective rise in temperature will occur within 15 to 20 minutes with microwave, and within 3 to 10 minutes with ultrasound. The area that may be treated with either modality is small. The use of these modalities must be discontinued if unpleasant sensations of heat occur.

Ultrasound or microwave may be indicated to supply deep heat in the treatment of bursitis, myositis, tenosynovitis, and tendinitis. Neither should be used in the presence of infection, malignant disease, peripheral vascular disease, acute hemorrhage, a metallic implant, or over a fracture site before callus has formed. Both should be used with caution over growing bone or over any bony surface that lies superficially beneath the skin surface. They should also be used with caution in the region of the eyes, over the testes, or over larger nerve structures. Deep heating modalities should never be used in the presence of an acute injury.

COLD THERAPY

Cold therapy has a more limited use than heat therapy, but it is occasionally of value because it causes vasoconstriction, with consequent decrease in local tissue blood flow, decrease in local metabolic activity, and decrease in local tissue temperature. These effects produce a decrease in edema or local swelling of the part. Ice bags and cold compresses are used extensively to minimize the local reaction in a part that results from acute trauma, such as sprains, fractures, or dislocations. If edema or local swelling can be minimized in an injured part by the use of cold therapy, the patient will respond more favorably to the range of motion and exercise program needed to return him to his pre-injury state of function. The local use of ice also seems to decrease muscle spasm and pain in chronic joint problems such as strains. It has been theorized that cold anesthetizes the skin and reflexly causes muscles to become relaxed and less painful. The use of cold therapy is contraindicated in the presence of peripheral vascular disorders.

Contrast baths (hot and cold) have some beneficial effect in the reduction of tissue edema. They are thought to produce alternating contraction and relaxation of blood vessels, with a significant increase in local blood flow. Contrast baths are used as follows: hot (110° to 115°) for 10 minutes, cold for one minute; hot for four minutes, cold for one minute; hot for four minutes, cold for one minute; hot for four minutes, cold for one minute; finish the baths with four minutes of hot water. Contrast baths are used for the relief of local pain and to effect a decrease in local tissue swelling.

MASSAGE

Massage is a therapeutic measure performed by a trained therapist. Its use should always be preceded by some form of heating.

Many physiological effects are attributed to massage. Its use seems to be followed by an increase in blood flow, which increases the interchange of substances between the cells and the bloodstream. External mechanical pressure increases the flow of lymph from tissue spaces into the venous circulation. The mechanical pressure of massage removes excess tissue fluid and decreases the likelihood of fibrosis. Connective tissue fibrosis responds to massage by the mechanical stretching and disruption of fibers by friction. Muscle nutrition improves following massage because the mechanical stimulation aids in removal of the extravascular fluids.

Two types of massage are generally utilized. Stroking (*effleurage*) is superficial and light. Compression (*petrussage*) consists of kneading a portion of a muscle or a group of muscles between the thumb, its eminence, and the fingers. The muscle is then compressed from side to side as the hand moves up the muscle in the direction of the venous flow.

Massage is indicated for the relief of pain, relaxation of muscle tension, improvement in local circulation, reduction of induration or edema, and the stretching of adhesions. Massage is contraindicated in the presence of acute inflammation, malignant tumors, and acute peripheral vascular disorders, such as phlebitis or thrombosis.

As mentioned previously, massage should be preceded by the use of local heat, as this will enhance the desired effects of the massage. Both heat and massage should be followed by an active or passive exercise program so that the maximum benefits of exercise can be obtained.

THERAPEUTIC EXERCISE

Therapeutic exercise is utilized to improve the balance and stability of the body. Its objectives are to improve coordination, to increase endurance and power, and to increase joint range of motion. Once an indication for therapeutic exercise has been identified and a purposeful goal established, the therapeutic exercise program must be carefully planned or the goal will not be reached. The exercise program should be on a graduated basis, tailored to the patient's needs as identified by periodic re-evaluation. A therapeutic exercise program can be successful only with a cooperative patient and an adequate prescription designed to improve what can be improved and to stabilize what cannot be improved.

The following types of exercises are available:

Passive. This is exercise that is accomplished by a therapist with no activity on the part of the patient. This form of exercise prevents joint contractures and maintains a normal joint range of motion. It is usually employed in a patient whose muscles are paralyzed or very weak.

Active Assistive. This form of exercise is usually the first step in a muscle re-education program. Strength can be obtained only by active contraction of the muscle involved on the part of the patient, with the therapist acting as an assistant by supporting the weight of the extremity so that gravity is eliminated or resistance overcome. This form of exercise not only helps to strengthen muscles but also aids range of motion and muscle coordination.

Active. This form of exercise is performed actively by the patient, who contracts the muscle with resistance and against the pull of gravity. Active exercise aids in increasing strength and improving function of the part. It may be started when a muscle is rated in the fair range

Resistive. This is an active exercise program with resistance added. It is usually carried out by applying manual resistance throughout the range of joint motion. Resistive exercise is used only when the muscle is rated good to normal. Its major purpose is to develop muscle strength.

Progressive Resistive Exercise (P.R.E.). This is essentially the same as resistive exercise, except that progressive resistance is added by means of weight varying from a light load to a load maximal for a muscle. The aim of this type of exercise is to increase the strength and endurance of the exercised muscle as quickly as possible.

AMBULATION

There are many devices available to assist a disabled patient to become ambulatory. The goal of rehabilitation is to enable the patient to become as independent as possible, either with or without the aid of a device. The type of device chosen and the length of time it will have to be used by the patient depend greatly upon the medical reason for disability. A patient with a fracture of a bone in the lower extremity is usually considered to have a temporary problem and is not as difficult to ambulate as a patient with paraplegia, which is a permanent problem. However, before an effort is made to ambulate a patient with either a temporarily or permanently disabling medical problem, it first must be determined that the patient has sufficient muscle strength and coordination to handle an ambulation program. If he does not, he must undergo an extensive exercise and conditioning program before ambulation can be realistically attempted. The standard ambulation aids are as follows:

1. Crutches (Metal or wood)
   a. Conventional
   b. Adjustable
   c. Lofstrand

2. Canes (metal or wood)
   a. Conventional (C curve or T top)
   b. Tripod
   c. Quadriped
3 Walkers (metal)

There are two methods in general use to measure a patient for crutches. One method is to measure from the patient's anterior axillary fold to the bottom of the shoe or heel and add an additional 2 inches to the measurement. The second method is to measure the patient from the anterior axillary fold to a point 6 inches lateral to the side of his foot. The handpiece of the crutch should be adjusted so that the elbow assumes a 30 degree flexion attitude with the wrist in extension. Lofstrand crutches, canes, and walkers can also be measured with the patient's elbow in a 30 degree flexion attitude with the wrist in extension.

Occasionally special adaptations become necessary because of problems existing in the upper extremities. These special adaptations can be modified by an orthotist for the individual patient and his problem.

There are seven different aided gait patterns, and the one selected should depend upon the patient's ability to take steps with either one or both of the lower extremities.

1. Four-Point Alternate Crutch Gait.   This gait has the following sequence: right crutch, left foot; left crutch, right foot. This is a simple gait that is used if weight bearing is allowed and if the patient can place one foot in front of the other. It is a safe gait pattern, as there are always three points of support on the floor.

2. Two-Point Alternate Crutch Gait.   This gait has the following sequence: right crutch and left foot simultaneously, followed by left crutch and right foot. This is a speeding up of the four-point gait, but it is not as safe, as only two points are supporting the body at one time.

3. Three-Point Crutch Gait.   In this gait pattern, both crutches and the weaker lower extremity start out, followed by the stronger lower extremity. This gait is used when one lower extremity cannot take full weight bearing and the other one can support the whole body weight. Orthopaedists frequently prescribe this gait for patients who have suffered lower extremity or pelvic trauma. The amount of weight borne on the affected extremity can be modified by allowing weight bearing to vary from simple touching down of the toes of the extremity to full weight bearing. The amount of weight borne on the extremity is usually monitored by the pain tolerance of the patient.

4. and 5. Tripod Crutch Gait.   This is used when a patient has no active means of placing one extremity ahead of the other, as would occur in paraplegia. There are two tripod gaits in use: the *tripod alter-*

nate (drug to) is first mastered, and then the *tripod simultaneous* (a faster, but not as safe, gait) is taught.

6. and 7. Swing Crutch Gait. There are two variations of this type of gait, the *swing to* gait and the *swing through* gait. Both are speedier modifications of the tripod gaits, but they require more energy output to balance safely.

In summary, walking aids, whether they be crutches, canes, or walkers, are utilized to assist the patient in becoming ambulatory. Each patient will have an aided gait tailored to fit his own problem. Whenever possible, at least two gaits should be taught, one to be used for speed and the other to be used for safety. It must be remembered that the use of walking aids greatly adds to the energy requirements of the patient. Older patients, and patients with medically debilitating illnesses, must be instructed with walking aids and gait patterns that are the least fatiguing.

THE REHABILITATION OF THE AMPUTEE

LOWER EXTREMITY AMPUTATION

The majority of amputations performed in civilian medical practice are of the lower extremities. The chief medical reasons for amputation in a civilian practice are peripheral vascular diseases, diabetes, and severe trauma. If amputation becomes necessary, the surgeon must make every effort to save as much limb length as possible for prosthetic fitting. It is difficult for a patient with a short stump to ambulate satisfactorily in a prosthesis, and the gait pattern developed is less cosmetically acceptable than the pattern developed by the patient with a long stump. An amputee will require a good stump and a comfortable, cosmetically acceptable prosthetic device to be rehabilitated satisfactorily. If at all possible, the surgeon should endeavor to save the knee joint. If an amputation is carried out above the knee, the prosthetic device must contain a mechanical knee joint, which adds another dimension to the prosthesis and is energy consuming and awkward for the patient.

At the present time, when amputation is performed for peripheral vascular disease or diabetes, it is more usual to be able to save the knee joint than not. This is a decided reversal of the earlier trend that has occurred only over the past two decades. One of the chief reasons for the reversal is the use of the rigid dressing technique of amputation surgery With this technique, the surgeon applies a cast in the nature of a patellar tendon bearing socket immediately after closing the amputation stump. The added resistance to swelling and the "mechanical pump set-up" combat edema and result in more rapid tissue healing.

The type of amputation performed and the prosthetic component required vary according to the amputation site, which is dictated essentially by the underlying disease or trauma.

Patients undergoing toe amputation need no special prosthetic device for ambulation. If amputation is required through the metatarsal or tarsal area of the foot, either a filling device or a special prosthesis will be necessary for the shoe.

Amputation through the ankle joint is called a Syme amputation. Its chief advantage is that the stump is end bearing, but the stump has a tendency to a bulbous shape that is cosmetically objectionable to most female patients. The prosthetic device used for a patient who has undergone a Syme amputation is called the Syme prosthesis. Along with most of the other lower extremity prosthetic devices, the Syme prosthesis has a S.A.C.H. foot (solid ankle, cushioned heel).

A below knee amputation level may vary from anywhere above the malleoli to 5 cm below the tibial plateau. The actual site of amputation below the knee will have to depend upon the level of available good skin and muscle. Ideally, a 15 cm. length stump should be sought in a below knee amputation. The prosthesis used for a patient with a below knee amputation is of the patellar tendon bearing, below knee type, with or without an added thigh lacer. The thigh lacer is necessary for patients with short or tender stumps, as it helps distribute the pressures about the stump and adds to stump comfort. It also serves as an added suspensory mechanism in a patient with a very short stump. The old conventional type of prosthesis (open ended) is still occasionally utilized, especially for those patients with distal stump pain, skin problems in the stump, or recurrent edema of the stump.

An above knee amputation should be performed anywhere from 10 cm above the knee joint to 10 cm. below the hip joint. The distance of 10 cm above the knee joint is required for the mechanical knee that is added to the prosthesis. Many types of knee mechanisms are available for the patient with an above knee amputation. The one most commonly used is called the *single axis constant friction knee*. The socket of the prosthesis is of the total contact design, and the top is quadrilateral in shape. This tends to shift most of the weight to the ischial tuberosity, with the remainder distributed peripherally about the stump. The prosthesis can be suspended by suction or a suctionless arrangement. A suction socket should not be used in conditions associated with skin changes, local edema, or skin ulceration. The patient with an above knee amputation cannot develop a gait as cosmetically acceptable as that of the patient with a below knee amputation. The energy required to propel an above knee prosthesis is much greater than the energy necessary to propel a below knee prosthesis.

Occasionally a patient will be seen who requires a hip disarticulation, hemipelvectomy, or hemicorporectomy. Prosthetic devices have been designed for these patients, and they consist of modifications of the Canadian hip prostheses and other types of pelvic support prosthetic devices. The energy necessary to propel these devices is even greater than the energy needed for the above knee prosthesis.

Upper Extremity Amputation

The objectives of upper extremity prosthetics are to give the patient prehension and to restore body image. As in lower extremity surgery as much length as possible must be maintained for better prosthetic fit. A patient with a below elbow amputation will generally function better than a patient with an above elbow amputation.

Prehension and cosmesis are difficult tasks to accomplish in the same terminal device. In most instances, a patient must have two devices, one for function (the hook) and the other for cosmesis (the hand).

As in the lower extremity, the prosthetic device for an upper extremity amputee will depend upon the level of amputation.

Partial Hand Amputation. These patients cannot be fitted with a prosthesis.

Wrist Disarticulation. These patients can become quite functional in a prosthesis, as they retain nearly full supination and pronation power in the prosthetic device. The terminal devices for this prosthesis, and for almost all other upper extremity prostheses, are either voluntary opening or voluntary closing devices, which are controlled by scapular abduction, shoulder flexion, or a combination of both. These motions are transmitted to the terminal device by a shoulder harness and a cable. Once the device is opened on a voluntary basis, terminal closing is supplied by rubber bands or spring loads. Voluntary closing devices allow the terminal devices to be locked at any angle of opening. However, a second motion is required to unlock the terminal device. The two terminal devices, the hook and the hand, are interchangeable, but most upper extremity amputee patients prefer the hook to the hand as it is lighter, more durable, and more suitable for manual labor. The hand is really for cosmetic purposes and is not designed for work.

Below elbow amputees with longer stumps can be fitted with the same prosthesis as those patients with wrist disarticulations. The Muenster prosthesis seems to work well for the patient with a short below elbow amputation stump. In this prosthesis, the socket extends posteriorly about the olecranon and fits closely about the biceps muscle. This arrangement suspends the prosthesis and eliminates the need for the elbow hinge and triceps cuff. It does, however, limit elbow flexion and extension, but this proves to be of little significance in a patient with a unilateral amputation.

An elbow disarticulation maintains desirable function, as these patients retain full internal and external rotation in the prosthesis. However, the prosthesis required is cosmetically objectionable to most female patients because of the bulk produced about the elbow by the addition of outside lock hinges. The elbow unit contains an alternating locking mechanism, with one controlled motion locking the elbow and the other motion unlocking the elbow. Terminal device control and elbow flexion are supplied by the same motions as occur in the wrist disarticulation prosthesis. In this instance, the housing is split so that when the elbow is unlocked, elbow flexion occurs. When the elbow is locked, the same control motion will produce terminal device operation.

The patient with an above elbow amputation can be fitted with the same prosthesis as is used by the patient with an elbow disarticulation, the prosthesis being modified only at the elbow unit and in its socket configuration. These patients will need a device to assist in rotation.

The patient who has undergone shoulder disarticulation may be fitted with a prosthesis that has the same basic units as those required by the patient with an above elbow amputation, but the socket must cover the scapular and pectoral muscles.

A patient undergoing forequarter amputation currently has no way of being fitted with a functional prosthesis. However, testing is now underway on a prosthesis for these patients, fitted with an externally powered device. At the present time, most patients undergoing forequarter amputation may use a light weight shoulder cup with a passive cosmetic arm if they so desire.

References

Barnes, G. H.: Skin health and stump hygiene. Artif. Limbs, 3:4, 1956.

Block, M. A., and Whitehouse, F. W.: Below knee amputation in patients with diabetes mellitus. Arch. Surg., 87:682, 1963.

Bloomberg, M. H.: Orthopaedic Braces. Philadelphia: J. B. Lippincott Co., 1964.

Burgess, E. M., and Romano, R. L.: The management of lower extremity amputees using immediate post surgical prosthesis. Clin. Orth. and Rel. Res., 57:137, 1968.

Ducroquet, R., Ducroquet, J., and Ducroquet, P.: Walking and Limping, A Study of Pathological Walking. Philadelphia: J. B. Lippincott Co., 1968.

Elftman, H.: Biomechanics of muscles with particular application to studies of gait. J. Bone and Joint Surg., 48-A:363, 1966.

Hoover, R. M.: Problems and complications of amputees. Clin. Orth. and Rel. Res., 37:47, 1964.

Klopsteg, P. E., and Wilson, T. D. (Eds.): Human Limbs and Their Substitutes. New York: McGraw-Hill, 1950.

Marmor, L. (Ed.): Amputations and prostheses. Clin. Orth. and Rel. Res., No. 37, 1964.

Rusk, H. A.: Rehabilitation Medicine, 3rd Edition. St. Louis: C. V. Mosby Co., 1971.

Sarmiento, A., Bella, J. N., Sinclair, W. F., McCollough, N. C., and Williams, E. M.: Lower extremity amputations: The impact of immediate post-surgical prosthetic fitting. Clin. Orth. and Rel. Res., No. 68, 1970.

Saunders, J. B. deC. M., Inman, V. T., and Eberhart, H. D.: The major determinant in normal and pathological gait. J. Bone and Joint Surg., 35-A:543, 1953.

Scott, M. G.: Analysis of Human Motion, A Textbook in Kinesiology. New York: F. S. Crofts and Co., 1942.

Swinyard, C. A., Deaver, G. G., and Greenspan, L.: Gradients of functional ability of importance in rehabilitation of patients with progressive muscular and neuromuscular diseases. Arch. Phys. Med., 38:574, 1957.

Syllabus on Heat in Physical Therapy, 7th Edition. Milton, Wis.: Burdick Co., 1969.

Thompson, R. G., et al.: Above-the-knee amputation and prosthetics. J. Bone and Joint Surg., 47-A:619, 1965.

Williams, M., and Lissner, H. R.: Biomechanics of Human Motion. Philadelphia: W. B. Saunders Co., 1962.

Glossary

Abduction: a movement by which a part of the body is drawn away from the mid-line of the body.

Active motion: movement occurring as a result of the patient's own muscular activity.

Adduction: a movement by which a part of the body is drawn toward the mid-line of the body.

Amputation: the removal of part or all of a limb by cutting through the bone.

Ankylosis: abnormal immobility or stiffness of the joint caused by fibrous or bony tissue bridging the joint space.

Antalgic gait: a self-protective limp due to pain and characterized by a short stance phase.

Arthrodesis: the operation by which fusion is obtained between the bony parts of the joint. This term may be used interchangeably with the words *fusion* and *ankylosis.*

Arthrography: x-ray examination of a joint performed after injection of a contrast material, usually either air or a radiopaque dye, for the purpose of visualizing an internal derangement.

Arthropathy: general term used to refer to any joint disease.

Arthroplasty: a reconstructive operation performed on a joint previously damaged by trauma or disease, designed to restore, as far as possible, the integrity and functional power of the joint.

Arthrotomy: the operation of cutting into a joint.

Aspiration: the act of withdrawing fluid material from a joint through a needle.

Bone grafting: the operation by which bone tissue is transplanted from one site in the body to another bone in order to give added strength to the recipient bone or to induce healing of a fracture nonunion.

Calcaneus: a deformity in which the foot is maintained in a position of dorsiflexion, so that with walking only the heel touches the floor (opposite of *equinus*).

Capsulotomy: the surgical cutting of a joint capsule.

421

Cavus: exaggeration of the longitudinal arch of the foot due to contraction of the plantar fascia or bony deformity of the arch.

Congenital: existing at or before birth.

Coxa: pertaining to the hip or hip joint.

Coxa valga: an increase in the femoral neck-shaft angle.

Coxa vara: a decrease in the femoral neck-shaft angle.

Crepitus: the crackling or grating sound or sensation produced by bone fragments or joint surfaces rubbing together.

Cubitus valgus: an increase in the normal carrying angle at the elbow.

Cubitus varus: a decrease in the normal carrying angle at the elbow.

Curettage: the surgical scraping of bone with a sharp cup-shaped instrument called a *curette*.

Debridement: the surgical cleansing of a wound to remove dead, devitalized, infected, or soiled tissue.

Disarticulation: the removal of a limb by cutting through a joint.

Dislocation: complete displacement of the bones forming a joint.

Displacement osteotomy: the operation of cutting a bone and shifting the fragments to change the alignment of the bone or to alter the weight bearing stresses applied to the associated joint.

Dorsiflexion: the movement of backward flexion or bending. When used in reference to wrist or ankle joints, it means extension of the joint.

Effusion: formation of abnormal amounts of synovial fluid within a joint cavity, resulting in distension of the joint.

Epiphysiodesis: the operation creating permanent premature closure of a growth plate.

Equinus: a physical deformity of the foot and ankle, in which the heel is elevated and the foot dropped forward into a plantar flexed position (opposite of *calcaneus*).

Eversion: turning the plantar surface of the foot outward in relation to the leg.

External rotation: turning the anterior surface of the limb outward or laterally.

Forefoot: the front part of the foot, consisting of the toes and metatarsal bones.

Fusion: has the same orthopaedic significance as the term *arthrodesis*.

Genu valgum: the orthopaedic term for "knock knee."

Genu varum: the orthopaedic term for "bowleg."

Hanging cast: a plaster cast designed and applied not only to immobilize a fracture but also to deliver a traction force through the "hanging effect" of its own weight. Used frequently for the treatment of fractures through the lower half of the humerus.

Hemarthrosis: the distension of a joint by blood lying free within the joint cavity.

Hemilaminectomy: the operation of removing a portion of the vertebral lamina in order to gain exposure to an underlying nerve root or intervertebral disc.

Hindfoot: the rear part of the foot, consisting of the talus and calcaneus.

Internal rotation: turning the anterior surface of the limb inward or medially.

Inversion: turning the plantar surface of the foot inward in relation to the leg.

Limp: an asymmetrical pathologic gait.

Midfoot: the middle part of the foot, consisting of the navicular, cuboid, and cuneiform bones.

Myopathy: a general term used to refer to any disease of muscles.

Neurectomy: the surgical excision of a part of a nerve.

Neuropathy: a general term used to refer to a degenerative or noninflammatory disease of a nerve or nerves.

Osteotomy: the surgical cutting of a bone.

Palmar flexion: a term used to denote the motion of flexion at the wrist causing the hand to be bent downward.

Passive motion: movement occurring by means of an external force, such as might be applied by an examiner.

Plantar flexion: a term used to denote the motion of flexion at the ankle joint causing the foot to be bent downward.

Pronation: when applied to the arm, the active turning of the forearm so that the palm of the hand faces downward; when applied to the foot, the combination of eversion and abduction, movements taking place in the tarsal and metatarsal joints and resulting in a "rolling over" of the longitudinal arch and an apparent "flat" foot.

Prosthesis: an artificial replacement for a part of the body that is diseased, damaged, or deficient. The term prosthesis also means an artificial limb.

Pseudarthrosis: a false joint formed when bone tissue does not successfully bridge a gap following an arthrodesis or fusion operation.

Recurvatum: a backward bending of a part or a joint.

Spica: a plaster cast applied in a figure-of-eight fashion, used to immobilize the trunk and an extremity, e.g., shoulder spica or hip spica.

Spinal fusion: the operation of fusing together two or more vertebral segments in order to eliminate motion between them.

Subluxation: partial displacement of the bones forming a joint.

Sugar-tong splint: a form of plaster immobilization useful in fractures of the wrist, forearm, humerus, ankle, and tibia. To immobilize the wrist or forearm, a continuous plaster splint is applied that begins just behind the metacarpal heads dorsally and extends along the dorsal aspect of the forearm, around the flexed elbow, and along the volar aspect of the forearm to end at the distal palmar flexion crease.

Supination: a turning of the forearm so that the palm of the hand faces upward.

Synovectomy: the operation of excision of the synovial membrane of the joint.

Tendon lengthening: the operation of lengthening a tightened or contracted tendon.

Tendon transplantation: the surgical relocation of the tendon of a normal muscle to another site to take over the function of a muscle permanently inactivated by trauma or disease.

Tenotomy: the surgical cutting of a tendon.

Total joint replacement: a special type of arthroplasty in which both sides of the joint are replaced by metal or plastic implants anchored to the bone by methyl methacrylate bone cement.

Valgus: in reference to a joint, the position assumed by the joint when the apex of the angle formed by the longitudinal axes of the component bones points toward the mid-line of the body; in reference to the foot, the term is usually applied to the heel and means that the heel is rotated outward on its longitudinal axis or everted.

Varus: in reference to a joint, the position assumed by the joint when the apex of the angle formed by the longitudinal axes of the component bones points away from the mid-line of the body; in reference to the foot, the term is usually applied to the heel and means that the heel is rotated inward on its longitudinal axis or inverted.

Index

Numbers in *italics* indicate illustrations; numbers followed by a "t" indicate tabular material.

425